The Jasper® Model for Children with Autism

The JASPER® Model for Children with Autism

Promoting Joint Attention, Symbolic Play, Engagement, and Regulation

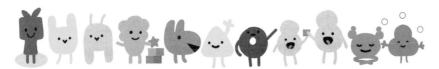

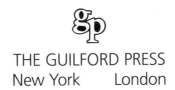

Connie Kasari, Amanda C. Gulsrud, Stephanie Y. Shire, and Christina Strawbridge

THE GUILFORD PRESS
New York   London

Library of Congress Cataloging-in-Publication Data is available from the publisher.

ISBN 978-1-4625-4756-2 (paperback) — ISBN 978-1-4625-4757-9 (hardcover)

JASPER is a registered trademark of Connie Kasari.

About the Authors

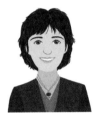

Connie Kasari, PhD, is Distinguished Professor of Human Development and Psychology in the Graduate School of Education and Information Studies and Distinguished Professor of Psychiatry in the Semel Institute for Neuroscience and Human Behavior at the University of California, Los Angeles (UCLA). Dr. Kasari is a founding member of the UCLA Center for Autism Research and Treatment. Her research aims to develop novel, tested interventions implemented in community settings. Recent projects include targeted treatments for early social communication development in infants, toddlers, and preschoolers at risk for or diagnosed with autism spectrum disorder (ASD), and for peer relationships in school-age children with ASD. She has led many multisite federally funded projects investigating the efficacy of interventions for children with ASD and other neurodevelopmental conditions. Dr. Kasari is on the science advisory board of the Autism Speaks Foundation and regularly presents to academic and practitioner audiences locally, nationally, and internationally.

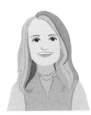

Amanda C. Gulsrud, PhD, is Associate Clinical Professor in the Division of Child and Adolescent Psychiatry at the David Geffen School of Medicine at UCLA and Clinical Director of the multidisciplinary UCLA Child and Adult Neurodevelopmental Clinic. Dr. Gulsrud is a clinical psychologist who specializes in ASD and the development of behavioral interventions across the lifespan. Her research focuses on the early identification and treatment of infants and toddlers with ASD and related neurodevelopmental disorders, using the JASPER intervention. She has played an integral role in the development and adaptation of JASPER for infants and toddlers, has worked closely with the team testing JASPER's effectiveness across a variety of settings, and is a collaborator on several current research trials using JASPER.

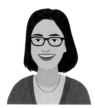

Stephanie Y. Shire, PhD, is Assistant Professor in Early Intervention and Early Childhood Special Education in the College of Education at the University of Oregon. Her research interests focus on the development, adaptation, and real-world effectiveness of intervention programs for children with ASD and other neurodevelopmental disorders, examined through community partnerships in both low- and high-resource settings. She is interested in the use of effectiveness–implementation hybrid designs to examine community practitioners' adoption of intervention strategies as well as children's development. Dr. Shire has played an integral role in the development and dissemination of the JASPER intervention. She has worked on studies focusing on classroom adaptation and deployment, JASPER for children who have minimal verbal language, and community implementation and training, including remote training strategies. She conducts JASPER training nationally and internationally.

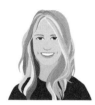

Christina Strawbridge is Research Associate in the Semel Institute for Neuroscience and Human Behavior at UCLA. Ms. Strawbridge joined the Kasari Lab in 2012 and spends most of her time writing about JASPER, in the form of training materials, clinicians' manuals, and websites. She played a key role in translating the in-person training program into systemized written instruction and headed up the writing and development of this book.

Preface

In my early years as a teacher of infants and toddlers with disabilities, I met a little girl with a perplexing set of symptoms that I now recognize to be autism spectrum disorder (ASD). At the time, we were confused by the inconsistency in her skills and her lack of interest in us. Why did she seem to learn something new one day but then not show the skill again? And most confusing to us was that she was not interested in playing with toys or engaging with others. It was 1982. Now, as an autism researcher and Professor of Human Development and Psychology and Psychiatry at the University of California, Los Angeles (UCLA), I have spent my career learning about the core features of autism and providing interventions for them. I often think back on this little girl, our lack of knowledge then, and how unprepared we were to help her and her family. Thankfully, much of the landscape has changed from these early days of intervention for children with autism.

The Problem

The developmental trajectories of children with autism in the 1980s were fairly dismal (DeMyer et al., 1973; Rutter, 1983). Nearly three-quarters of children were entering school with few or no spoken words. By the mid- to late 1990s, it was widely recognized that developing language by the time a child entered kindergarten was a powerful predictor of an individual's best outcome, yet progress remained slow for many of these children. The intervention approaches of the 1980s were highly structured and behavioral. They focused on teaching discrete language and cognitive skills, often out of context, and not within the natural flow of interactions. The interventionist had a target skill he wanted the child to learn, and the child repeated the skill a number of times until she reached a set criterion. Once the skill was in place, the interventionist attempted to generalize it across people, contexts, or situations. Though this was the primary approach of the day, it was not effective for all children, with a staggering number reaching school age without functional language.

Other problems emerged as well. First, these discrete skills did not easily transfer into the child's everyday world. Children remained dependent on the prompts of others and were unable to use their new skills spontaneously and independently. Second, this structured approach to teaching was at odds with the way children naturally learn. Whereas typically developing children learn through play and social interactions, children with ASD were spending many hours per week sitting at a table, in an unnatural environment, repeating skills over and over again. Third, these approaches did not focus on the many other aspects of development that give a child a voice in this world, such as *spontaneous* communication, engagement, independence, and flexibility.

Children with autism were not taught the foundations of social interaction or given the tools to learn these skills from their environments. With the emphasis placed on discrete actions, we were still missing the glue that binds these skills together and makes them meaningful. The question, then, was how could we improve?

The Right Targets

In 1985, a few years after meeting the little girl above, I was a postdoctoral scholar in Marian Sigman's lab at UCLA. At the time, Dr. Sigman was perhaps the foremost developmental researcher in the field of ASD. I had the great fortune to be in the lab at the same time as Peter Mundy and just after Judy Ungerer, both developmental psychologists with expertise in early typical development that they applied to social communication and play of young children with ASD. We conducted many experimental studies investigating the key differences in the development of children with ASD compared to typically developing children and those with other developmental delays aside from ASD.

Our team was concerned about the significant delay in language for young children with ASD, and we wondered if any of the prerequisite communication skills in typical development emerged in ASD as well. From these early studies, we learned that children with ASD in fact have specific challenges in early social communication, namely, joint attention, a skill that develops before children learn to use spoken language. Joint attention refers to the active sharing of a focus on an object or activity between two people. It involves one person directing or sharing the other's attention by looking, pointing, showing, giving, or commenting about the object or event. Children with ASD showed the fewest joint attention gestures when compared to other children who were at the same language and cognitive level. However, within the group of children with autism, those children who showed more joint attention gestures had greater spoken language skills (Mundy, Sigman, & Kasari, 1990).

Thus, joint attention became a central topic of focus during my postdoctorate studies in Sigman's lab. Core challenges in joint attention are commonly discussed today, but this approach was rather novel at the time. Mundy expanded the application of the Early Social Communication Scales (ESCS), a measure for joint attention and other aspects of social communication, to children with ASD. Studies using the ESCS drew attention to the unique strengths and weaknesses in the social communication skills of children with autism and helped to isolate joint attention as a significant missing link in language development for children with autism.

Ungerer, also a postdoctoral scholar with Sigman, studied similarities and differences in the play behavior of children with ASD. Play was theorized to be important for development, as it predicts language and social development in typical children. She created measures of independent and social play and found very specific differences in the play of children with ASD compared to other children of similar developmental ages. Children with ASD displayed the ability to play with toys as they were meant to be used (e.g., rolling a truck or putting shapes in a shape sorter), yet they showed delays in symbolic play acts, such as taking on pretend roles or pretending dolls were alive. They struggled with the imaginative, flexible, and spontaneous nature of play and also had difficulty engaging in social play (reciprocal play with others). This early foundational work on the play and social communication development of children with ASD led to our understanding of the targets we needed to improve and shaped the next phase of my career, where I began to test interventions.

The Intervention

The beginnings of JASPER (the joint attention, symbolic play, engagement, and regulation intervention) started coming together in 1997, when I created a study to teach joint attention and play to preschoolers with ASD. In this study, we separated joint attention and play into two separate interventions—one that taught joint attention skills and the other that taught play skills—and we compared these interventions with the best-informed treatment at that time, discrete trial training (DTT; Lovaas, 1987). DTT is based on applied behavior analysis (ABA). Treatment targets are broken into small, manageable steps, and activities are simplified to maximize successful responses (Smith, 2001). A major active ingredient of this approach involves teaching discriminations between stimuli and providing systematic reinforcement (Smith, 2001). This leads to a highly structured, adult-led intervention that is usually disconnected from natural contexts to reduce distraction.

All the children in the study received DTT for many hours per week (6 hours per day, 5 days per week). We substituted 30 minutes of DTT for our play and joint attention intervention, thus controlling for the overall amount of intervention each child received. When the study was completed, we found that both the joint attention and the play interventions improved language significantly more than the DTT program alone (Kasari, Paparella, Freeman, & Jahromi, 2008). The joint attention intervention also improved joint attention skills more than the other interventions, and the play intervention improved play to a greater extent than the other interventions. In other words, when joint attention and play were specific targets of the intervention, these skills improved in children with ASD (Kasari, Freeman, & Paparella, 2006).

This was an exciting moment in our research, as we recognized that a brief and targeted intervention could have significant effects on children's language outcomes. When children were tested a year later (Kasari et al., 2008), 5 years later (Kasari, Gulsrud, Freeman, Paparella, & Hellemann, 2012), and even 10 years later (Gulsrud, Hellemann, Freeman, & Kasari, 2014), both the play and joint attention interventions improved children's language more than the DTT program alone.

One unexpected finding was that children who received the joint attention or the play intervention had more social engagement with their parents, though their parents were not taught the intervention as part of the study (Kasari et al., 2006). We hypothesized that joint engagement, measured by the length of time that child and parent spent in a shared activity with each other, was the common element between the two experimental interventions and was perhaps why the children in these two groups had similar growth in language outcomes compared to the group who received only DTT. Furthermore, children were more regulated with greater engagement. These data provided valuable information for combining the joint attention and play interventions into one integrated intervention, which was then named JASPER for the relevant intervention targets (Joint Attention, Symbolic Play, Engagement, and Regulation).

The Results

After putting the pieces of JASPER together into one intervention approach, I launched into a series of studies to advance our understanding of how and when JASPER improved child outcomes. We conducted short-term studies (3–6 months) to determine if we could see changes quickly, if at all, and we tested both the proximal and distal effects of the intervention. We started by testing outcomes of preschool-age children working directly with interventionists. After this early success, we expanded our approach to coaching caregivers, teachers, and paraprofessionals, and working in community clinics, homes, and schools. We assessed the effects for children from infancy to early school age, minimally to highly verbal, and those with intellectual disability. We tested JASPER against other viable interventions, alone and when blended with additional interventions.

After more than 10 randomized controlled trials in our laboratory as well as by other researchers in independent laboratories, what we have discovered can be summarized below:

1. ***Change is possible.*** In a short period of time change is evident on the core social communication challenges of autism.

2. ***Change is important.*** Improvements in core challenges of joint attention and play have downstream effects on cognition and language.

3. ***Change is developmental.*** Children with autism are a heterogeneous group. Gains are very fast with some children, and much slower with others. The outcomes are not the same for all children, but even small changes can be helpful.

4. ***JASPER has flexible application.*** JASPER is a comprehensive social communication module that pairs well with other therapies. This flexibility allows JASPER to be readily incorporated into diverse environments, such as inclusion and special education classrooms as well as everyday activities in the home, and combined with other treatments for additional personalization.

5. ***JASPER has active ingredients.*** When parents use a JASPER strategy of imitating the child and engaging with adequate pacing (mirrored pacing), they are better at achieving longer periods of joint engagement than if they did not use this strategy (Gulsrud, Jahromi, & Kasari, 2010). When interventionists use JASPER strategies and increase joint engagement with children, children are more likely to initiate joint attention gestures, and increased use of joint attention gestures results in better language skills downstream (Shih, Shire, Chang, & Kasari, 2021).

Research studies about early intervention are imperative. This area of research is on a fast-moving train—new models are constantly being developed, and new studies appear. However, there are a couple of things to remember when evaluating research evidence. First, while there are many interventions available for children with autism, most have never been rigorously tested (meaning we do not have evidence that the intervention itself is better for a child than whatever the child has access to currently, if anything at all). Sometimes it is clear the intervention did not work. A caution here is that just because a study has been published does not mean it has statistical or clinical significance. It is essential to read the papers for yourself. As well, no intervention operates the same for every child. Some children will make incredible gains, while others make much slower progress. Often this has to do with where children begin, and we must be both hopeful and realistic about what we can accomplish with any intervention (Georgiades & Kasari, 2018).

Second, most children with autism have never been in a research study. Studies include and exclude certain children, depending on their model and the research questions. In JASPER we have conducted studies with children who are often left out of research, including children living in low-resourced communities, who have minimally verbal language, and who are nondominant in language and culture. As the field continues to evolve, we should have more information on which interventions are best for which children and their families.

Because we have conducted multisite studies within the United States and have trained people in countries outside of the United States, we have discovered the amount of detail required for caregivers, interventionists, and educators to execute JASPER at a high level of accuracy. This has allowed us to train and disseminate JASPER broadly.

Conclusion

Here we are, more than 20 years after those initial studies on joint attention and play, and we have come a long way. The intervention landscape today is much different than it was when I met the little girl in the early 1980s. We now know much more about ASD, including how to identify and diagnose children in early childhood. Far fewer children are minimally verbal, and we have more to offer in terms of effective interventions. We have seen firsthand the positive impact intervention has made on the many children and families we have worked with over the years. With our research into how JASPER works for a variety of different learners and settings, we are poised for the future. This future involves more detailed study of the various ways that JASPER can support the development of children with ASD, while helping others, like yourself, access this information. Our hope is that this book will serve as a helpful guide as you work to support families and children with ASD.

CONNIE KASARI

Acknowledgments

Like the research, the writing of this book took many years. JASPER is both systematic and highly individualized, requiring flexible application for each child. While we have been teaching this method for many years through in-person training and feedback, the process is quite different to convey in writing, where the information is presented linearly and without individualization. Through many years of research trials and feedback from training others in JASPER, we refined our teaching methods and are excited to deliver a book that captures both the methodical and flexible nature of this intervention. We have many people to thank for where we are today.

First, I (C. K.) want to recognize the many early contributors to JASPER. Marian Sigman and Peter Mundy planted the seeds of JASPER by involving me in their careful theoretical, experimental, and longitudinal studies on the development of joint attention and play. First-generation implementers of JASPER were my graduate students, Stephanny Freeman, Tanya Paparella, and Lavada Minor. Over the years many, many graduate students and research assistants have implemented JASPER in multiple studies; they made the studies possible. There are also many excellent trainers who travel distances near and far and spend endless hours training and supporting their students with good humor.

I also want to thank my coauthors. Amanda Gulsrud, my former graduate student, has worked alongside me in many research trials over the years and keeps us focused on the "big picture" of intervention science—one that prioritizes both the family and the child. Stephanie Shire, also a former graduate student, has been brilliant in her adaptation, deployment, and training of JASPER across many places, people, and varied levels of children. She has been a champion for the most underserved and underrepresented children we see. And Christina Strawbridge has kept pushing us along, writing and coordinating everyone and everything! She transformed our packet of strategies into the book it is today. We would not be at this point without her dedication to the project.

Next, all four of us want to thank Karie Del Solar for the JASPER design. From the shape characters, to background doodles, to the logo, she captured the playfulness of JASPER and the uniqueness of children on the spectrum. We are lucky to work with someone so talented, passionate about this intervention, and patient in working with us. We also want to express our thanks to our talented illustrator, Arielle Trenk. After drawing so many illustrations, she is practically an expert in laying out a JASPER environment. Her enthusiasm for character design was a perfect match for representing a diverse group of children. Her work can be found at *www.arielletrenk.com*.

Beth Donati and Alyssa Lu, two JASPER interventionists and trainers, did a tremendous amount of work in the development of this book. Ms. Donati wrote exercises and examples, integrated feedback from readers, and edited the content many times over. She fleshed out the troubleshooting sections of the book and clarified the layering of our strategies for a broad group of readers. In addition to skillful editing, she also designed many of the supplementary materials, including checklists, summaries, and visuals to integrate the content with our current training program. Ms. Tan wrote many of the chapter exercises, updated the forms, and provided diverse examples in the text. Her insight and writing were particularly helpful in layering the information across the communication chapters and in developing the ACT Troubleshooting Framework.

In addition, there were many students who read the manuscript over the years, contributed examples, and improved the overall clarity and organization. We are grateful as well for the training groups who read early drafts of the manuscript, tested the exercises, and provided feedback, especially Lisa Baker Worthman and her team of senior trainers and practitioners in the Department of Health and Community Services in the Government of Newfoundland and Labrador. We are especially indebted to their commitment and feedback. Many people at The Guilford Press were also instrumental in guiding us through this process, including Rochelle Serwator, Anna Brackett, and Naomi Burns. We owe special thanks to Barbara Watkins as well, who read our early drafts and provided valuable feedback that guided our writing process.

Finally, we want to thank the many children with autism we have worked with over the years, along with the families, teachers, and community members who support them. We have learned so much from these individuals and are grateful that they have let us work alongside them. These are courageous children who deserve a louder voice in this world (whether that voice is verbal or augmented), and we hope to continue learning how to provide an environment more inclusive of neurodiversity. It is not our intention to provide a "cure," or make children conform or "fit in" to someone else's expectations, but rather to meet children where they are, build on their strengths, and learn to support their needs. We hope that this book accomplishes that goal and that you will join us in our efforts.

Contents

The **Jasper**® Model for Children with Autism

PART I

INTRODUCTION TO JASPER

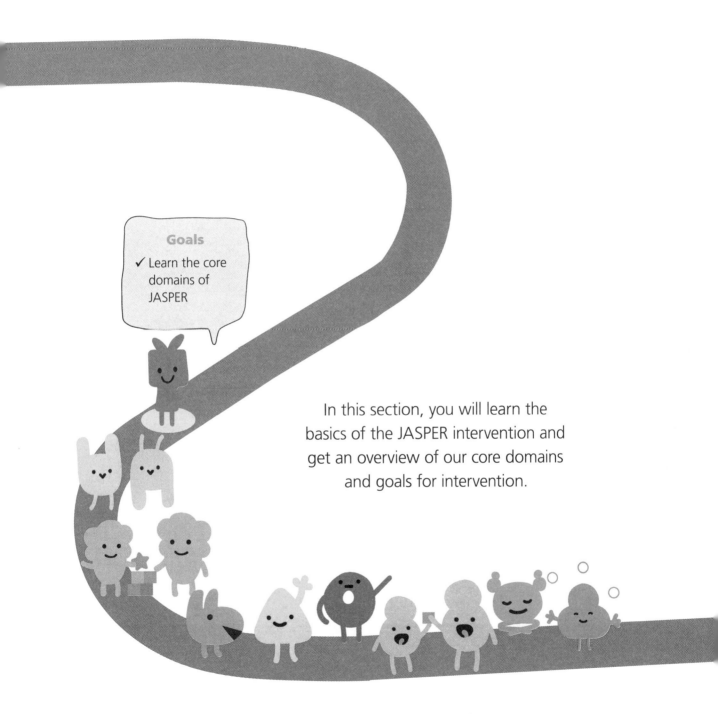

Goals

✓ Learn the core domains of JASPER

In this section, you will learn the basics of the JASPER intervention and get an overview of our core domains and goals for intervention.

CHAPTER 1

What Is JASPER?

1.1 Introduction

This book presents in-depth information about the Joint Attention, Symbolic Play, Engagement, and Regulation (JASPER) intervention, which addresses the core challenges we observe in children with autism spectrum disorders (ASD). JASPER is a targeted, modular intervention in the domain of social communication and included in the broader category of naturalistic developmental behavioral interventions (NDBIs; Schreibman et al., 2015). JASPER aims to improve children's relationships with people (through joint attention and engagement) and interactions with objects (through development of play), while helping children maintain and modulate their affect and behavior (through regulation strategies). In this chapter, we introduce the features of JASPER, including a brief overview about how to implement the intervention, assess the child, and apply strategies to address core domains. These topics are addressed in more detail in chapters to come.

1.2 Intervention Details

Before we begin, we will provide a quick example of what JASPER looks like in a session. JASPER is taught through the child's natural learning context, play. Prior to starting intervention, the interventionist assesses the child's play and communication skills, identifies developmentally appropriate targets, and selects motivating toys that build upon the child's current skill level. Here is a fictional example of what you might see if you were observing a JASPER session (see Figure 1.1).

> *A small play area is set up to promote the child's engagement and regulation. There is a table in the corner of the room, with some building materials partially built into a house and extra pieces off to the side and a set of toy fruit pieces with a knife and bowl. On the floor, cardboard bricks are partially stacked into a tower adjacent to a handful of small animal figures.*

The environment is set up to facilitate a smooth transition into the session by providing motivating and developmentally appropriate toys arranged and ready for the child. The goal is for the child to show interest in a toy and begin playing.

> *The adult and child step into the room and the adult exclaims, "We have so many fun toys today!" The child moves toward the table, picks up a block, and adds it to the house. The adult follows suit by adding a block to the house and moves the fruit out of the way, so they can focus on building the house.*

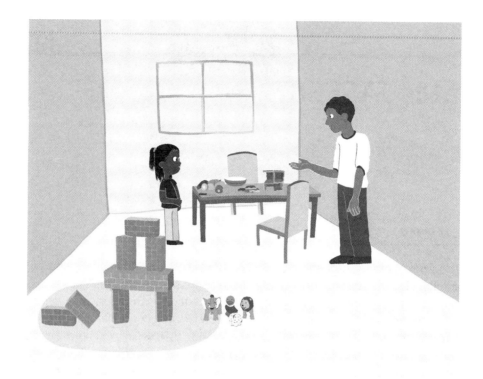

FIGURE 1.1. The JASPER session is set up with play choices for the child.

The child and adult begin to create a play routine. These routines are densely packed with opportunities to foster the child's play ideas and communication and to support the child's engagement and regulation.

> *After the adult and child build the block house together, the adult puts some chairs and small people onto the table. The child picks up a figure of a boy but does not know what to do with it, so the adult picks up a figure and puts it into the house while commenting "People," with a big smile. The child follows in and comments, "House," as she puts a figure inside. The adult responds, "Big house!" and they continue taking turns putting people into the structure. After a few turns, the child starts to stand up from the table. Noting her waning engagement, the adult moves a few blocks closer and the child starts to build a second story for the house. The adult quickly follows in again while pairing his turns with simple comments.*

The adult is responsive to the child in the interaction. When the child decides to put some people in the house, the adult reinforces this idea and follows along, imitating the actions and adding on to the child's communication. When the child loses engagement, the adult helps the child get back on track. The adult also facilitates opportunities for the child to work toward new play and communication skills.

> *As they complete the house, the adult adds more related materials to the environment to continue growing the routine. The child starts adding animals to the house. As the adult takes*

his turn, he shows a dog to the child and says, "Puppy." They continue to add new steps and communication opportunities until the child is done playing with these toys. The adult makes the other toy options clear, the child makes another choice, and they begin to create a new routine.

Throughout the routine, the adult ensures that there are clear opportunities for new play and communication skills. There are extra materials in the environments for the child to add new steps, and the adult capitalizes on motivating moments to help the child use new skills. The adult creates an environment that encourages the child's ability to initiate and provides additional strategies when the child needs more support to build skills in play, communication, engagement, and regulation. In the sections that follow, we will provide additional details about the intervention.

1.2.1   Objectives

The objectives for each JASPER session are to increase (1) the child's time regulated and jointly engaged in a shared activity with a social partner; (2) the diversity, flexibility, and complexity of the child's spontaneously initiated play skills; and (3) spontaneous initiations of both nonverbal and spoken (and/or augmented) language for the purpose of joint attention, requesting, and overall intentional communication.

1.2.2   Participants

The intervention is most commonly delivered one-on-one with an interventionist and a child with ASD. It is designed for children 12 months of age through early childhood and older children who have minimal spoken language. JASPER strategies may also be relevant and effective for children with other developmental disorders who experience challenges in the areas of engagement, regulation, communication, and play skills.

    This book is primarily written for practitioners who have received some prior training with children with autism, such as clinicians, educators, early interventionists, clinical psychologists, applied developmentalists, special educators, and speech–language pathologists. JASPER has also been successfully implemented by caregivers, paraprofessionals, and other community members. Those who wish to implement the intervention must go through training and reach fidelity with a certified JASPER expert. Additional information is on our website *www.jaspertraining.org*.

1.2.3   Setting

JASPER takes place in the child's home, school, clinic, or other community setting. Ideally, sessions range from 45 to 60 minutes but vary based on the age and ability of the child. Some children may need to start with a shorter session and work up to longer sessions, particularly infants, toddlers, children new to intervention, and those with frequent episodes of dysregulation.

1.2.4   Adaptations

This book focuses on one-to-one implementation between an interventionist and a child; however, it is meaningful to note that JASPER has also been tested with other implementers and specific subgroups of children. Several studies have been conducted teaching caregivers to implement

JASPER with their children who are toddlers (Kasari, Gulsrud, Paparella, Hellemann, & Berry, 2015; Kasari, Gulsrud, Wong, Kwon, & Locke, 2010), preschoolers (Kasari et al., 2014b), or older and minimally verbal children (Kasari et al., 2014a). We have taught teachers and paraprofessionals to implement JASPER in small groups (Chang, Shire, Shih, Gelfand, & Kasari, 2016) or one to one (Lawton & Kasari, 2012; Shire et al., 2017). We have also implemented JASPER with an augmentative and alternative communication (AAC) support (Kasari et al., 2014a), and in dyadic peer-to-peer groups (Shire, Shih, Bracaglia, Kodjoe, & Kasari, 2020a). After learning to deliver the intervention directly with children, there are also opportunities to learn to coach others to use JASPER, supporting caregivers to use the strategies at home with their children or teachers to use the strategies in classrooms with their students, or to train other interventionists and trainers. This training is beyond the scope of this book, but information can be obtained from our website.

1.2.5 Materials

All that is needed for a session is a small space to play, a child-sized table and chair, toys at the child's developmental level, and containers to keep the toys organized (e.g., bags, bins, or shelves within reach). If the child uses an AAC system, then the system should be present during the session. Visual supports, positive behavioral supports, and other systems of support can be incorporated as well.

1.3 Intervention Framework

In this section, we explain the JASPER approach, including its extensive evidence base and its place within the field of early interventions for children with ASD.

1.3.1 Evidence-Based

JASPER is evidence-based. By this, we mean it has gone through rigorous testing and has been shown to be efficacious. The JASPER intervention has been tested in 10 published randomized controlled trials by our research team, as well as other independent research teams involving nearly 500 children with ASD over the course of 20 years. Many other trials are currently underway. Altogether, these trials demonstrate gains in children's time jointly engaged in play activities with others (noticing both the partner and the shared activity; Kaale, Fagerland, Martinsen, & Smith, 2014; Kaale, Smith, & Sponheim, 2012; Kasari et al., 2006, 2010, 2014b, 2015), initiations of joint attention (e.g., Kasari et al., 2010, 2014b), and language (e.g., Kasari et al., 2008), and in play level (e.g., Kasari et al., 2014b) and play diversity (e.g., Kasari et al., 2010). Short-term longitudinal follow-ups find that most children maintain these skills, and long-term follow-ups find maintenance of social communication skills as well as language and cognitive gains (Kasari et al., 2012). As you can see in Figure 1.2, the research leading up to JASPER started with experimental studies exploring the characteristics of ASD in the mid-1980s and early joint attention and play studies in the late 1990s. Subsequent work focused on translating this work into community settings. JASPER has made significant strides to make intervention accessible to those in the community who need it most, starting with caregiver-focused interventions in the early 2000s, and then leading into teacher-implemented interventions, adaptations for minimally verbal children, and extensions into community health systems and international settings. For a more comprehensive list of JASPER evidence, see the annotated bibliography on this book's companion website.

JASPER Intervention Research Timeline

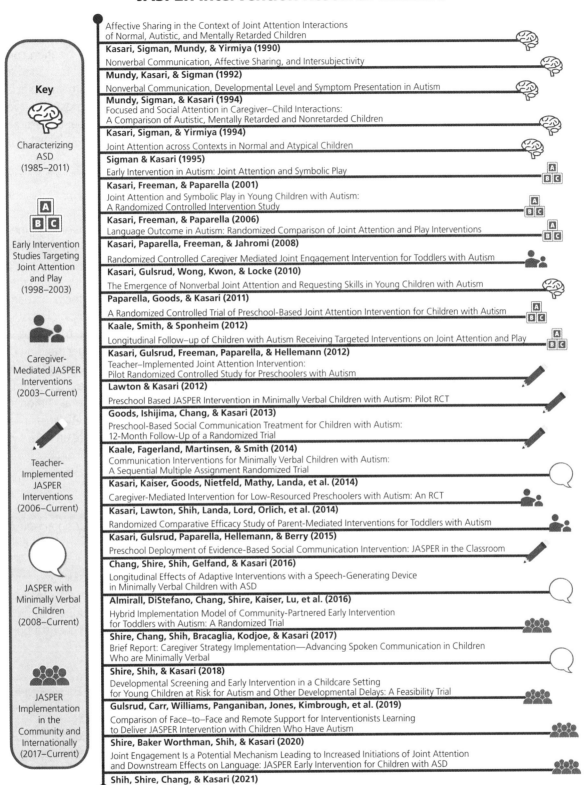

Key

Characterizing ASD (1985–2011)

Early Intervention Studies Targeting Joint Attention and Play (1998–2003)

Caregiver-Mediated JASPER Interventions (2003–Current)

Teacher-Implemented JASPER Interventions (2006–Current)

JASPER with Minimally Verbal Children (2008–Current)

JASPER Implementation in the Community and Internationally (2017–Current)

Affective Sharing in the Context of Joint Attention Interactions of Normal, Autistic, and Mentally Retarded Children
Kasari, Sigman, Mundy, & Yirmiya (1990)

Nonverbal Communication, Affective Sharing, and Intersubjectivity
Mundy, Kasari, & Sigman (1992)

Nonverbal Communication, Developmental Level and Symptom Presentation in Autism
Mundy, Sigman, & Kasari (1994)

Focused and Social Attention in Caregiver–Child Interactions: A Comparison of Autistic, Mentally Retarded and Nonretarded Children
Kasari, Sigman, & Yirmiya (1994)

Joint Attention across Contexts in Normal and Atypical Children
Sigman & Kasari (1995)

Early Intervention in Autism: Joint Attention and Symbolic Play
Kasari, Freeman, & Paparella (2001)

Joint Attention and Symbolic Play in Young Children with Autism: A Randomized Controlled Intervention Study
Kasari, Freeman, & Paparella (2006)

Language Outcome in Autism: Randomized Comparison of Joint Attention and Play Interventions
Kasari, Paparella, Freeman, & Jahromi (2008)

Randomized Controlled Caregiver Mediated Joint Engagement Intervention for Toddlers with Autism
Kasari, Gulsrud, Wong, Kwon, & Locke (2010)

The Emergence of Nonverbal Joint Attention and Requesting Skills in Young Children with Autism
Paparella, Goods, & Kasari (2011)

A Randomized Controlled Trial of Preschool-Based Joint Attention Intervention for Children with Autism
Kaale, Smith, & Sponheim (2012)

Longitudinal Follow–up of Children with Autism Receiving Targeted Interventions on Joint Attention and Play
Kasari, Gulsrud, Freeman, Paparella, & Hellemann (2012)

Teacher–Implemented Joint Attention Intervention: Pilot Randomized Controlled Study for Preschoolers with Autism
Lawton & Kasari (2012)

Preschool Based JASPER Intervention in Minimally Verbal Children with Autism: Pilot RCT
Goods, Ishijima, Chang, & Kasari (2013)

Preschool-Based Social Communication Treatment for Children with Autism: 12-Month Follow-Up of a Randomized Trial
Kaale, Fagerland, Martinsen, & Smith (2014)

Communication Interventions for Minimally Verbal Children with Autism: A Sequential Multiple Assignment Randomized Trial
Kasari, Kaiser, Goods, Nietfeld, Mathy, Landa, et al. (2014)

Caregiver-Mediated Intervention for Low-Resourced Preschoolers with Autism: An RCT
Kasari, Lawton, Shih, Landa, Lord, Orlich, et al. (2014)

Randomized Comparative Efficacy Study of Parent-Mediated Interventions for Toddlers with Autism
Kasari, Gulsrud, Paparella, Hellemann, & Berry (2015)

Preschool Deployment of Evidence-Based Social Communication Intervention: JASPER in the Classroom
Chang, Shire, Shih, Gelfand, & Kasari (2016)

Longitudinal Effects of Adaptive Interventions with a Speech-Generating Device in Minimally Verbal Children with ASD
Almirall, DiStefano, Chang, Shire, Kaiser, Lu, et al. (2016)

Hybrid Implementation Model of Community-Partnered Early Intervention for Toddlers with Autism: A Randomized Trial
Shire, Chang, Shih, Bracaglia, Kodjoe, & Kasari (2017)

Brief Report: Caregiver Strategy Implementation—Advancing Spoken Communication in Children Who are Minimally Verbal
Shire, Shih, & Kasari (2018)

Developmental Screening and Early Intervention in a Childcare Setting for Young Children at Risk for Autism and Other Developmental Delays: A Feasibility Trial
Gulsrud, Carr, Williams, Panganiban, Jones, Kimbrough, et al. (2019)

Comparison of Face–to–Face and Remote Support for Interventionists Learning to Deliver JASPER Intervention with Children Who Have Autism
Shire, Baker Worthman, Shih, & Kasari (2020)

Joint Engagement Is a Potential Mechanism Leading to Increased Initiations of Joint Attention and Downstream Effects on Language: JASPER Early Intervention for Children with ASD
Shih, Shire, Chang, & Kasari (2021)

FIGURE 1.2. JASPER intervention research timeline.

1.3.2 Targeted and Modular

JASPER is targeted and modular. It is *targeted* in that it focuses on the social communication core challenges of ASD and *modular* in that it can stand alone as an intervention or it can be added to the child's ongoing intervention programs. While it is comprehensive within the domain of social communication, it does not specifically address a wider range of outcomes, such as cognitive, motor, and academic skills (though these may be indirect outcomes) over a longer period of time.

1.3.3 Naturalistic Developmental Behavioral Intervention

JASPER, included in the broader category of NDBIs, is a blended approach of developmental and behavioral principles (Schreibman et al., 2015). It works within a natural, developmental framework, while also incorporating explicit teaching strategies drawn from behavioral theory (Skinner, 1957). Like most NDBIs, JASPER takes place in a *naturalistic* context, specifically play routines. This allows the child to experience natural contingencies within a developmentally appropriate learning environment. Sessions are child led as much as possible and structured to promote social engagement. JASPER is *developmental* in all areas of the intervention. The core domains focus on early skills that are critical to the development of play, engagement, and social communication. Using data from our assessments, we identify each child's current developmental level. We then apply a developmental framework to set appropriate goals and track progress. With our understanding of the child's current level, we support the growth of new skills by embedding opportunities to learn and initiate these skills throughout different contexts and routines in a JASPER session. Within these opportunities, we use *behavioral* strategies and principles, such as using natural reinforcement, modeling, and prompting to help a child achieve success. When challenging behaviors arise, we hypothesize the function (i.e., motivation) of the child's behavior in order to create an effective plan to respond.

The Child as Initiator

In JASPER, children are expected to share their own thoughts and ideas, that is, *spontaneously initiate,* within the interaction. It is not sufficient for the child to respond to the prompts and bids of another. To help achieve this, the adult models the role of a supportive "playmate" and conversational partner. For instance, instead of choosing the activity, teaching a discrete skill, and then removing the toy once the task has been completed, the adult actively leaves room for the child to make choices and share ideas, responds to the child's initiations, and provides support to help the child play productively and stay engaged. Thus, the adult adjusts the type and level of support based upon the needs of the child in the moment.

1.4 Domains

JASPER aims to facilitate growth in social communication skills across four domains: *joint attention* (the *JA* in JASPER; targeted in conjunction with other social communication skills), *simple to symbolic play* (the *SP* in JASPER), *engagement* (the *E* in JASPER), and *regulation* (the *R* in JASPER; see Figure 1.3). All of these domains are core challenges for children with ASD, closely linked to social communication and predictive of later language development. We will provide a brief introduction here, and each domain will be discussed in detail in Chapter 2.

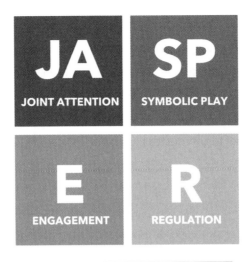

FIGURE 1.3. Four domains of JASPER.

1.4.1 Joint Attention and Social Communication Skills

JASPER aims to teach joint attention, among other social communication skills. *Joint attention* is the coordination of attention between objects and people for purposes of sharing. In our early research studies, we learned that children with ASD have specific challenges in joint attention. In one study, joint attention skills alone correctly classified the majority of children with ASD compared to children with general developmental delays or typical development (Mundy, Sigman, Ungerer, & Sherman, 1986). While the majority of children with ASD demonstrated delays or differences in their joint attention skills, the more joint attention skills children demonstrated, the better their language skills were when tested at the same time, and a year later (Mundy et al., 1990). We target other social communication skills as well, including both nonverbal and verbal modes of requesting.

1.4.2 Simple to Symbolic Play

Another primary goal of JASPER is to teach play, as children with ASD often have delays and differences in this domain when compared to typically developing peers. Play is a universal way for children to learn about the world and provides an important context to teach social communication and language skills. To teach play, we assess the child's current developmental play level, choose a play target based on the child's mastered play level, and then systematically work toward higher, more symbolic levels of play. The intervention follows a hierarchy of play skills (adapted from Ungerer & Sigman, 1981; Lifter, Sulzer-Azaroff, Anderson, & Cowdery, 1993). In all, there are 16 play levels that follow a typical developmental framework (more about this in Chapter 2). While teaching specific play skills, we also focus on the social aspects of play as a developmentally appropriate context for learning.

1.4.3 Engagement

JASPER also aims to improve the child's engagement with others. *Engagement* is a state of being connected with objects and/or people, with higher states of engagement involving more coordination between objects and people. We follow the developmental model of engagement that Adamson, Bakeman, and Deckner (2004) have described for typically developing children. Engagement is an important domain in JASPER, given that children must be engaged in order to learn. It is in the highest state of engagement, *joint engagement,* that children coordinate between objects (such as toys) and people. In this state, they can notice the actions and words of others in the context of the shared activity. Because children with ASD show delays in establishing and maintaining states of joint engagement, JASPER places great emphasis on the child's ability to initiate and ultimately to coordinate the interaction, as measured by play and communication initiations.

1.4.4 Regulation

JASPER stresses the importance of emotion and behavior regulation, as children with ASD have greater difficulty regulating, compared to their typically developing peers (Konstantareas & Stewart, 2006). *Regulation* is a process of appropriately monitoring, evaluating, and modifying a range of emotions, responses, and behaviors to a given context. A child is regulated if she is calm, attentive, and amenable to learning. Rich episodes of play, communication, and engagement are only possible if a child is regulated. While there is much that we do to promote regulation, we recognize that it is common for dysregulation and challenging behaviors to arise. This becomes a concern when the behaviors interfere with the child's ability to participate effectively in the interaction. Therefore, it is imperative to both promote regulation and respond to dysregulation.

1.5 Assessment

Intervention targets are set during initial assessments using the *Short Play and Communication Evaluation* (SPACE; Shire, Shih, Chang, & Kasari, 2018). The SPACE is a brief play-based tool designed to identify the child's mastered and emerging skills and to set intervention targets for social communication (verbal and nonverbal joint attention and requesting), play, engagement, and regulation. The SPACE is based and validated on longer research instruments (Structured Play Assessment and Early Social Communication Scales; Ungerer & Sigman, 1981; Mundy et al., 2003) and has been used in community partnered research to track change over time (Shire et al., 2017; Shire et al., 2020a). Using this information, the interventionist selects developmentally appropriate play materials at the child's mastered and targeted social communication and play levels. The child's progress is recorded on a separate tracking log each session, and additional assessments can be conducted every 3 months or so. See Chapters 3, 4, and 18 for additional information.

1.6 Strategies

We have many strategies to support the child's engagement, regulation, play, and communication. In Chapters 5–17, you will learn the ins and outs of each strategy, as well as how each strategy works together to create a whole that becomes the JASPER approach. These strategies are introduced in Figure 1.4, and a more detailed list is provided in Appendix A. In addition to the strategies, we will introduce the JASPER characters, which serve as visual reminders of the key strategies and components of the intervention.

CORE STRATEGIES	
Environmental Arrangement	Environmental arrangement is the process of setting up and maintaining all aspects of the physical space to support the child and limit distractions. It includes the layout of the room, the child, toys, and even yourself. **Chapter 7**
Imitating and Modeling Play	Imitation is the act of repeating and responding to the child's productive play skills. Modeling is the act of demonstrating a developmentally appropriate skill when the child needs support to play productively. **Chapter 9**
Establishing Play Routines	Play routines are the context for teaching our targets and goals. Routines include developmentally appropriate toys, two active play partners, repeated practice, and a combination of familiar and flexible steps. **Chapters 5 and 10**
Expanding Play Routines	Expanding is the process of adding new steps to an established play routine. We prepare the environment to support the child to initiate new ideas, and we provide support to increase play diversity and complexity as the routine grows. **Chapter 11**
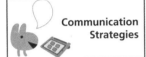 **Communication Strategies**	Many strategies support communication, such as imitating and expanding the child's initiations and modeling developmentally appropriate words and gestures about the play routine. For some children, we also include an AAC device. **Chapters 12, 13, and 14**
Programming	Programming is the process of providing explicit and systematic opportunities for the child to practice joint attention and requesting skills. We use a prompting hierarchy as needed to help the child successfully use the targeted skill. **Chapter 13**
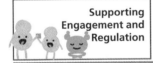 **Supporting Engagement and Regulation**	Many JASPER strategies support engagement and regulation. We prepare the environment, set the child up for success in the session, and try to get ahead of challenges before the child loses engagement or becomes dysregulated. **Core Strategies and Chapter 8**
TROUBLESHOOTING	
ACT Framework	We provide a three-step process for troubleshooting: Assess the situation, Create a plan, and Test for success (ACT) to address challenges during the session. **Chapter 8**
CONDITIONAL STRATEGIES	
Conditional Play and Communication Strategies	When children need more support to make progress, we use a prompting hierarchy and introduce additional strategies to promote productive play. **Chapters 8 and 17**
Conditional Engagement Strategies	If the child loses engagement, such as becoming object engaged, we layer in specific strategies to help the child reconnect and return to a higher state of engagement. **Chapter 15**
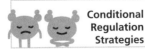 **Conditional Regulation Strategies**	If the child has significant or reoccurring periods of dysregulation, we identify the function of the child's behavior and create a plan to provide a tailored response. **Chapter 16**

FIGURE 1.4. List of JASPER strategies.

1.6.1 Layers of Support

Beyond learning each individual JASPER strategy, the interventionist must coordinate all the strategies together and choose the right strategy for the right moment. JASPER provides three layers of support: core strategies, the ACT framework for troubleshooting, and conditional strategies.

1. *Core strategies.* The core strategies provide the basis of the intervention and include strategies to reinforce the child's behaviors (e.g., imitation) and subtle forms of support to show the child new skills (e.g., environmental arrangement, modeling). We use the core strategies throughout the session to set the child up for success, maintain engagement, model new skills, and respond to challenges.

2. *ACT framework for troubleshooting.* We provide a three-step process for troubleshooting: Assess the situation, Create a plan, and Test for success (ACT). We refer to this as the ACT framework. It can be used to troubleshoot challenges progressing toward our core domains.

3. *Conditional strategies.* The conditional strategies offer more explicit forms of support and are only implemented in select cases after using core strategies and troubleshooting. They include a prompting hierarchy for play and communication, as well as strategies to improve regulation and engagement.

In JASPER, we rely heavily on core strategies and are more selective in using the conditional strategies. Ideally, we begin by using the core strategies. If we notice challenges, we troubleshoot using the ACT framework. We then choose to try a new balance of core strategies or begin to introduce some conditional strategies (see Figure 1.5). Through this process, we tailor support to help children reach their goals.

1.7 Conclusion

This book includes 18 chapters broken up into seven main parts: Introduction to JASPER, Setting Targets, Preparing for Session, Play, Communication, Troubleshooting, and Conclusion (see Figure 1.6). Throughout the book, we provide additional materials to support learning, such as exercises, case examples, and illustrations, as well as checklists, forms, and tables. The children and clinicians we reference are entirely fictional. While they often build on common scenarios we have encountered over the years, any resemblance to names, individuals, or events is purely coincidental. Answers and explanations for each exercise can be found in Appendix B. If you are interested in learning JASPER, we encourage you to read this book and sign up for JASPER training. Those

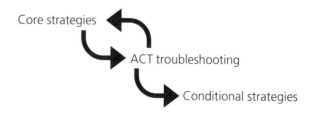

FIGURE 1.5. When providing support in JASPER, we begin with core strategies, move into troubleshooting, and then return to core strategies or incorporate conditional strategies.

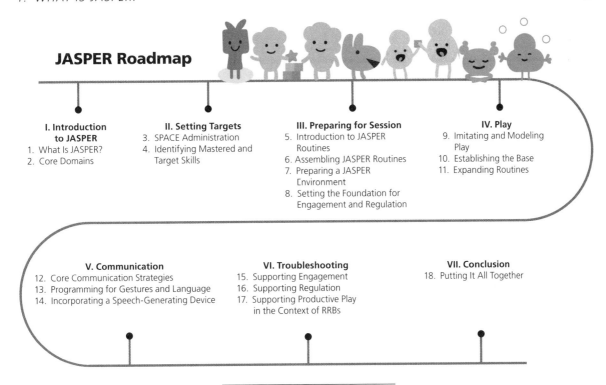

FIGURE 1.6. JASPER roadmap.

who would like to become certified to deliver JASPER must attend an official JASPER training and reach fidelity on practice cases. The most challenging part in learning any intervention is in putting the strategies together into something meaningful and individualized to the child. As you read, we encourage you to reflect on your previous experiences and think of a specific child to practice setting targets and applying strategies. As you are first learning, it is difficult to apply everything at one time, but as you move through training, receive feedback, and gain experience, it will become easier to find balance and integration among key concepts.

A note on terminology. In this book, we alternate between masculine and feminine pronouns and use the person-first descriptor "child with autism" or "child with ASD." We have made these choices to promote ease of reading and not out of disrespect toward readers who identify with other personal pronouns (e.g., they/them) or identity-first descriptors (e.g., "autistic" or "autistic child") as terminology has not yet been settled at this time of writing. We sincerely hope that all persons regardless of age, race, gender, or identity will feel included. In the following chapters, we will expand on the topics discussed here, starting with core domains.

CHAPTER 2

Core Domains

2.1 Introduction

In the last chapter, we introduced the four components of our JASPER acronym: Joint Attention, Symbolic Play, Engagement, and Regulation. We will now look closer at each domain and outline our goals for improvement. This information will help prepare you to identify specific intervention targets for each child and apply the strategies in chapters to come. We will start with the domain of *engagement*. Engagement provides a foundation for learning a variety of skills during the session. Next, we will introduce *play*, from the simple to symbolic levels. We match the child's developmental play level and support the acquisition of new play skills. Then, we will introduce *social communication,* in particular joint attention. Social communication is taught within the context of play and is an expression of joint engagement. Finally, we will discuss the core domain of *regulation,* recognizing that children need support to reach a state in which they are ready to learn. In addition to the core domains, we will discuss the importance of *child initiations* as a key element of improvement across our goals. We will also discuss *restricted and repetitive patterns of behavior* (RRBs), interests, or activities. Figure 2.1 illustrates the order in which the four core domains are discussed in this chapter. Although we present each domain separately in the sections that follow, we think of them as interconnected. Improvements in any one domain will likely lead to improvements in the others, and we encourage you to consider them collectively when entering each session.

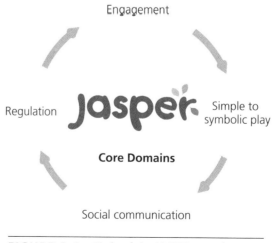

FIGURE 2.1. Circle of the JASPER core domains.

2.2   Engagement

Engagement establishes a frame of reference for children to learn. When children are engaged, they learn more, spend more time connected with others, and are better able to understand the world around them. The ability to engage with others is also critical for developing other skills, like social communication and play. Yet children with autism show greater difficulty engaging with objects and others. Thus, our goal is to help children engage at higher levels for longer periods of time and to learn to coordinate engagement with others. The strategies to support engagement are discussed in Chapters 8 and 15.

2.2.1   States of Engagement

Engagement can change moment by moment. It is not a fixed skill but rather a fluid and flexible state. All children can become more or less engaged based on the circumstances of the day, environment, and for a variety of other reasons relating to their energy level, mood, or interests. Researchers who study engagement of young children have identified six different engagement states that may fluctuate during interactions: unengaged, onlooking, person engaged, object engaged, supported joint engaged, or coordinated joint engaged (Bakeman & Adamson, 1984; Adamson et al., 2004). These states of engagement range from the least engaged, *unengaged,* to the most sophisticated form of engagement, *coordinated joint engaged* (see Figure 2.2).

Unengaged

When a child is unengaged, she is not interacting with objects, people, or events. She is not focused on anything, not a person or an object. In this state, the child may be bored, unsure of what to do, or upset. The child might wander around the room, look out the window, or show signs of distraction or disconnection. If the child does not attend to any toys or participate in the interaction for an extended period of time, as is illustrated in Figure 2.3, then she is considered unengaged. Unengagement can happen any time and may occur when the child is merely daydreaming or when the child is bored or disinterested in what is going on around her.

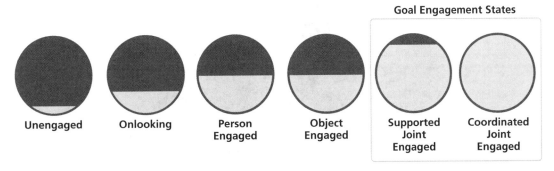

FIGURE 2.2.   The engagement states progress from unengaged up through supported and coordinated joint engaged.

Engagement States

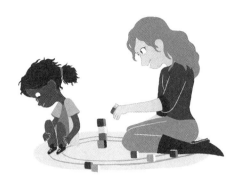

Unengaged State

The child is looking away from the toys and the adult. She is not playing an active role in the interaction.

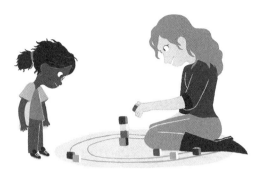

Onlooking State

The child is watching the adult stack the blocks but is not actively playing.

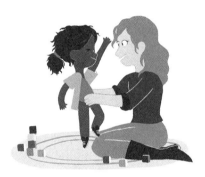

Person Engaged State

The child is interacting with the adult in an activity that does not require objects.

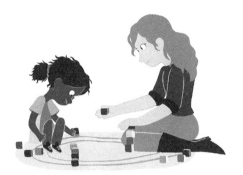

Object Engaged State

The adult tries engaging the child by handing her a block, but the child is solely focused on her own blocks.

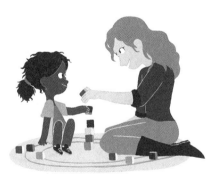

Joint Engaged State

The child looks up at the adult while she is stacking blocks, indicating a sense of togetherness in the interaction.

FIGURE 2.3. Engagement states.

Onlooking

When a child is onlooking, he is watching someone or something else but is not actively playing or involved in an activity. For example, the child is standing to the side watching other children on the playground, or the child is watching the adult stack blocks but does not join in, as illustrated in Figure 2.3. Some children in this state may be taking in information in order to learn new skills, while others may remain as observers because they do not understand what is going on or know how to engage.

Person Engaged

When a child is person engaged, she is solely focused on another person. The focus of attention is the person, and there are no objects involved. Some examples include singing songs, playing peek-a-boo, or playing "chase" with another person. In Figure 2.3, the child is playing with the adult without the involvement of objects. In typical development, this is the primary state for infants under 6 months of age before they have discovered objects (Bakeman & Adamson, 1984).

Object Engaged

When a child is object engaged, he plays exclusively with objects. He is not engaging in social behavior and is solely focused on the objects in front of him. For example, a mother tries to get the child to roll the ball down a ramp, but the child does not respond and continues to roll the ball on the floor. Even if others are playing with the same toys or are sitting next to the child who is object engaged, the child remains focused on his own toys and actions and cannot yet shift attention easily between the person and objects. In Figure 2.3, the child is playing with blocks but shows no awareness or signs of interest in the adult and does not respond to others' efforts to participate. In typical development, this state is common midway through the first year of life.

Joint Engaged

When a child is jointly engaged, she interacts with both a person and a shared object at the same time as in Figure 2.3. This level of engagement requires active participation and interaction among the child, another person, and an object. The child shows indicators she is "with" the person by her behaviors. In this state, the child might initiate ideas (e.g., making choices, taking actions, initiating joint attention gestures, or speaking spontaneously) and demonstrate awareness of the adult (e.g., imitating the other person's play action or language, taking turns in the play, or responding to the other's ideas or prompts). This is distinct from indicators of compliance (see Box 2.1). In typical development, joint engagement begins to emerge toward the latter end of the first year of life and becomes critical to a child's learning of language.

   The state of joint engagement requires active participation between the child and another person. It can be *supported* by the person or *coordinated* by the child. When children are learning to engage, they rely more heavily on the other to support the interaction.

   • In a state of **supported joint engagement**, the child shows a few clear signals of togetherness with the adult, but these may be fleeting or largely in response to the adult's behaviors; there may be instances of looking at the adult's face, talking together, or even explicitly directing the actions of the adult. For example, if an adult and a child are playing with blocks, the child

---

BOX 2.1. Compliance Is Not the Same as Joint Engagement

A state of joint engagement is distinct from indicators of compliance or "on-task" behaviors that other interventions might measure. It might be easy to confuse the two constructs, as the child may seem "engaged" when displaying compliance. A child washing her hands after being requested to do so or being attentive to a task is not the same thing as being jointly engaged. Instead, we find that children are often engaged during these tasks.

---

might take a block when the adult hands her one or she may wait for the adult to take his turn. Children in this state may not use eye contact, but they will still indicate that they are aware of interacting with someone else (e.g., imitating the adult's language or play action). This state is the predominate state from 18 to 36 months and the state where many of the child's language skills are learned (Adamson et al., 2004).

• In a state of ***coordinated joint engagement***, the child initiates and maintains the interaction with limited support from the adult, demonstrating he can initiate and respond easily to communication about an object or event and the person. The child might initiate ideas, lead the interaction, and make decisions about what happens during play. Or he might use eye contact, gestures, or language to interact with and respond to the adult. A child in this state, for example, may tell the adult that the animals are hungry, pretend to feed an animal, and then give the adult a piece of food to feed an animal.

In supported joint engagement, the other person more heavily scaffolds this state, but it is clear the child is aware of the person and objects by his communicative behaviors, and in coordinated joint engagement, the child has very clear communicative signals of intent and connection and may be driving the interaction more than the person. For an overview of the engagement states, see Figure 2.3. Practice identifying the engagement states using Exercise 2.1 before you move on.

EXERCISE 2.1. **Engagement States**

Match the description of the interaction to the child's engagement state.

Description of interaction	Engagement state
1. You and the child hold hands and sing "Old MacDonald" while swaying back and forth.	A. Unengaged
2. You and the child are playing with dolls. The child notices you brush a doll's hair and brushes another doll's hair.	B. Onlooking
3. The child wanders around the room.	
4. You and the child are stacking blocks. The child looks up at you before stacking a block onto a tower. The child then gives you a block and you stack another block on the tower.	C. Person engaged
	D. Object engaged
5. The child places a figure in a bus. As the child looks for another figure, you place a figure in another bus. The child quickly puts three more figures in the bus and then lies down to watch the wheels as he pushes the bus away.	E. Supported joint engaged
6. You put some toy furniture in front of the child. The child watches as you put all the furniture in a house.	F. Coordinated joint engaged

2.2.2 Developmental Framework of Engagement

Typically developing children follow a clear developmental progression through the more advanced states of engagement outlined above. Very young infants start out solely focused on another person, frequently in face-to-face interactions in the first 6 months of life. Midway through the first year, often after children can sit up and take stock of the environment around them, children become very interested in objects. At this developmental state, children are often solely focused on objects or solely on the person; they cannot easily shift between the two. Toward the latter end of the first year of life, children begin to enter states of joint engagement, as they can now shift their attention more smoothly between people and objects and begin to communicate a mutual interest in an object or event with the person. By 18 months of age, typically developing children spend two-thirds of a playful interaction in a state of joint engagement. While they may spend some time in the lower states of engagement (for example, only person engaged or only object engaged), the majority of interactions are spent jointly engaged. Half of the interaction is spent in supported joint engagement, with a smaller percentage (16%) spent in coordinated joint engagement (Adamson et al., 2004). Research has indicated that it is in the state of *supported* joint engagement that children spend the most time between 18 and 36 months, and where most of their language skills are learned (Adamson et al., 2004).

Children with ASD, on the other hand, do not spend as much time coordinating joint engagement compared to their typically developing peers. Whereas a typically developing child spends about 20% of an interaction coordinating engagement by 30 months, a child with ASD might spend only 5% coordinating engagement at the same age (Adamson et al., 2004). A child with autism is also more likely to be unengaged or object engaged with engagement states changing very frequently, even every few seconds in your first interactions, compared to minutes for typically developing children (Adamson et al., 2004). There is also a notable difference in the quality of engagement in children with ASD. Whereas typically developing children are naturally quite social and interactive, children with ASD show fewer indicators or symbols of "togetherness," and it may be difficult to gain the child's attention or connect on a social level. The use of these "symbols" in interaction also represents developmental advancement for the child. For example, a typically developing child might talk, look up, share a play idea, or give the play partner a toy. Conversely, a child with ASD may use fewer symbols of acknowledgment, perhaps only pausing to acknowledge the other person's turn and showing less responsiveness to the play partner overall. Research studies have confirmed that staying engaged in sustained interactions is important to the development of communication and language skills, and thus, a critical developmental task for all children (Adamson et al., 2004; Bruner, 1983; Tomasello & Todd, 1983).

2.2.3 Goals for Engagement

Our goal for engagement in JASPER is to increase the amount of time a child spends in a high-quality state of joint engagement. This means we want to see longer episodes of joint engagement (supported and coordinated), fewer fleeting episodes of engagement, and greater use of symbols while engaged. Thus, our goal is to increase the coordination of shared attention, shared ideas, and togetherness.

- *Increased duration of joint engagement.* We aim to increase the amount of time children spend jointly engaged with others and to decrease unengaged, onlooking, and object engaged states. The goal is to increase the frequency at which moments of joint engagement occur, build upon these moments, and sustain them for longer periods of time.

- *Increased coordination through initiations.* In order to coordinate the interaction and enter the highest states of engagement, the child must be able to initiate ideas of his own, not just follow the adult. Through play and communication initiations, the child attempts to include the adult into the interaction and fosters a sense of togetherness. See Box 2.2 for more information on the importance of child initiations.

Understanding the distinction between initiations and responses is critical to the success of the intervention. Intervention approaches often define these skills differently, and JASPER takes a stricter line than most. Take a moment to learn more about how we define these skills in Box 2.2 and practice identifying them in Exercise 2.2.

BOX 2.2. **A Note on Child Initiations**

Critical to our core domains is the distinction between *initiations* and *responses*. In order to engage successfully with others, children must be able to participate in dynamic interactions that involve back-and-forth exchanges, with the participants seamlessly switching between the roles of initiating and responding. The initiator might share something interesting, ask a question, make a request, and so forth; in turn, the responder can interact with what was shared and then wait for the other person to respond or add a new thought of his own. In JASPER, we want children to be fluent in both of these roles, initiating and responding. While responding to others remains important and is also targeted in JASPER, children with ASD have much greater difficulty initiating social and communicative interactions compared to responding, and thus it becomes an important goal for improvement (Mundy et al., 1986). There has been some confusion in the literature on what constitutes an initiation; thus, we will take a moment to draw distinction between these roles.

In JASPER, we define *initiations* as spontaneous and internally motivated actions or communications. When we refer to initiations, we mean that the act is spontaneous, not prompted, and has a clear intent (not random). By contrast, *responses* occur in reaction to the actions or communication of another person. When we refer to responses, we mean that the action or communication is prompted or motivated by another person, directly follows the action or communication of another person, or is externally influenced. Consider the following scenario: The adult holds up a ball and a truck, and says, "Which one do you want?" Many intervention programs would consider the child's choice in this context as an initiation. Yet JASPER takes a more strict definition of initiations and considers this a response, because the child's answer occurs in reaction to the adult's question. If, however, the child announces that he wants to play with the ball spontaneously, without being asked or prompted, we would consider this an initiation. While there will be moments when the child imitates play or communication, our strategies and targets are geared toward supporting the child's spontaneous initiations.

Children can initiate across engagement, play, and communication. Here are a few examples of initiations within each of these different domains. Though we provide examples of these separately, it may be helpful to note that they are interconnected, with initiations of joint engagement often expressed through play and communication.

- Initiation of joint engagement
  - The child invites the adult to play by handing the adult a toy compass while holding up a treasure map. The adult and child then take turns pointing out areas on a treasure map while laughing and talking with each other.
  - The child picks a ring stacker to play with, puts a ring on, and looks at the adult expectantly, waiting for the adult to take a turn.

- Initiation of play
  - The adult and child are cutting toy fruit. The child begins putting the pieces of fruit into a bowl and then pretends to cook it in the oven to make pie.
  - After the adult and child have taken turns stacking rectangle sticking blocks on top of one another, the child brings over nesting boxes and begins to stack them on top.

(continued)

BOX 2.2 *(continued)*

- Initiation of communication

    ○ When a figure falls off the play swing set, the child looks up at the adult and says, "He's hurt!" (Initiating joint attention)

    ○ The child tries to open a jar of balls. Unable to open it on his own, the child then hands the jar to the adult and says, "Bah." (Initiation to request)

Understanding the distinction between initiations and responses is critical to the success of the intervention. Take a moment to identify initiations in Exercise 2.2.

EXERCISE 2.2. **Initiation or Response?**

Identify whether the child provides a response or an initiation in the following scenarios.

1. The child notices the blocks that were placed on the table. The child stacks a block.	Response	Initiation
2. The child is putting pieces in a puzzle. You ask, "What is it?" The child says, "Animals!"	Response	Initiation
3. You and the child are taking turns pretending to eat a cake. The child shows a slice to you and says, "Cake!"	Response	Initiation
4. You ask, "What do you want?" as the child reaches across the table. The child presses "pepperoni" on the AAC.	Response	Initiation
5. You and the child take turns putting cookies into a jar; then the child puts cookies into a box.	Response	Initiation

---

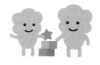

2.3 Simple to Symbolic Play

Play is one of the most meaningful contexts for early learning, yet it is a core challenge for children with ASD. Children with ASD show core challenges in not only symbolic, or "imaginary" play, but also the social and motivational aspects of play. Our goal in JASPER is to increase the complexity and diversity of the child's play skills and increase spontaneous initiations of play ideas. We introduce our framework for supporting play here and will cover key strategies for developing play in Chapters 9–11.

2.3.1 Play Levels

We group play into four main categories: simple, combination, presymbolic, and symbolic. The first three groupings fall under functional (concrete) play, while only the last is symbolic (imaginative). This is illustrated in Figure 2.4. Each of these broad categories of play is broken up into more specific play levels. The list of play levels is adapted from the work of Ungerer and Sigman (1981) and Lifter et al. (1993). Although these four categories of play are presented as separated and

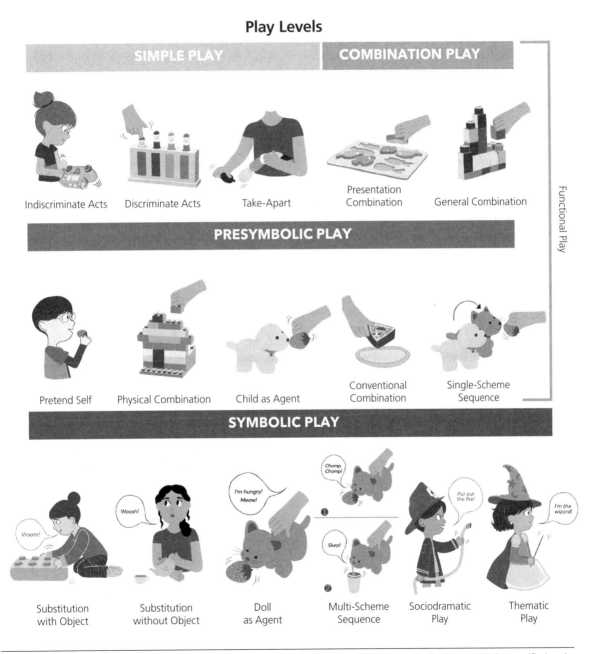

FIGURE 2.4. Play emerges from functional to symbolic with each main category, including multiple specific levels.

ordered, the specific play levels build upon each other, often clustering and overlapping in the child's development.

Simple Play

In simple play, children begin to explore objects and their functions. They are either working toward or beginning to show purposeful acts. Some examples of simple play actions include banging a toy, squeezing a stuffed animal, rolling a ball, and dumping toys out of a bucket. The specific levels within simple play are *indiscriminate acts, discriminate acts,* and *take-apart.*

- **Indiscriminate acts.** Children often first engage with objects *indiscriminately.* They may mouth, bang, and drop toys repeatedly. In Figure 2.4, the child repeatedly shakes the bus. These play acts are not unique to the object and may rely on sensory aspects of play (e.g., the child mouths all toys in the same way). While this is the first level of object play, it is not one we explicitly target in JASPER since most children will be at an age to at least learn actions at the next play level—discriminate acts.
- **Discriminate acts.** *Discriminate acts* consist of single play actions with an object. This often involves cause-and-effect actions. In this play level, the child differentiates among objects. Some examples include dropping a ball down a ramp and rolling a car. In Figure 2.4, the child pushes the button on a pop-up toy.
- **Take-apart.** In *take-apart* play, items that were once together are separated. Some examples include taking puzzle pieces out of the board, removing a cup from a stack of cups, and taking shapes out of a shape sorter. In Figure 2.4, the child takes apart snap-and-lock beads.

Early Combination Play

At the earliest levels, combination play involves putting one object into another in a way that is meaningful and logical. One object has a clearly designated place, such as a puzzle piece into its corresponding spot on a puzzle board or a geometric shape into its correct shape-sorter slot. The child may stack blocks or place blocks into a bucket, but the combination does not "represent" anything in particular. Specifically, early combination levels include *presentation combination* and *general combination.*

- **Presentation combination.** In *presentation combination,* items are combined or put together in their specific, designated spots. Some examples include putting pieces into a puzzle (see Figure 2.4), nesting cups, stacking rings on a peg, and putting coins through a slot into a piggy bank.
- **General combination.** In *general combination* play, items are combined in any fashion. There is no "correct" way to combine the materials. Some examples include stacking with blocks (see Figure 2.4), stacking materials, and putting objects in a dump truck.

Presymbolic Actions and Combinations

In presymbolic levels, play begins to take on a pretend quality but is still considered functional rather than symbolic. This emerging pretense appears when play acts are taken to the self, when play acts are taken to another person or an inanimate object, and when objects are combined in ways representing conventional and culturally expected actions (e.g., putting a bed in a house). These types of presymbolic actions and combinations often emerge concurrently. (We will explain this overlapping emergence of skills in greater detail in Chapter 4, as you set targets and choose toys for routines.)

• **Pretend self.** In *pretend-self* play, the child engages in familiar actions directed toward himself or another person in the room. Some examples include pretending to eat a piece of toy food, extending a brush to one's own or another person's hair, holding a phone to one's ear, and putting a hat on one's own head or another person's head. In Figure 2.4, the child pretends to take a bite of a toy strawberry.

• **Physical combination.** *Physical combination* play consists of putting items together with a clear indication that the child is making "something" or creating a familiar object, place, person, or animal. The child may or may not verbally tell you what the item is but should show you in some way that he intentionally built something. Examples include using magnetic tiles to build a car or using blocks to make a chair or airplane. In Figure 2.4, the child constructs a house out of blocks.

• **Child as agent.** *Child as agent* play consists of the child extending actions seen in the pretend-self play level to toy figures such as dolls, puppets, and animals. In this play level, the child is the agent taking action on the objects (e.g., the child feeds the dog a toy strawberry as seen in Figure 2.4, or the child brushes the doll's hair). This is still a functional level of play, in contrast to the upcoming symbolic level of doll as agent in which the child pretends the doll is alive (e.g., child pretends that the dog is eating the strawberry). This is a subtle but significant difference in development.

• **Conventional combination.** With *conventional combination* play, items are put together based on an awareness of customs, conventions, or experiences. Some examples include placing a cup on a saucer, placing pretend food on a plate (see Figure 2.4), using a spoon to make a stirring motion in a cup, putting a chair next to a table, and placing a pillow on a bed.

• **Single-scheme sequence.** In a *single-scheme sequence,* the child extends one child-as-agent play-level action to more than one figure in direct succession. Some examples include extending a piece of toy food to one doll and then to another doll (see Figure 2.4), or brushing one doll's hair and then another's.

Symbolic Play

Symbolic play involves the representational use of objects, such as pretending one object represents another. For example, a sponge represents a piece of food or a pile of blue blocks represents an ocean. Symbolic play also includes pretending that dolls and animals are alive and pretending that children themselves can take on real-world or fantasy roles. Symbolic play is distinct from presymbolic play in that the play demonstrates true imagination. In presymbolic play, the child performs actions on the doll; in symbolic play, the child pretends that the doll is alive or pretends to be the doll. We often rely on the child's language or the context in which the play act is occurring as a second indicator to determine whether the play act is symbolic.

• **Substitution with object.** In *substitution with object,* the child pretends one object is something else, usually indicated by communication (e.g., sound effects or words) on the child's part to suggest that the child is performing a substitution. For example, the child places a block to his ear and says, "Hello!" (block as a phone), or the child pushes a block while making an engine noise (block as a car; see Figure 2.4).

- **Substitution without object.** In *substitution without object,* the child pretends to represent something without the presence of an object. In other words, the child pretends something is there when it is not. For example, the child pretends to give her play partner "money" while playing restaurant, stirs a bowl while saying, "Soup," as if there is actually liquid in the bowl, or pretends to pour tea out of a pot while making a *shhh* sound (see Figure 2.4).

- **Doll as agent.** At the *doll as agent* play level, the child takes on the role of the figure, pretending that the doll is alive. Some examples include having a doll eat dinner, a dinosaur fly, and a farmer figure drive a tractor. Children will often use language (e.g., "We're running!"), or sound effects (e.g., snoring sounds) to indicate the symbolic nature of play. The child might also help the figure use and manipulate objects (e.g., holding a tool in the doll's hand to fix the bridge) or speak as the doll (e.g., pretending to be a pirate and saying, "Let's go find the treasure"). In Figure 2.4, the child takes on the role of the cat as she pretends to eat the strawberry, saying, "I'm hungry! Meow!"

- **Multi-scheme sequence.** A *multi-scheme sequence* is a sequence of doll-as-agent actions. The sequence appears to mimic a story with one figure. For example, a doll walks to the park, goes down a slide, pushes a friend on the swing, walks home, and then lies in bed and snores. In Figure 2.4, the child takes on the role of the cat, pretending to take a bite of the strawberry, saying, "Chomp, chomp!" and then taking a drink from the cup, saying, "Slurp!"

- **Sociodramatic.** In *sociodramatic* play, the child is enacting a familiar role such as a caregiver or teacher. Some examples include the child playing house or playing restaurant. In Figure 2.4, the child pretends to play the role of a firefighter.

- **Thematic.** *Thematic play* is similar to *sociodramatic* play, but it extends to fantasy characters rather than familiar roles. The actions and roles can be highly creative. Some examples include playing a superhero or a fairy. In Figure 2.4, the child pretends to be a wizard.

Exercise 2.3 provides examples matching particular play actions to their corresponding play levels.

EXERCISE 2.3. **Play Levels**

Match the following play acts to their corresponding play level.

Play act	Play level
1. Pretend a tissue is a blanket	A. Indiscriminate
2. Put a ring on a peg	B. Discriminate
3. Put a chair at a table	C. Take-apart
4. Place a figure on a slide	D. Presentation combination
5. Make a figure hold a cup to take a drink	E. General combination
6. Shake "salt" over play food (no object in hand)	F. Pretend self
7. Tap a block on a table	G. Physical combination
8. Take rocks out of a dump truck	H. Child as agent
9. Stack shapes	I. Conventional combination
10. Put a toy phone to ear	J. Single-scheme sequence
11. Place two figures in a bed	K. Substitution with object
12. Make a figure walk then drive a car	L. Substitution without object
13. Pretend to be a mommy	M. Doll as agent
14. Push a train back and forth	N. Multi-scheme sequence
15. Make a zoo out of blocks	O. Sociodramatic
16. Pretend to be a superhero	P. Thematic

2.3.2 Developmental Framework of Play

In typical development, play emerges rapidly and in a predictable sequence of play skills. By 2½–3 years old, most children have developed the social skills and play skills to maintain the highest levels of symbolic play (Lillard, Pinkham, & Smith, 2011). At first, children engage with objects *indiscriminately*, between 4 and 6 months of age. Around 9–12 months, they begin exploring how these objects work and start to play more intentionally. They might begin with simple actions such as rolling a ball or knocking down a tower. In the second year of life, play becomes more deliberate with children starting to combine objects. Soon after, children's play takes a distinctive turn toward interacting and building with objects in ways that seem more "pretend." For example, they might "pretend" to feed themselves or build with blocks to make a "house." They may put a cup on a saucer and bring a cup to their lips to drink or extend the cup to a doll. Despite appearing more pretend-like, these actions are still considered presymbolic. Between the ages of 18 and 36 months, children begin to play symbolically. In this stage, children come up with many new ideas, create more complex play stories, and mix play acts across the various play categories. By 48 months, children plan and act out elaborate play stories (e.g., pretending to be pirates going on a treasure hunt), assign roles and actions ("I'll be the pirate and you hide the treasure"), and use objects as substitutes in their environments in creative ways (pretending pebbles are the treasure; Lillard, 2015; Ungerer, Zelazo, Kearsley, & O'Leary, 1981). Play is also social, with each child contributing to the interaction. Together, children generate ideas and respond to the ideas of the other, they talk about what they are doing with the toys, they use the toys to build something or carry out a developing story, and there is a sense of playful togetherness marked by smiles and laughter. In moments of disagreement, they problem-solve together, check their emotions, and learn from one another. Throughout the play, they are naturally practicing skills such as creativity, troubleshooting, and communication.

Children with ASD often play at less sophisticated levels of play than their typically developing peers (Mundy et al., 1986; Sigman & Ungerer, 1984). For example, a 4-year-old child with ASD may be learning to stack blocks (general combination) while typically developing children of the same age are playing house (sociodramatic). Additionally, the hurdle between functional play and symbolic play can be particularly difficult, as children with ASD tend to play in a more concrete manner rather than abstract (Jarrold, Boucher, & Smith, 1996; Rutherford, Young, Hepburn, & Rogers, 2007). For example, a child may have an easier time stacking blocks (general combination) compared to building an airplane out of the blocks (physical combination). The child may be very comfortable "giving dolls life" in contexts he may have experienced himself, such as bath time or getting on the bus to go to school; however, the child may be less comfortable with more abstract ideas, such as having the dolls dress up like astronauts and fly to the moon. Play may also include repetitive play acts, rigidity and resistance to change, restricted interests, difficulty developing an interest in toys, and difficulty sharing play with others (Kasari & Chang, 2014).

2.3.3 Goals for Play

In JASPER, our goal is to increase the complexity, diversity, and overall quality of the child's play initiations.

- *Increased initiations in play.* We want to see the child spontaneously and creatively thinking of and executing new play ideas. After all, the definition of play is that the child engages with objects and toys in spontaneous, creative ways that originate in his own ideas and preferences.

- *Increased diversity in play.* Diversity refers to the range of play skills within a single level. For example, if the child plays at a *conventional combination* level, we would want her to show many different types of *conventional combination* skills: putting the cups on the saucers, food on the plates, pillows on the bed, chairs next to the table, stop signs next to the road, and so on. The importance of diversity is often overlooked and underestimated. It is not a race to the highest skill. In order to build complexity, we must build diversity as well.

- *Increased complexity of play skills.* Complexity refers to increases in the child's play level (e.g., moving from *pretend-self* to *child as agent* play). The goal is not to target the highest play level first but rather to build the child's skills sequentially, starting at the child's "mastered" (e.g., fluent) play level and filling in missing skills along the way. Although symbolic play is our ultimate goal given its relations to cognition, we do not target these skills until the child has developed the skills that precede them (Lillard et al., 2011).

2.4   Social Communication

Another core domain in JASPER is social communication. Social communication is a core challenge in ASD, and one of the two diagnostic criteria for ASD. We highlight joint attention in our acronym (the JA in JASPER) and in our intervention, as this is a particular area of challenge for children with ASD (Mundy & Sigman, 1989); however, we work toward many skills to create a comprehensive social communication repertoire. Our goal is to improve the core aspects of social communication, not just the frequency of the child's language, but also the overall quality, diversity, complexity, and flexibility of the child's communication skills. This includes both verbal and nonverbal skills within the functions of joint attention and requests, as described below. We will focus on communication in Chapters 12–14.

2.4.1   Joint Attention Skills

Children use joint attention to socially connect and share with others. As you may recall from Chapter 1, joint attention is the coordination of attention between objects and people for the purpose of sharing. Joint attention is not just one skill but a cluster of skills that help the child communicate about his experiences with others. In JASPER, we focus on the following joint attention (JA) skills: *responding to joint attention, coordinated joint looks, showing, pointing, giving,* and *language.*

- ***Responding to joint attention.*** The child shifts his gaze to follow the adult's initiation of joint attention.
- ***Coordinated joint look.*** The child looks from the adult to the object or event and back to the adult or vice versa (e.g., object–adult–object or event–adult–event) to share (see Figure 2.5).
- ***Joint attention show.*** The child extends his arm and holds up an object to the adult to call attention to something the child finds interesting (see Figure 2.5).
- ***Joint attention point.*** The child extends his arm and points his index finger to share an experience or highlight something surprising or interesting (see Figure 2.5).
- ***Joint attention give.*** The child hands an object to the adult to share an action or experience with someone else (see Figure 2.5).
- ***Joint attention language.*** The child uses spoken or augmented words to comment on an object or event to share something interesting (see Figure 2.5).

We want the child to be able to use a combination of these skills—eye contact, gesture, and language—to share something with another person. Once children start using joint attention, these combinations naturally start to occur, especially in the case of eye contact. These joint attention skills are illustrated in Figure 2.5.

2.4.2   Requesting Skills

Children use requesting skills to express a want or need to others. Although there are many ways children might communicate their wants and needs, we focus on the following skills: eye contact, reaching, pointing, giving, and language.

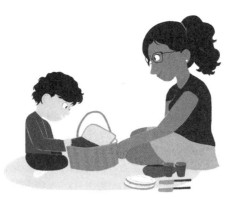

Joint Attention Skills

Context: The child looks in the picnic basket and discovers a toy.

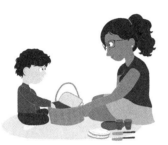

Coordinated Joint Look

The child uses eye contact to share his discovery with the adult.

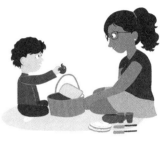

JA Show

The child holds up the apple to show it to the adult.

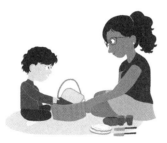

JA Point

The child points to share his excitement about what is inside.

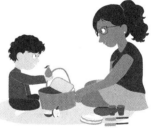

JA Give

The child gives a pear to the adult as if to say, "This is for you!"

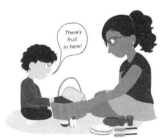

JA Language

The child says, "There's fruit in here," to share the moment with the adult.

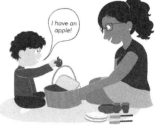

JA Combination

The child looks, shows, and says, "I have an apple!" to share the experience with the adult.

FIGURE 2.5. Joint attention skills.

- *Eye contact to request.* The child looks between an object and a person to express a want or need (see Figure 2.6).
- *Requesting reach.* The child extends her arm out to ask for an object (see Figure 2.6).
- *Requesting point.* The child extends her arm and points her index finger to ask for something she wants or needs help with (see Figure 2.6).
- *Requesting give.* The child hands an object to another person to ask for help operating or fixing it or to indicate that she is finished and wants the adult to remove the object (see Figure 2.6).
- *Requesting language.* The child uses spoken or augmented words to ask for something from the adult—for example, "I want juice" (see Figure 2.6).

The child may start out with only one skill (eye contact or language without eye contact), but the goal is for the child to eventually combine several communicative skills using eye contact, language, and gestures to communicate a want or need. These requesting skills are illustrated in Figure 2.6.

2.4.3 Distinguishing between Joint Attention and Requesting Skills

Requesting and joint attention skills are often confused, likely because many of the individual communication skills can be used for either function. For example, a child could point to *share* or to *request*. When unclear, we rely on the social context and other communication indicators (e.g., body language, affect) to interpret the child's intent. Take a moment to complete Exercise 2.4 below, which offers practice distinguishing these skills.

EXERCISE 2.4. **The Difference between Joint Attention and Requesting**

Identify whether the child demonstrates a joint attention or a requesting skill.

Description of child's skill	Function	
1. The child points to the tall rocket you built together.	Requesting	Joint attention
2. The child looks around after building a road and presses "truck" on her speech-generating device.	Requesting	Joint attention
3. The child puts a train on the tracks and then gives you a train to put on the tracks.	Requesting	Joint attention
4. The child holds up two halves of a toy tomato he wants to stick together and says, "Help."	Requesting	Joint attention
5. The child points to the castle you are building together and says, "Want blocks."	Requesting	Joint attention
6. The child holds up a piece of fruit and says, "Look, apple!"	Requesting	Joint attention

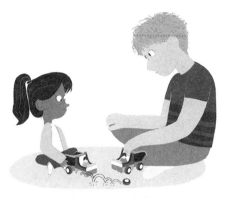

Requesting Skills

Context: The child and adult are playing with cars. The wheel falls off the child's car.

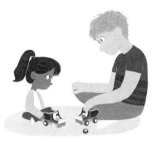

Eye Contact to Request

The child looks to the adult for help, as if to say, "Can you help?"

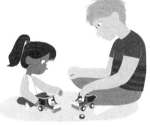

Requesting Reach

The child reaches out her hand to request for the wheel.

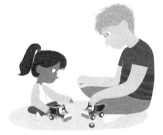

Requesting Point

The child points to the wheel that is out of reach to ask the adult to give it to her.

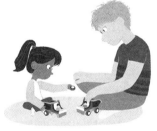

Requesting Give

The child gives the wheel to the adult to ask for help to fix it.

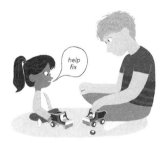

Requesting Language

The child says, "Help fix," to ask the adult to fix the broken wheel.

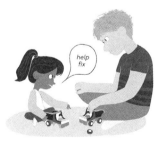

Requesting Combination

The child looks, points, and says, "Help fix," to ask for help to fix the wheel.

FIGURE 2.6. Requesting skills.

2.4.4 Developmental Framework of Social Communication

In typical development, communication is primarily a social activity. Typically developing children use gaze and gestures to interact with others long before they learn to "talk" with spoken words. In the first year of life, children learn to follow others through gaze and gestures (responding to joint attention), as well as share attention using these same nonverbal methods (initiations of joint attention; Mundy & Newell, 2007). Using nonverbal means to communicate intentionally with others has been found to be very important to the later development of spoken language (Tomasello & Todd, 1983). Studies show that early nonverbal joint attention skills, such as following another's gaze, showing, and pointing, are related to language development and predict both concurrent and future language skills for children with ASD (e.g., Kasari et al., 2008; Mundy et al., 1990).

Children with autism often show delays in the development of both nonverbal and spoken social communication skills. This impacts the child's awareness of others and ability to share thoughts and needs with others. While typically developing children gain a full repertoire of nonverbal joint attention and requesting skills by about 20 months of age (Paparella, Goods, Freeman, & Kasari, 2011), children with ASD demonstrate very few joint attention behaviors (e.g., coordinating gaze or using gestures) and tend to master requesting skills prior to, rather than concurrent with, joint attention skills (Mundy & Sigman, 1989). These gaps in the early development of social sharing behaviors uniquely distinguish children with ASD from children with other developmental disabilities (e.g., Mundy et al., 1986; Shumway & Wetherby, 2009).

These delays often result in unclear patterns of communication. For example, children with ASD may use limited or no eye contact when they communicate and may display unclear or atypical gesture use, such as showing an object to themselves or not clearly extending an index finger to point. Children may also scream or cry to communicate what they need instead of using functional language. They may also display atypical forms of communication, such as leading an adult by the hand to access an item they desire. When the child's bids are ambiguous, not clearly directed at others, repetitive, poorly articulated, or otherwise unclear, it can be much more difficult for even careful observers to understand the child's message. This can lead to frustration and dysregulation in the child.

2.4.5 Goals for Social Communication

Our goal is for children with autism to communicate both nonverbally and verbally to request what they need and to share with others. Critical to this goal is the ability to coordinate all of these skills together in a natural way.

- ***Increased initiations of communication.*** Although we support the child around responding to the adult as needed, we are focused on encouraging the child to share her thoughts, ideas, and requests spontaneously with others.
- ***Increased use of joint attention and requesting.*** Whereas some approaches may target communication skills separately (i.e., first requesting skills and then joint attention), we set specific targets for both communication functions for each child simultaneously (as you expect to see in typical development). For children with ASD, joint attention and requesting skills may develop in a unique order (Paparella et al., 2011). We identify skills that emerge out of sequence and support the development of missing skills.
- ***Increased combinations of nonverbal and verbal means of communication.*** In JASPER, nonverbal communication is as meaningful of a target as is verbal communication. We work

on gesture use, even if the child is already using language. Even highly verbal children benefit from targeting nonverbal skills in conjunction with their language, as gestures can help to clarify ambiguous social bids.

2.5 Regulation

Regulation is the process of appropriately monitoring, evaluating, and modifying a range of emotions, responses, and behaviors to a given context (Figure 2.7). It is an important precursor for learning (Graziano, Reavis, Keane, & Calkins, 2007; Trentacosta & Izard, 2007). We know that when a child is not regulated, it is difficult for him to engage (Jahromi, Bryce, & Swanson, 2013) and to learn. Therefore, a focus on regulation is essential in order to meet our goals. Regulation and related behaviors are discussed in more detail in the section that follows, and strategies are discussed in Chapters 8 and 16.

2.5.1 Dysregulation

Issues with regulation arise when certain behaviors, emotions, or lack of attention interfere with the child's ability to learn—for example, when a child throws or swipes toys off the table out of frustration or becomes so upset that she is no longer able to continue the interaction. In these cases, the child has entered a state of dysregulation. *Dysregulation* manifests as difficulty controlling and modulating emotional responses, which then affects the child's interactions with others (Figure 2.8). Dysregulation is often accompanied by a wide range of observable behaviors, such as crying (Cole, Martin, & Dennis, 2004). These behaviors signal dysregulation, but they might also serve as a tool for self-regulation or be idiosyncratic responses to distress (e.g., the child is thumb sucking, tapping, rocking, or swaying to manage discomfort; Cole et al., 2004). The child might also have patterns of behaviors that are not directly related to a feeling of distress (e.g., the child screams to get what she wants even though she is not upset, because she has found this to be a successful strategy in the past).

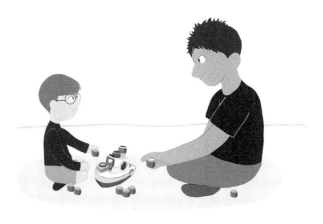

FIGURE 2.7. The child is regulated and happily playing.

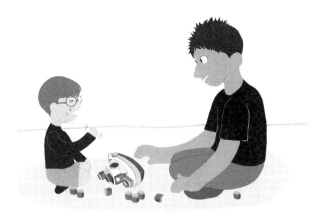

FIGURE 2.8. The child is crying and dysregulated because his boat fell over.

Functions of Behavior

When dysregulation behaviors occur repeatedly or at a high level of intensity, it may be necessary to troubleshoot an appropriate response. In these more difficult cases, we assess the *function of the behavior,* that is, the message the child's behavior is sending. There are four common functions of behavior: social attention, avoidance, access, and automatic (Cooper, Heron, & Heward, 2007; Fisher, Piazza, & Roane, 2011).

- *Social attention.* The behavior occurs to obtain or increase attention from another person. This could be rewarding social attention (e.g., praise, imitation) or punitive social attention (e.g., scolding, correction).
- *Avoidance/escape.* The behavior occurs to avoid or stop interacting with something or someone. For example, these behaviors may occur in order to avoid a demand, a less preferred activity, or an unpleasant place.
- *Access.* The behavior occurs to obtain something desired or preferred (such as a toy, an activity, a reward, or a treat).
- *Automatic/sensory.* The behavior itself is immediately rewarding and self-reinforcing, and often seems to fulfill a sensory need (i.e., feels, looks, tastes, or sounds good).

Methods for understanding and responding to these functions of behavior will be further discussed in Chapter 16.

2.5.2 Developmental Framework of Regulation

For typically developing children, regulation strategies begin in infancy and grow more sophisticated as the child ages. At first, caregivers play a primary role in responding to and managing children's needs, and they naturally fade support as children learn self-regulation strategies on their own (Thompson & Goodman, 2010). Caregivers often start with more physical and active strategies to comfort the child and transition to more passive strategies as children mature, such as redirecting the child's attention or verbally explaining the situation (Grolnick, Kurowski, McMenamy, Rivkin, & Bridges, 1998). Over time, children learn the strategies that have been modeled to them and are able to take on more responsibility for their emotional state. The use of self-soothing strategies (e.g., thumb sucking) decreases, and they are replaced by more sophisticated strategies. By preschool age, children are more confident in selecting and applying appropriate self-regulation strategies (e.g., distracting themselves or shifting their attention to something more pleasant; Feldman, Dollberg, & Nadam, 2011; Morris et al., 2011; Raver, Blackburn, Bancroft, & Torp, 1999). In typical development, there may be moments of frustration or sadness. Even moderate and significant forms of dysregulation are a normal part of childhood. For example, a child may scream or throw toys to test the limits in getting what he wants or to avoid an unwanted demand. Over time, children learn to navigate these negative experiences (Gross et al., 1997; Thompson & Goodman, 2010). Eventually, episodes of dysregulation become less frequent and severe (Gross et al., 1997).

For children with ASD, dysregulation can be greater in type and degree (Sofronoff, Attwood, Hinton, & Levin, 2007). Children with ASD may have limited opportunities to learn regulation strategies from others due to their challenges with engagement (Kasari et al., 2010), and they may have fewer or less clear communication skills (Mazefsky & White, 2014), which makes it more difficult to express their wants and needs. Because of this, it can be challenging for caregivers to anticipate, interpret, and respond to daily challenges in the life of their child. Caregivers report their children with ASD as being more temperamental, slower to adapt, less persistent, less able to focus and shift attention, and more easily distracted when compared to typically developing matched peers (Bailey, Hatton, Mesibov, Ament, & Skinner, 2000; Capps, Kasari, Yirmiya, & Sigman, 1993; Konstantareas & Stewart, 2006). Because of these challenges, children with ASD often need more support to stay regulated and engaged. This is especially true in the context of intervention, when demands are continuously placed on the child in order to support skill development.

2.5.3 Goals for Regulation

The goal for regulation in JASPER is to sustain appropriately modulated affect and attention to the task. We usually think of children as either being regulated (marked by attention, behavior, and affect) or experiencing varying degrees of dysregulation. Thus, our goal is for the child to spend more time in a learning state with fewer interfering behaviors and episodes of dysregulation.

- *Longer periods of regulation.* We want the child to spend longer periods of time in a regulated state, thus providing more opportunities for meaningful moments of sharing and learning. It is often unrealistic to expect children with ASD to be fully regulated (and engaged) for the entire session, but you can improve their readiness to learn by supporting both regulation and engagement.
- *Fewer episodes of dysregulation.* In each session, we want the child to experience fewer episodes of dysregulation. If the child becomes dysregulated, we put supports in place to help the child return to a regulated state. Overall, we aim to reduce episodes and behaviors that may interfere with the child's ability to learn (see Box 2.3 for a note on restricted and repetitive patterns of behavior).

2.6   Conclusion

There is a complementary relationship among the JASPER domains. Engagement and regulation are crucial for learning play and communication, and the strategies that support play and social

BOX 2.3. **A Note on Restricted and Repetitive Patterns of Behavior**

Restricted and repetitive patterns of behavior (RRB), interests, or activities are usually present in children with ASD and are a defining feature of the diagnosis (DSM-5; American Psychiatric Association, 2013). Thus, we will take a brief look at these behaviors, how they might appear in session, and our goals when they arise.

RRBs may manifest as repetitive actions on objects, repeated movements or sounds, rigidity, restricted interests, or under- or overstimulation to sensory input (DSM-5; American Psychiatric Association, 2013). We also see RRBs in the form of language scripts and echolalia. Notably, these types of behaviors often occur in typical development, but to a lesser extent. A typically developing child may enjoy organizing her trains by color but still remains flexible and engaged, whereas a child with ASD may insist on maintaining the trains in a particular order and may be resistant to interruptions or attempts from others to join in the play.

As RRBs are a defining feature of ASD, we encounter them frequently during sessions. They may be subtle and occur in the background, or they may be so intrusive that it is difficult for the child to interact with others. Sometimes repetitive behaviors may appear to be play actions, such as the repetitive opening and closing of doors on a car. For example, in Figure 2.9, the child persistently spins the wheels on the bus instead of taking a more complex action, such as driving the bus or putting figures inside. RRBs may limit your ability to work toward play diversity, particularly if the child has a very rigid idea of how the toy should be used or for your role in the routine. These behaviors may also make it difficult for the child to engage and can lead to increased dysregulation.

Here are some signs that the child's actions are becoming inflexible, repetitive, or rigid:

- Child becomes increasingly object engaged.
- Child begins to repeat play steps excessively, and the adult may feel as though child is "stuck" on one step or toy.
- Child organizes materials (e.g., lines up, matches, sorts the toys) instead of playing with them.

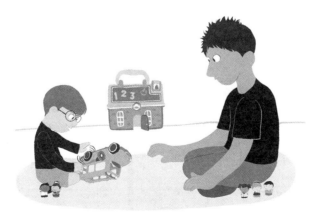

(continued)

FIGURE 2.9. The child spins the wheels of the bus repetitively without taking any productive play acts.

BOX 2.3 (continued)

- Child's affect changes or is inappropriate to the situation.
- Child has fewer social initiations (looking at partner, communicating appropriately).
- Child turns away from the play partner.
- Child consistently rejects the play partner's ideas.
- Child becomes increasingly dysregulated.

When we encounter repetitive or rigid behaviors in the context of a JASPER session, our goal is to maintain a high-quality interaction, reduce interfering behaviors, and increase flexibility over time. By doing so, we support our other play, communication, engagement, and regulation goals, as it can sometimes be difficult for the child to make progress when RRBs are present. RRBs will be discussed further in Chapters 6, 9, 11, 16, and 17.

communication in turn support the child's regulation and engagement states. Thus, we think of the domains as interconnected, with improvements in one domain naturally leading to improvements in the others. This is important to keep in mind as you continue reading. JASPER is a highly individualized approach. The most successful interventionists are those who are able to see the interplay among the domains, find a balance among the goals, and tailor their support to the child's needs in the moment (see Figure 2.10). In the next few chapters, we provide details on how to assess the child's skills and set individualized intervention targets in each domain.

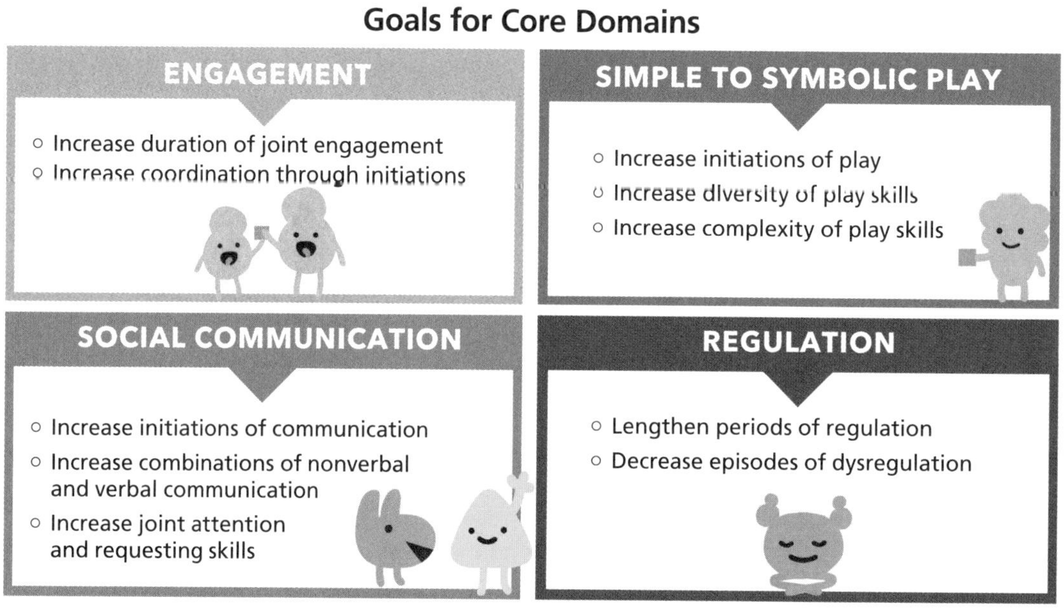

Goals for Core Domains

ENGAGEMENT
- Increase duration of joint engagement
- Increase coordination through initiations

SIMPLE TO SYMBOLIC PLAY
- Increase initiations of play
- Increase diversity of play skills
- Increase complexity of play skills

SOCIAL COMMUNICATION
- Increase initiations of communication
- Increase combinations of nonverbal and verbal communication
- Increase joint attention and requesting skills

REGULATION
- Lengthen periods of regulation
- Decrease episodes of dysregulation

FIGURE 2.10. Goals for core domains.

PART II

SETTING TARGETS

In this section, you will learn how to use the Short Play and Communication Evaluation (SPACE) to set intervention targets for the child.

Goals

✓ Assess the child's spontaneous play and communication skills

✓ Set developmentally appropriate targets for core domains

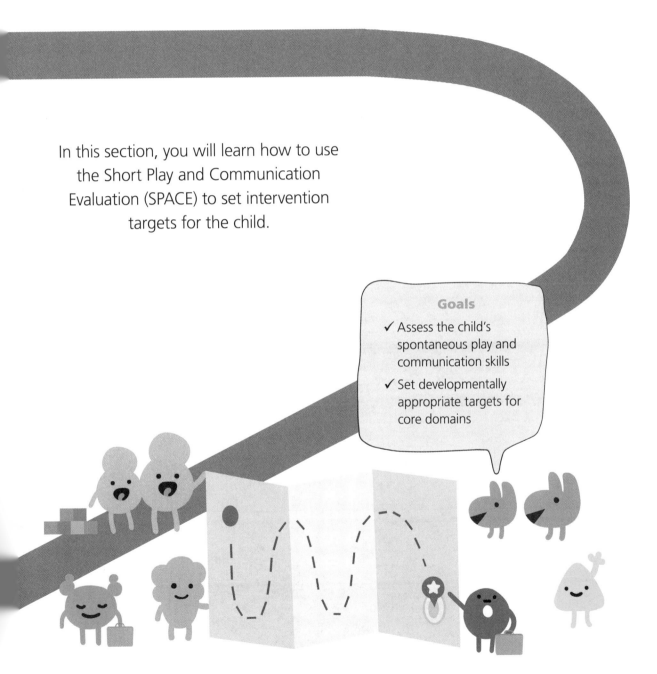

CHAPTER 3

SPACE Administration

3.1 Introduction

The core domains of social communication, play, engagement, and regulation present themselves differently for each child with ASD. Given the diverse abilities that children with ASD display, a personalized approach to intervention is necessary to support the unique strengths and challenges of each child. As a JASPER interventionist, you will get to know the child, identify his profile of skills, and adjust your support strategies to match each need. The most accurate way to evaluate the child's current skill set is to conduct an assessment before the first session. For this intervention, we use the Short Play and Communication Evaluation (SPACE), developed by Shire, Shih, Chang, and Kasari (2018). The SPACE measures the child's capacity across the core domains of engagement, regulation, play, and social communication. It also provides an opportunity to get a "first read" on how the child performs in other areas as well (such as environmental needs, play preferences, social connectivity, and readiness to learn). With this body of information, you will choose specific targets for the intervention and prepare for the strategies to come.

3.2 SPACE Information

The SPACE is designed to identify the child's spontaneous skills and determine appropriate intervention targets for young children with ASD. The assessment is delivered in the context of play and takes approximately 15 minutes to administer. To begin, the child sits in a chair at a table with the SPACE materials within view but out of reach. The activities are presented one at a time, and the child has opportunities to request the toys throughout the assessment. Each activity provides opportunities for the child to demonstrate play and communication skills. The child is also evaluated based on her ability to remain regulated and engaged. You will use Form 3.1 (SPACE Data Collection and Targets, pp. 67–68) to record the child's skills throughout the assessment. The information gathered from the SPACE will determine the intervention targets discussed in the following chapter.

3.2.1 Objectives

The SPACE captures a wealth of information about the child in the following domains.

Engagement and Regulation

For the domains of engagement and regulation, you will identify the amount of time the child spends in a state ready to learn (see Chapter 2 for detailed definitions and descriptions of these states). We will evaluate the following states:

- *Joint engagement.* The total amount of time the child spends connected in a shared activity while socially connected with a partner.
- *Regulation.* The total amount of time the child spends in a calm and focused state, ready to learn.

Play and Communication

For the domains of play and communication, you will identify the types and frequencies of *spontaneous* skills. The skills are considered "spontaneously initiated" if the child performs them without explicit or implicit instruction, prompts, models, or demands (see Chapter 2 for detailed descriptions of each of these skills and Box 3.1 for additional information on why we target initiations). We will evaluate the following skills within the domains of play and communication:

- *Play skills.* Spontaneously initiated actions with toys (see Table 3.1 in Section 3.5).
- *Nonverbal joint attention.* Spontaneously initiated eye contact and gestures to share an object or event with another person.
- *Joint attention language.* Spontaneously initiated language (including all functional modes of communication such as spoken and augmented words) to share an object or event with another person.
- *Nonverbal requests.* Spontaneously initiated eye contact and gestures to meet a want or need.
- *Requesting language.* Spontaneously initiated language, including all functional modes of communication such as spoken words and augmented words (e.g., words generated via speech device, picture exchange, sign language) to meet a want or need.

3.2.2 Activities

The SPACE is not a preset kit for purchase. We provide a list of materials that provide a number of opportunities for play actions at each of the developmental play levels as well as specific opportunities for social communication. The assessor can choose to assemble the recommended materials or substitute items with toys they have available to simulate this structure. The toys selected must be different from those used for JASPER to avoid "practicing" discrete actions during intervention and "testing" those actions during assessment. Prepare the following materials for the SPACE using the guidelines in Section 3.2.3:

BOX 3.1. **Why Do We Count Only Spontaneous Initiations?**

Children with ASD can often imitate what they see and hear but have a harder time initiating these skills on their own. In the SPACE, we want to find out what skills the child can demonstrate independently. The skill does not count if the child sees or hears it performed first or if the child is instructed to act with a model, a verbal prompt, or a physical prompt.

Toy Set 1: Blocks, Truck, Shape Sorter, and Puzzle (see Figure 3.3 in Section 3.3.2)

- 8–10 small blocks
- Dump truck with hinges (large enough to fit some of the blocks)
- Chunky wood or peg puzzle with six to eight pieces (preferably with animals or people)
- Shape sorter with six to eight shapes (present the shape sorter with the lid on)
- Opaque box or bag
  - The box or bag should be large enough to obscure some of the toys in this toy set. Choose a few pieces of one toy (e.g., puzzle pieces or blocks) and place them in the box or bag before the assessment. This will be used later to provide an opportunity for the child to request or share.

Toy Set 2: Barn, Food, Furniture, and Figures (see Figure 3.4 in Section 3.3.2)

- Furniture: two chairs, table, bed that fits both dolls, two pillows, blanket, tissue (to serve as a substitute blanket)
- Two dolls that fit the furniture
- Small barn
- Two animals that fit in the barn
- Cookie toy with six to eight Velcro pieces and Velcro cookie tray
- Two forks, two knives, two spoons
- Two plates, two cups
- Brush or comb
- Opaque box or bag
  - The box or bag should be large enough to obscure some of the toys in this toy set. Choose a few pieces of one toy (e.g., furniture) and place them in the box or bag before the assessment. This will be used later to provide an opportunity for the child to request or share.

Bubbles or Balloons (see Figure 3.5 in Section 3.3.2)

- Two-piece bubble container with wand and container, *or*
- Balloons of the same color, two per administration

Cartoon Pictures (see Figure 3.6 in Section 3.3.2)

- Three different cartoon pictures
- The pictures should include visual scenes similar to a picture book with several images or actions the child can observe, as opposed to a single character, image, or action. This provides more objects of interest for the child to notice.

Windup Toy (see Figure 3.7 in Section 3.3.2)

- Small windup figure (preferably animal or person figure)

Ball (see Figure 3.8 in Section 3.3.2)

- Small- to medium-sized ball

3.2.3 Setup

The SPACE is typically administered with the child seated in a chair at a table. The toys are placed on a second table or a shelf within the child's view but out of the child's reach (see Figure 3.1).

Environment (see Figure 3.1)

- Table
- Two chairs (one for the child and one for the adult)
- Shelf or second table for the toys
- Form 3.1 (SPACE Data Collection and Targets, pp. 67–68)
- Pen or pencil
- Video-recording equipment (if necessary)
- Augmentative and alternative communication (AAC) device
  - If the child frequently uses an AAC system to communicate (e.g., speech generating device, picture communication symbols), ask the child's caregiver or teacher to have it available for the assessment.

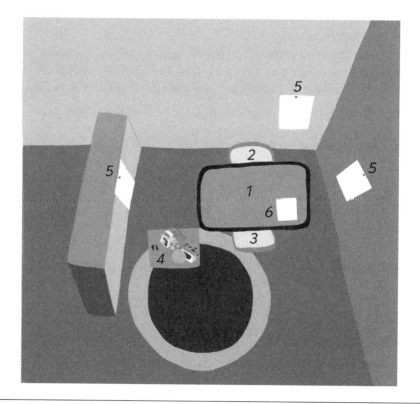

FIGURE 3.1. The SPACE is set up to include (1) table, (2) chair for the child, (3) chair for the adult, (4) toys on a small table or shelf next to the assessor, (5) three different cartoon posters, and (6) the SPACE Data Collection and Targets Form.

Instructions for Setup

1. Set up a small table with two chairs, one for the assessor and one for the child (see Figure 3.1, Items 1–3).
   - The assessor should sit directly across the table from the child.
   - Arrange the assessment so that the child's chair is in the corner of the room. This prevents the child from easily wandering off. You can also add a barrier, such as the bookshelf in the illustration, to create a smaller area.

2. Place the toys on a small table or shelf next to the assessor (see Figure 3.1, Item 4).
   - The toys should be visible to the child but intentionally out of the child's reach both as the child transitions into the room to get seated and when the child is sitting at the table. The presentation of toys creates opportunities for the child to request throughout the assessment.
   - Keep the toys visible. Toys should be fully taken apart and organized to be easily transferred onto the table.

3. Hang three different cartoon pictures on the wall out of the child's reach (see Figure 3.1, Item 5).
   - To the child's left
   - To the child's right
   - Behind the child and slightly to the left or right

4. Keep Form 3.1 (SPACE Data Collection and Targets) and a pen or pencil on hand to record the child's skills throughout the assessment (see Figure 3.1, Item 6). Box 3.2 includes additional tips for tracking skills.

3.3 SPACE Implementation

The following sections explain how to conduct the SPACE, which skills to look for during each activity, and how to ensure you are providing your child with clear opportunities to demonstrate skills.

BOX 3.2. Additional Support Tracking Skills

When first learning the SPACE, the assessor may find it difficult to administer the assessment and record the child's skills at the same time. Here are some options to ensure an accurate recording of skills:

- Conduct the assessment while a second person fills out the form.
- Video-record the assessment and fill out the form as you watch the video later.
- Code the assessment live and compare against a second coder.

3.3.1 Steps

Follow the steps below to conduct the SPACE. *Do not model, prompt, or play with the toys.* If the child imitates or responds to a model or prompt, it is not tallied as a spontaneous skill.

1. Invite the child to play.
   - Gesture to the toys with an *open palm* and say, "Let's play!" (see Figure 3.2).
   - Do *not* point to the toys. This is considered a gesture model for a *point to request*. If the child points in response, the skill does not count.

2. *Pause* to give the child an opportunity to request a toy.
   - Make sure the toys remain out of reach.
   - If the child requests a toy, bring that toy and the rest of the set forward first.
   - If the child does not request, choose any one of the toys to begin the assessment.

3. Give the child a fair opportunity to play with the toys and demonstrate skills before you move on. Do not rush through the sets.
   - Make sure the child notices and has the opportunity to interact with all of the toys within each set.
   - Organize and rearrange the toys in front of the child as necessary to highlight toys the child may have overlooked, while remaining careful not to prompt the child.

4. Know when to move on to the next activity.
   - The amount of time you spend on each activity will vary. When the child has noticed and explored all the materials in the set and is no longer demonstrating new skills or begins to repeat the same actions, this is typically a good indicator that it is time to move on.
   - Continue presenting each set, one at a time, until you have presented all of the materials.

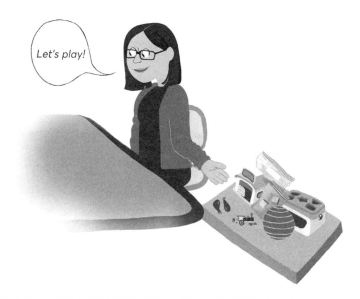

FIGURE 3.2. The assessor gestures to the toys with an open palm to invite the child to play.

- Give the child opportunities to request in between each set.
- Follow the child's toy choice whenever possible and within reason.
- If the child does not request, select the next activity.
- You are not required to present the toys in a particular sequence. Present the materials in an order that maximizes the child's initiations (see Section 3.3.3).

5. Be mindful of the time. You must present *all* the materials in approximately 15 minutes (some assessments will be shorter for younger players and may be longer for children with lots of play skills). Find a balance between giving the child time to demonstrate skills and knowing when to move on to the next set. For example, you may present a toy a second time at the child's request; however, if the child continues to engage in the same actions with that toy, you are not obtaining new information about the child's skills. In this case, you may choose to give the child a brief opportunity to play with the toy a second time and then move on to new toys.

6. When the child completes the final activity, signal that it is time for the assessment to end.
- Try to end on a positive note. You can praise the child for staying seated or playing with the toys.
- If you promised access to a reward for playing, then follow through.
- If the child is dysregulated, help the child regulate before leaving the assessment area to end on a positive note.

3.3.2 Instructions for Activities

The following activities can be administered in any order. Introduce them in the order the child requests. Ensure that the child is given enough opportunity to play with all the items in each set.

Toy Set 1: Blocks, Truck, Shape Sorter, and Puzzle

This activity provides opportunities for requesting, joint attention skills, and demonstration of play skills across all play levels. While these toys can be used in presymbolic and symbolic ways, they primarily target skills at the simple and combination levels. Place the items for the activity on the table and give the child an opportunity to play with them or communicate about them (see Figure 3.3). Items should be placed on the table deconstructed (e.g., take all of the puzzle pieces out of the puzzle board) so that each child has an equal opportunity to play with the activity. It is preferable to present the entire set at one time, so that the child can combine the toys. However, if this is overwhelming for the child, you can introduce one toy at a time (e.g., first puzzle and then shape sorter, etc.) until all the toys are out on the table. Organize the materials to help the child access each toy. If the child does not notice the opaque bag or box, follow the instructions below.

INSTRUCTIONS FOR OPAQUE BOX OR BAG

The purpose of the box or bag is to obscure some of the toys in order to create an opportunity for the child to initiate joint attention. For example, the child might notice something interesting in the bag once he opens it and excitedly share it with the adult. We try to preserve this moment of surprise by giving the child the opportunities to open the bag without the adult jumping in too quickly.

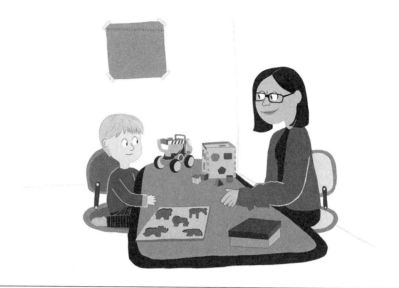

FIGURE 3.3. Presentation of Toy Set 1 with blocks, truck, shape sorter, and puzzle.

1. Place the closed bag or box of obscured toys on the table in front of the child among the other materials from Toy Set 1. *Pause* approximately 5 seconds.
   - If you place the puzzle pieces in the bag, make sure the child has access to the puzzle board as well; otherwise the child will not be able to take any play acts with the pieces.
2. If the child does not show interest in the bag or box, partially unzip or open it. If the child still does not open it, fully open it.
3. If the child still does not engage with the toys, take the objects out of the container.

EXAMPLES OF TARGET SKILLS

Toy Set 1 provides opportunities for a variety of skills. A few examples follow:

Play Skills

- Pushing truck (discriminant act)
- Fitting puzzle pieces into board (presentation combination)
- Stacking up shape-sorter pieces (general combination)
- Building a "chair" (physical combination)
- Pretending an animal puzzle piece is driving the truck (doll as agent)

Requesting Skills

- Giving the assessor a shape that is difficult to fit in the sorter (give to request)

Joint Attention Skills

- Taking blocks out of the box and showing the assessor (JA show)
- Pointing and commenting on each animal puzzle piece (JA point and language)

Toy Set 2: Barn, Food, Furniture, and Figures

This toy set, illustrated in Figure 3.4, gives opportunities to demonstrate play skills across a variety of play levels, including higher levels such as presymbolic and symbolic. The child may communicate about these toys as well. Place the items for the toy set on the table, and give the child an opportunity to play or communicate about them. Like the previous toy set, toys should be presented deconstructed (e.g., do not set the chairs up at the table); it is preferable to have the entire set on the table at one time, so that the child can combine them. However, if the large number of toys is overwhelming for the child, you can choose to divide this set. If you divide up the toys, make sure the figures are present with both the barn toys (figures, barn, and furniture) and the food toys (figures, food, plates, cups, and utensils; see Box 3.3). The order of presentation within the set does not matter. Make sure the child notices and has enough time to play with all the items. If the child does not notice the opaque bag or box, follow the same "Instructions for Opaque Box or Bag" listed under Toy Set 1.

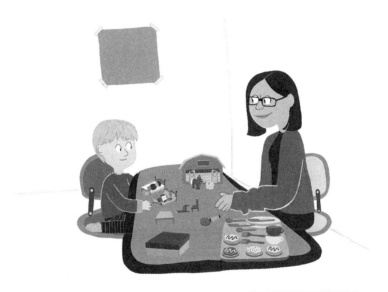

FIGURE 3.4. Toy Set 2 with barn, food, furniture, and figures.

BOX 3.3. **Why Do We Need Figures?**

Figures allow the child to demonstrate higher levels of play. For example, rather than only being able to pretend to eat with the plates and utensils (pretend self), the child can also feed the figures (child as agent) and have the figures eat with the plates and utensils (doll as agent). This is also why we suggest the windup toy and the puzzle include animals or people so that children may use these toys as additional agents.

EXAMPLES OF TARGET SKILLS

Toy Set 2 provides opportunities for a variety of skills. A few examples follow:

Play Skills

- Putting Velcro frosting on top of cookies (presentation combination)
- Setting animal in barn (child as agent)
- Seating two dolls in chairs (single-scheme sequence)
- Mixing (conventional combination) a cup of "juice" (substitution without object)

Requesting Skills

- Giving bag or box for help opening it (requesting give)

Joint Attention Skills

- Holding up a figure to show the adult (joint attention share)
- Handing the adult a spoon to eat with (joint attention give)

Bubbles or Balloon

The presentation of the bubbles or balloon provides opportunities for the child to demonstrate joint attention or requesting gestures, gaze, and language. Once you blow the bubbles or blow up the balloon, the goal is for the child to initiate joint attention to share her excitement. She may also *reach* or *point to request* for access or another repetition (i.e., more bubbles, blow up the balloon again) or give to ask for help to activate the toy. Choose to include either bubbles or a balloon in the assessment, not both. The assessor may consider the child's motivation and age when making this choice. For example, balloons can be a safety hazard for younger children and the sounds may be aversive to others. The bubbles or balloon should be presented twice according to the instructions below. If the child requests more, honor the request and present once more.

INSTRUCTIONS

1. Place the balloon or bubbles in the center of the table in front of the child and let the child explore it. This provides an opportunity for the child to share excitement (e.g., comment or hold up and show you the toy) or request help to activate the toy (e.g., give you the toy and look at you). Do not recruit the child's attention (e.g., gasp and wait).

   Depending on whether you choose the bubbles or balloon, move on to the corresponding Step 2 below.

Instructions for the Bubbles

2. Blow the bubbles and then place the tightly sealed container in front of the child. *Pause.* Wait for the child to initiate to share or request. [*Note.* Pausing is an important part of the assessment. Children sometimes need more time to communicate, so it is important to pause and leave room for the child to initiate or respond. We describe pauses in more detail in Section 3.3.3.]

3. Respond to the child's communication (e.g., in response to a point to request, hand the child the bubble wand to allow the child to try to activate the bubbles).

4. Playfully take back the bubble container and wand. At this point, you can choose, depending on the skills you are still hoping to see: Blow the bubbles again and hold the wand and bottle out of reach (to target reach or point to request), or blow the bubbles again, close the bottle tightly, and then place it in the middle of the table again (to target give to request). *Pause* and wait for child to communicate. Consider the skills you are still looking to see from the child at this point in the assessment:

- Blowing the bubbles typically evokes joint attention skills.
- Holding the wand and container out of reach typically evokes gaze, reach/point, and/or language to request.
- Placing the bottle on the table typically evokes a requesting give to ask for help to activate the bubbles.

5. If the child communicates, respond appropriately by fulfilling the request or responding to the child's joint attention. If the child does *not* initiate, blow the bubbles again and *pause.*

6. Present this sequence at least two times.

Instructions for the Balloon

2. Once the child has adequate opportunity to explore the deflated balloon, playfully take it back and blow up the second balloon. (There are two balloons of the same color to avoid sharing germs. Keep your balloon separate, and give the child the extra balloon when he requests.)

- Hold the balloon up out of the child's reach and *pause* (see Figure 3.5). The child may look, gesture, or comment to share the balloon with you.
- Do *not* tie the balloon, as you will let the air out next.

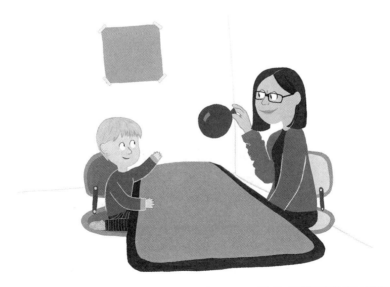

FIGURE 3.5. The assessor holds a blown-up balloon out of reach to evoke communication skills.

3. Slowly release air from the balloon. (You can allow the balloon to make a silly sound if the child finds it funny and not upsetting.)

- *Pause* and wait for the child to initiate to communicate. This moment will likely lead to gaze, gesture, or language to ask for the balloon.

4. If the child communicates, respond appropriately by fulfilling the request or responding to the child's initiation to share. If the child does *not* initiate, blow the balloon up again and *pause*.

EXAMPLES OF TARGET SKILLS

The bubbles or balloon provide opportunities for a variety of skills. A few examples follow:

Requesting Skills

- Looking up at the balloon (requesting eye contact)
- Handing the adult the balloon for help (requesting give)

Joint Attention Skills

- Blowing the bubbles and saying "Bubble!" (joint attention language)

Joint Attention Points to Pictures

Demonstrate a series of three distal wall points, as illustrated in Figure 3.6. Point to cartoon pictures in the order listed below. The primary goal is to measure the child's ability to respond to the assessor's bids for joint attention by shifting his gaze to follow the point.

The three points include:

- Left across: Cross your *left* arm across your body to point to the *right*.
- Right across: Cross your *right* arm across your body to point to the *left*.
- Behind: Using either arm, bend your elbow and point to the picture behind the child.

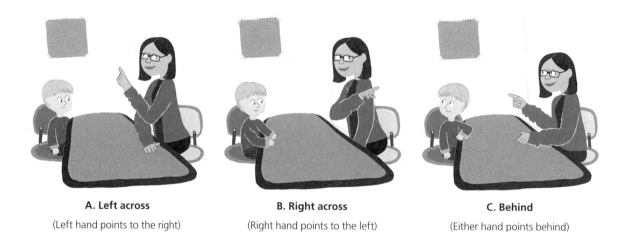

| **A. Left across** | **B. Right across** | **C. Behind** |
| (Left hand points to the right) | (Right hand points to the left) | (Either hand points behind) |

FIGURE 3.6. The assessor uses clear points while maintaining her gaze toward the posters.

(Bend your elbow to make sure that the child can see your point. If you fully extend your arm, your point might be out of the child's line of sight.)

INSTRUCTIONS

1. Call the child's name twice (e.g., "Joey, Joey!") as you point to a picture on the wall. Do *not* say "Look."

2. Hold your gaze *in the direction* of your point and *pause* approximately 3 seconds for the child to respond or initiate.

- Look in the direction of your point, *not* at the child. (If you are looking at the child, you are not giving the child an opportunity to follow your gaze. Looking back and forth between the child and the picture also provides additional cues for the child to shift his gaze.)

- During this pause, the goal is for the child to respond by shifting his gaze toward the direction of your point (response to joint attention). In addition, the child may communicate to share by looking back at you and gesturing or commenting about something he sees.

3. After the pause:

- If the child does *not* respond, label what you are pointing to in the picture: "Joey, Joey!" (*Pause.*) "It's a lion!"

- If the child responds by commenting, respond appropriately: "Joey, Joey!" (*Pause.*) Child responds, "Lion!" Respond appropriately: "It's a lion!"

EXAMPLES OF TARGET SKILLS

The points provide opportunities for a variety of skills. A few examples follow:

Responding to Joint Attention

- Following the adult's gaze
- Following the adult's point

Initiating Joint Attention

- Commenting on the picture (joint attention language)
- Pointing to something new in the room (joint attention point)

Windup Toy

The primary goal of the windup toy is to evoke coordinated joint looks, JA gestures, and language (see Figure 3.7). This toy also provides additional opportunities for the child to request.

INSTRUCTIONS

1. Activate the windup toy in one corner of the table, *well out of the child's reach,* and *pause.* The child may use gaze, gesture, or language to share the toy with you as it moves.

- Do *not* give the windup toy to the child first.

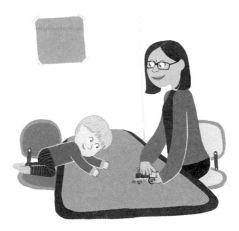

FIGURE 3.7. The assessor activates the wind-up toy out of the child's reach to evoke communication skills.

2. Once the toy stops moving, *pause*. If the child requests for access to the toy, respond immediately and give her the toy.

- You are only required to present the windup toy once; however, you may present it again if the child requests.
- Try to give the toy to the child in response to the child's communication (e.g., the child begins to reach for the toy), rather than allow the child to grab the toy off the table or out of your hand. Grabbing does not count toward the communication skills we are looking for in this assessment.

EXAMPLES OF TARGET SKILLS

The windup toy provides opportunities for a variety of skills. A few examples follow:

Requesting Skills

- Pointing to the windup toy across the table (requesting point)
- Looking at the windup toy and saying, "Do it again!" (requesting language)

Joint Attention Skills

- Looking at the windup toy after it is activated, looking at the adult, and then looking back to the windup toy (joint attention look)
- Holding the windup toy out for the assessor to see (joint attention show)

Ball

The primary goal of the ball is to see whether the child will demonstrate a JA give, specifically whether the child will roll the ball to you.

INSTRUCTIONS

1. Place the ball in the middle of the table and hold your hands out as though you are ready to catch the ball. *Pause* and wait expectantly, as shown in Figure 3.8.

- Do not rush this step. Allow the child a few seconds to explore the ball and roll it to you.

2. If the child gives or rolls the ball to you, take a couple of turns rolling the ball back and forth. If the child does *not* roll the ball to you, lean in and wait expectantly for the child to roll the ball to you.

- If the child notices that you are waiting and still does not roll the ball to you, model rolling the ball to the child so the child understands the expectation. Take a few turns rolling the ball back and forth if the child responds. If there is no response, put the ball away.

- Make sure you provide the child adequate opportunity to notice you and then share with you *before* you model. The child only gets credit for a JA give if she initiates rolling the ball. If the adult models rolling first, the child's response does not count.

EXAMPLES OF TARGET SKILLS

The ball provides opportunities for a variety of skills, including the following:

Play Skills

- Rolling the ball back and forth (discriminate play)
- Bouncing the ball up and down (discriminate play)

Joint Attention Skills

- Sharing the ball with the adult (joint attention give)
- Coordinating gaze between the ball and the assessor (joint attention look)

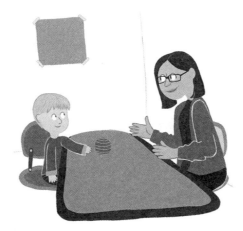

FIGURE 3.8. The assessor presents the ball and holds her hands in a ready-to-catch position.

Person Engagement Activity (Optional)

If the child shows little interest in the toys or needs support to regulate or engage, an optional activity that focuses on person engagement can be incorporated into the assessment. Person engagement activities are brief and completed without objects; examples include tickle games, big motor games (e.g., swinging), and songs (e.g., "Itsy Bitsy Spider," or "Row, Row, Row Your Boat"). This can be especially useful for children who are unfamiliar with the assessment environment and are not engaging with the toys. It also provides an additional opportunity for the child to demonstrate requesting skills within a motivating context.

INSTRUCTIONS

1. Indicate the start of the game by saying, "Let's sing a song" or "Let's play a game."

2. Sing a few lines of a song or tickle game. *Pause* and wait for the child to initiate a request for you to sing again.

3. Repeat song or tickle game.

4. Provide two to three opportunities for the child to initiate a request for you to continue.

3.3.3 Provide Clear Opportunities for Initiations

The best way to help the child demonstrate spontaneous skills is to follow the administration guidelines closely, as outlined above. Included below are some additional tips and tricks to optimize the child's performance without prompting or modeling.

Consider Engagement and Regulation

Introduce the activities in an order that is conducive to the child's regulation and engagement.

- Start with something you suspect the child will find fun and engaging.
- Be strategic about when you introduce toys that are more motivating to the child (e.g., windup, balloon, or bubbles). You can use them when the child's attention begins to wane. Similarly, you can reintroduce a favorite toy as needed to motivate the child.
- Present the points when the child is most likely to be engaged. Avoid presenting the points last, as children are often less engaged toward the end of the assessment.

Consider the Environment

Rearrange the environment and reduce distractions.

- Keep the toys organized. Do not dump everything into a pile and expect the child to sort through it.
- Keep the table free of clutter, especially the area in front of the child.
- Group the toys together (e.g., put shapes next to the shape sorter) without showing the child any explicit play acts (e.g., do not put chairs to the table).

Move objects closer to the child (as needed).

- Help the child notice all the toys by moving some toys closer (e.g., if the dolls or animals are hidden among the toys, move them directly in front of the child). If the child does not notice or have access to all the toys, she may miss opportunities to show all her play skills.
- Do not show the child how to use the toys or prompt the child in any way, as these skills do not count.

Do Not Rush through the Pauses

It is often difficult for children with ASD to initiate. Pauses provide clear opportunities for the child to demonstrate a skill.

- Be clear with each pause. Watch and wait for communication.
- Do not pause so long that you lose the child's interest and attention (often three seconds or less).
- If the child does not act, you can simply move on.

Adjust the Wait Time

Adjust the wait time based on the child's abilities and needs.

- If the child quickly loses engagement or becomes dysregulated, wait only a couple seconds when you pause or present a toy choice.
- If the child is likely to communicate or request a toy, or if the child has longer periods of regulation and engagement, allow for longer pauses to give the child a chance to communicate.

Hold the Items Well Out of the Child's Reach When Waiting for a Request

When creating an opportunity for a request using the bubbles or balloons and windup toy, the items must be held well away from the child's reach. If the child can grab or take the toy, then you lose the opportunity to see the child use gestures or words to request the toy. This is important throughout administration and also as child is transitioning into the room at the beginning of the assessment.

Prioritize Skills You Have Not Yet Seen

Balance the activities based on the skills you are trying to evoke.

- If the child has already demonstrated many instances of a skill, you can spend less time providing opportunities to evoke that skill.
- If the child has not yet demonstrated a skill, spend more time on the activities that evoke those skills. For example, during the balloon, if the child has not yet demonstrated a point to request, you might choose to hold the balloon out of reach to provide an additional

opportunity to point. If the child has not yet demonstrated a give to request, you might choose to put the balloon back on the table to provide additional opportunities to give.

Be Fun, Positive, and Social!

You will not play with the child during the assessment, but you can still be an active, exciting, and enjoyable partner in the interaction. If you do not create a positive social environment, the child will be less likely to enjoy the interaction and will be less likely to demonstrate play skills and communicate.

- Provide a warm and inviting presence with your affect and tone.
- Respond to all the child's communication (including eye contact) by smiling, praising the child, commenting on what the child is doing, and imitating the child's functional communication.
- Do not sit in silence. This should be a comfortable environment for the child to share.

3.4 Common Questions

In the section below, we address common questions regarding the SPACE.

Can I talk during the assessment?

Yes! To help create a social and warm environment for the child, you should be responsive to the child's communication and play skills. You may comment and talk about what the child is doing with the toys (e.g., "Wow, that's a good idea!" or "That is so cool!"). *Avoid* language that leads the child to use specific play or communication skills.

- ***Avoid language that implies acts at higher play levels.*** For example, the child places a doll in the bed and then puts a blanket over the doll and says, "Blanket." You respond by saying, "The doll is sleeping."
  - *Issue*: By suggesting the doll is sleeping, you have implied that the doll has life (doll as agent), a higher play level than simply placing a doll in the bed (child as agent).
  - *Instead*: Imitate the child's language (e.g., "Blanket!"), comment on the action itself, or offer praise.
- Here is another example of language that implies a higher play level. The child makes a scooping action with a spoon and pretends to eat. The child looks at you but does not say anything. In response, you say, "Wow, you're eating soup!"
  - *Issue*: By suggesting the child is eating soup, you have implied (and possibly) prompted a substitution. If the child says, "Soup," the act must be considered prompted and the child will not receive credit for a symbolic play act (substitution without object).
  - *Instead*: Comment on the child's action (e.g., "Scoop!") or offer praise (e.g., "Great idea. That looks so fun!").

- ***Avoid actively recruiting the child's attention or trying to evoke skills.*** For example, you should not gasp or look back and forth between the child and the windup toy while you are waiting for the child to communicate.
  - *Issue*: By using eye contact, sounds, or facial expressions to get the child to request or share, you are implicitly prompting the child.
  - *Instead*: Stay quiet during moments when you are waiting for the child to use skills. Respond to the child's initiations rather than trying to evoke skills.
- ***Avoid teaching the child new words.*** For example, the child picks up the puzzle piece and you immediately name it (e.g., "Giraffe!").
  - *Issue*: When you model commenting language for the child, the child's response is not counted, since any imitated words are not considered spontaneous.
  - *Instead*: Wait to see what the child says, or make general comments (e.g., "Good idea!"). Try using language that is more complex than what the child would say on her own (e.g., "Oh, you put them inside!") to avoid modeling words kids might use to comment.

Can I use gestures to communicate?

Do *not* use gestures (e.g., point, show, give) during the assessment, since your gestures act as a prompt and a model. The child does not receive credit for imitated gestures.

Can I play too?

Try not to actively play with the child. Do *not* show the child how to play with the toys or imitate the child's actions unless the child asks you to play. Instead, use general commenting language and praise to maintain a positive social environment. Your goal is to be responsive, engaging, and positive without playing with the materials.

Can I help the child if she is not playing?

If the child is not playing with the toys after you have provided sufficient time and opportunity, consider the ideas below. In general, you should try to use the least intrusive form of support necessary to help the child play.

- Make sure the table is not cluttered and there is a clear area in front of the child to play. (It may be necessary to limit the number of items, so the child has clear choices. Once she starts playing, you can move additional pieces into her environment.)
- Move interesting toys closer to the child and shift toys that the child has not played with directly in front of the child.
- Remove items that cause object-focus or repetitive behaviors (e.g., visual inspection, banging). (Refer to Chapter 6, Section 6.2.3, for signs of productive vs. interfering actions.)
  - You may use some behavioral strategies to help manage challenging situations (such as supporting transitions) during the SPACE. For example, you may provide the child with a verbal warning and visual countdown in order to remove an item, as needed.
- Simply orient a toy toward the child or hand the child a piece.

- Provide a general verbal prompt (e.g., "Let's play!").
- For young children, it can be helpful to have caregiver present, especially if this is one of your first interactions with the child. In this case, explain the purpose of the assessment and ask the caregiver not to prompt the child.

Can I fulfill requests outside of the context of the assessment?

Fulfill requests if you can (as long as they do not distract from the assessment) and then quickly redirect the child back to the assessment. If the request is a method to escape the interaction (e.g., child repeatedly requests to be "all done"), use your own clinical judgment (i.e., your prior experience and intuition) to determine whether to respond or redirect. Motivating activities and items may be great options as reinforcers for participation in the assessment (e.g., "First play and then snack").

Can I repeat a toy?

If the child asks to repeat a toy, you can bring it forward and continue to record the child's skills, as long as the toys are used productively and appropriately. If the child continues to request for the same toy numerous times, you may need to move on to the next set due to the time constraints of the assessment. Use your best judgment. You can also use the requested toy as a reinforcer and redirect the child to the other activities (e.g., "First play and then balloon").

What if the child is not using a skill I know she can?

If the child does not use a skill you believe she already knows, there may be a few reasons:

- The child only knows how to use the skill to respond, not initiate.
- The child may not be fully comfortable using the skill, because it is not yet mastered.
- The child is simply having an "off" day. This might be a sign that the child is not completely comfortable in this new setting.

Simply record the skills as you see them in the SPACE. If it is clear later during intervention that the child has fully developed a skill, you can adjust your targets accordingly.

3.5 SPACE Forms

The following forms and table are also required for the assessment:

- *Form 3.1 (SPACE Data Collection and Targets, pp. 67–68).* Use this form to record the child's skills during the SPACE and to set intervention targets. (Instructions for setting targets are discussed in Chapter 4.)
- *Table 3.1 (SPACE List of Most Common Play Acts by Level, p. 61).* Use this table as a reference to identify the play levels that correspond to various play acts.
- *Form 3.2 (SPACE Administration Fidelity, p. 69).* Use this form to establish reliability as you learn to administer the SPACE.

TABLE 3.1. SPACE List of Most Common Play Acts by Level

Instructions:

● Use this list as a guide to identify the play level associated with each play act.

● The child might demonstrate play acts that are not on this list. (See Chapter 2, "Core Domains," for more information identifying play levels.)

Play level	Play act
Simple	Push truck (discriminate)
	Open and close doors on the barn (discriminate)
	Take blocks out of truck (take-apart)
	Take pieces out of puzzle (take-apart)
Combination	Put pieces in puzzle (presentation combination)
	Put cookie on Velcro tray (presentation combination)
	Put frosting on cookie base (presentation combination)
	Put shapes in shape sorter (presentation combination)
	Stack furniture (general combination)
	Stack cookies (general combination)
	Stack or build with blocks (general combination)
	Put blocks in truck (general combination)
	Stack puzzle pieces (general combination)
Presymbolic	Put cup or spoon to mouth (pretend self)
	Put cookie to mouth (pretend self)
	Brush to own hair or assessor's hair (pretend self)
	Build structure out of blocks (physical combination)
	Put figure in bed (child as agent)
	Put figure in barn (child as agent)
	Put figure in chair (child as agent)
	Put cup or spoon to figure (child as agent)
	Put cookie to figure (child as agent)
	Put spoon in cup (conventional combination)
	Put cookies in cup or on plate (conventional combination)
	Place blanket on bed (conventional combination)
	Place pillow on bed (conventional combination)
	Place chair at table (conventional combination)
	Mix with spoon on the plate or in the cup (conventional combination)
	Take one child-as-agent act with two figures (single scheme)
Symbolic	Pretend the tissue is a blanket (substitution with object)
	Pretend to cook something in the cup or on the plate (substitution without object)
	Pretend to make the truck horn "beep" (substitution without object)
	Pretend the figure sleeps or snores (doll as agent)
	Pretend the figure walks (doll as agent)
	Pretend the figure eats or drinks (doll as agent)
	Perform a sequence of two unique doll-as-agent acts with one figure (multi-scheme)
	Pretend to be a baker (sociodramatic)

3.6 Scoring Instructions

After conducting the SPACE, you will have a better sense of the child's ability to initiate skills. Some initiations may be clear (e.g., the child holds up a figure and says, "Go to the barn!"), while others may be subtle (e.g., the child looks at a new toy she wants to explore and looks at you). In this section, we will help you to identify and record the child's skills.

3.6.1 Recording Skills on the SPACE Data Collection and Targets Form

Record the skills you observe during the assessment on Form 3.1 (SPACE Data Collection and Targets). Live data collection is the most efficient method to capture data for the SPACE assessment. Research has shown that community-based assessors, including classroom teachers, have learned to collect high-quality data while administering the SPACE with high fidelity (Shire et al., 2018). Remember to record only the child's *spontaneous initiations* of play, gestures, and language. If the child uses a skill to imitate the adult or in response to a prompt, do *not* record that skill.

Total Time in Joint Engagement (Column 1)

- After the assessment, circle the total amount of time the child spent in supported or coordinated joint engagement during the assessment.

Total Time Regulated (Column 2)

- After the assessment, circle the total amount of time the child spent in a regulated state during the assessment.

Joint Attention Skills (Column 3)

RESPOND to JA Points

- During the assessment, tally the number of times the child responded by shifting his gaze when the assessor pointed to the pictures on the wall.
- After the assessment, circle the total number of times the child responded to the points.
- Do *not* record gestures or language that the child used to respond as separate instances of joint attention. But *do* record unique initiations that follow.
- For example: You point and say, "Benny, Benny!" Benny looks, points, and says, "It's a lion" in response. (This is recorded as a response.) Then Benny spontaneously points to another picture and says, "It's a giraffe!" (This is recorded as a spontaneous gesture and language.) Altogether, you would record one instance of response to joint attention, one spontaneous JA point, and one instance of JA language.

LOOK, SHOW, POINT, and GIVE to Share

- During the assessment, tally the number of times the child used each skill.
- After the assessment, circle the total number of times the child used each skill.
- Do *not* score unclear or partial gestures; only record those that are clear and fully formed.
- Do *not* record gestures that the assessor modeled, especially in the case of the ball activity. For

example, if the assessor modeled rolling the ball, do not record the child's imitation of rolling the ball back.

LANGUAGE to Share

- After the assessment, circle "yes" if the child used spontaneous language to share or "not yet" if the child did not use spontaneous language to share.

Requesting Skills (Column 4)

LOOK, REACH, GIVE, and POINT to Request

- During the assessment, tally the number of times the child used each skill.
- After the assessment, circle the total number of times the child used each skill.
- Do *not* record unclear gestures; only record those that are clear and fully formed.

LANGUAGE to Request

- After the assessment, circle "yes" if the child used language to request or "not yet" if the child did not use language to request.

Combines Eye Contact, Gestures, and Language (Column 4)

- After the assessment, circle "request" if the child frequently used eye contact, a gesture, and language simultaneous to request. For example, while the child is holding the windup toy, he looks at the assessor, says, "Help!" and holds out the windup toy to give to request.
- Circle "joint attention" if the child combined these skills to share or comment. For example, during the bubbles, the child looks at the assessor, JA points to a bubble, and says, "It popped!"
- Circle "not yet" if the child did not frequently combine skills.

Language Level (Column 5)

- After the assessment, circle the child's language level. The language level is based on the child's mean length of utterance (MLU), that is, the average number of words the child used within each utterance (using either spoken or augmented language). Use Exercise 3.1 to practice identifying the child's language level.

EXERCISE 3.1. **SPACE Language Level**

Circle the child's language level given the following words or phrases spoken during the SPACE.

Words used	Child's language level
Barn, elephant, boy in, Old MacDonald, in, cookie, door, cow, out	No words
	Partial/approximations
	One word
	Two words
	Phrases
	Sentences

Play Skills (Page 2)

Identify the sophistication of the child's spontaneous play skills and the number of unique types of play acts the child demonstrated in each play category (see Table 3.1).

- During the assessment, tally the number of different types of play acts the child used at each level (e.g., rolls car, stacks four blocks, and puts three pieces into a puzzle = three different types of play acts: one type at take-apart, one type at presentation combination, and one type at general combination).
- After the assessment, circle the total number of different types of play acts. (Use Exercise 3.2 to practice.)

EXERCISE 3.2. **SPACE Play Acts**

Circle the number of play types the child demonstrated for each play level during the SPACE given the following description.

Play acts demonstrated	Scoring		
• Stacks three blocks	General combination		
• Puts two blocks into the barn	Not yet	1–2 types	3+ types
• Puts the spoon to own mouth			
• Stacks four cookies on top of each other			
• Puts two blocks into the dump truck	Pretend self		
• Pretends to eat a cookie	Not yet	1–2 types	3+ types

Notes

The SPACE also provides an opportunity to get a "first read" on the child in several areas that we do not measure individually. Record additional observations in this section. These observations will give you a better picture of the child's development, help you identify necessary supports, and prepare you for the strategies to come. Here are examples of information you may choose to record.

Environment and Supports

- Needed or existing behavioral supports (difficulty with transitions)
- Needed or existing environmental supports (distractions in the room)
- Needed or existing physical supports (difficulty staying seated, low tone)

Play

- Specific play acts the child demonstrated
- Pace of play (fast or slow, many or few steps)
- Toy preferences
- Flexible or rigid play style
- Repetitive play actions, nonfunctional play with toys, distracting toys

Joint Attention or Requesting Eye Contact and Gestures

- Partial, unclear, emerging skills

Language

- Words and phrases used to request or share
- Rate of communication to respond, request, or share (fast, slow, immediately, after a pause)
- Word approximations
- Needed or existing communication supports (picture exchange system, speech-generating device)

Regulation and Engagement

- Rigid and repetitive behaviors, sensory-seeking behaviors
- First signs and possible triggers of dysregulation
- Repetitive play actions, interfering actions with toys, distracting toys

Affect and Personality

- Upbeat or low affect
- Bored or motivated
- Not interested in play or happy to play
- Not interested in people or happy to engage with people

3.6.2 Instructions for the SPACE Administration Fidelity Form

Use the SPACE Administration Fidelity Form (Form 3.2) to evaluate the quality of administration and determine which areas need to be improved. Reaching fidelity is necessary because this ensures that each child receives equal opportunities to demonstrate skills. The assessor is considered reliable after receiving a passing score of 90% with three different children who are representative of the population the individual plans to assess. If you are interested in becoming a certified SPACE assessor, a qualified trainer must evaluate your assessment and rate your fidelity form. See our website, *www.jaspertraining.org,* for more information.

3.7 Conclusion

The SPACE is an important tool for measuring the child's skills and setting targets. We recommend repeating the SPACE frequently (e.g., after 2–3 months) to ensure that the child is making progress and that your targets are on track. You will also evaluate the child's skills informally throughout the intervention using the data collection methods in Chapter 18. In the next chapter, you will use the data gathered from the SPACE to set appropriate targets for the intervention.

FORM 3.1. **SPACE Data Collection and Targets Form**

Child: _____ Adult: _____ Date: _____

Instructions:
- Record the overall quality of joint engagement and regulation and then set targets for each state.
- Tally and circle communication skills and then set targets for these skills.
- Use page 2 to record the child's play skills and targets.
- Record only *spontaneous initiations* of skills (*not* imitated or prompted responses).

DATA COLLECTION				
Joint engagement	Regulation	Joint attention skills	Requesting skills	Language (MLU)
None	None	RESPOND to JA points *Not yet 1 2 3*	LOOK to request *Not yet 1 2+*	No words
Fleeting moments	Fleeting moments	LOOK to share *Not yet 1 2+*	REACH to request *Not yet 1 2+*	Partial/ approximations
Sustained intervals	Sustained intervals	SHOW to share *Not yet 1 2+*	GIVE to request *Not yet 1 2+*	1 word
1–2 minutes	1–2 minutes	POINT to share *Not yet 1 2+*	POINT to request *Not yet 1 2+*	2-word combinations
Several minutes	Several minutes	GIVE to share *Not yet 1 2+*	LANGUAGE to request *Not yet Yes*	Phrases
Most of the interaction	Most of the interaction	LANGUAGE to share *Not yet Yes*	COMBINES eye contact, gesture, and language *Not yet Request Joint attention*	Sentences

JOINT ENGAGEMENT AND REGULATION TARGETS					
Joint engagement:	Fleeting moments	Sustained intervals	1–2 minutes	Several minutes	Most of the interaction
Regulation:	Fleeting moments	Sustained intervals	1–2 minutes	Several minutes	Most of the interaction

COMMUNICATION TARGETS					
Joint attention:	Respond*	Look*	Show	Point	Give	Coordinate skills
Requesting:		Look*	Reach	Give	Point	Coordinate skills
Language:	Diversity: _____		Complexity: _____		

*If chosen, also choose a *gesture* target (show, point, or give).

(*continued*)

	DATA COLLECTION OF PLAY SKILLS		
Simple	Indiscriminate *None 1–2 types 3+ types*	Discriminate *Not yet 1–2 types 3+ types*	Take-apart *Not yet 1–2 types 3+ types*
Combination	Presentation combination *Not yet 1–2 types 3+ types*	General combination *Not yet 1–2 types 3+ types*	
Presymbolic	Pretend self *Not yet 1–2 types 3+ types*	Physical combination *Not yet 1–2 types 3+ types*	Child as agent *Not yet 1–2 types 3+ types*
	Conventional combinations *Not yet 1–2 types 3+ types*	Single-scheme sequence *Not yet 1–2 types 3+ types*	
Symbolic	Substitution with object *Not yet 1–2 types 3+ types*	Substitution without object *Not yet 1–2 types 3+ types*	Doll as agent *Not yet 1–2 types 3+ types*
	Multi-scheme sequence *Not yet 1 2 types 3+ types*	Sociodramatic *Not yet 1–2 types 3+ types*	Thematic *Not yet 1–2 types 3+ types*

PLAY TARGETS
Mastered play level: _____   Target play level: _____
Remember to increase the quality of the skills too!
Diversity   Flexibility   Creativity

Notes:

SPACE Administration Fidelity Form

Child: _____ Adult: _____ Rater: _____

Date of assessment: _____ Date of rating: _____

Instructions:
- Mark "Yes" if the adult used the strategy appropriately and according to JASPER guidelines.
- Mark "No" if the adult did not use the strategy appropriately and according to JASPER guidelines.
- Mark N/A if the adult did not have an opportunity to use the strategy during session.
- Additional notes can be taken on the back of the form.

Action during the assessment		Yes	No
1. Adult provides full set of correct materials.			
2. Adult begins assessment by gesturing with an open palm and saying, "Let's play!" and then pauses for child to make toy selection.			
3. Adult helps child notice and engage with all materials through environmental arrangement.			
4. Adult avoids modeling play acts and avoids providing verbal or physical prompts related to the toys.			
5. Adult uses appropriate supports for engagement and regulation.			
Blocks, truck, shape sorter, and puzzle set		**Yes**	**No**
6. Adult introduces occluded box or bag of toys and waits for child to open box and explore toys.			
7. Adult allows child enough time to play with all materials in set.			
Barn, food, furniture, and figures set		**Yes**	**No**
8. Adult introduces occluded box or bag of toys and waits for child to open box and explore toys.			
9. Adult allows child enough time to play with all materials in set.			
Balloon or bubbles		**Yes**	**No**
10. Adult places balloon or bubbles in center of table and gives 2–4 presentations.			
11. Adult pauses and provides opportunity for child to spontaneously initiate requests (eye contact, point, give, language) and does not prompt child to return balloon or bubbles to the adult.			
Points to pictures		**Yes**	**No**
12. Adult completes set of 3 distal points. Adult's points are fully formed and do not extend past the elbow. Adult holds gaze with point and does not look back at child. Adult implements points in correct order (left across, right across, behind).			
13. Adult calls child's name twice while pointing to picture. Adult pauses and waits for response, and then labels picture.			
Windup toy		**Yes**	**No**
14. Adult activates windup toy on corner of table (out of the child's reach), pauses, and allows child opportunity to request toy or share excitement.			
Ball		**Yes**	**No**
15. Adult places ball in center of table to start and holds out hands as if ready to catch ball. Adult pauses and waits for child initiation.			
16a. If child rolls ball, adult rolls it back and forth a couple of times. OR 16b. If child does not roll ball, adult rolls it once to child and then removes it if child is not interested in rolling it back and forth.			

Person engagement activity (if included)	N/A	Yes	No
17. Adult starts with invitation, such as "Let's sing a song" or "Let's play a game."			
18. Adult pauses for child to request and then repeats song.			
Scoring			
Total "Yes": _____ of _____ Percentage Fidelity (passing rate = 90%): _____%			

CHAPTER 4

Identifying Mastered and Target Skills

4.1 Introduction

In this chapter, we explain how to select developmentally appropriate intervention targets given the information acquired from the SPACE (see Chapter 3). For every child, you will set targets for the following domains: joint engagement, regulation, play, language, joint attention gestures, and requesting gestures. Once the child acquires a target, you will move on to the next skill within that domain. Each child progresses at a different rate. You may not reach the highest skills in each category; however, you should see regular indicators of improvement as the intervention progresses.

4.2 Setting Targets

Use Form 3.1 (SPACE Data Collection and Targets) from the previous chapter to set developmentally appropriate targets for the intervention. In JASPER, we set *targets* in small, attainable increments, one step higher than the child's current developmental level. For example, if the child starts with indiscriminate acts, we target the next level of simple play (discriminate acts), then the next level in simple play (take-apart), and so on. We do not target higher skills in a domain before the child has acquired the preceding levels. This ensures that the targets are realistic and attainable for the child.

4.2.1 Indicators of Mastery and Emergence

To set targets, you must have a clear sense of which skills are mastered, which skills are emerging, and which skills are absent. A *mastered* skill is a skill the child has already learned and is able to use spontaneously. An *emerging* skill is a skill that the child can demonstrate but is not yet fully comfortable using or is using infrequently. See Figure 4.1 for indicators of emerging and mastered skills.

Frequency is often a clear sign of mastery, but it is not always a reliable indicator on its own. You must consider the overall quality of the skill as well. For example, if the child points to request several times, but only partially extends his finger after a considerable delay, the skill is probably not yet mastered. Similarly, if the child only imitates the skill but never spontaneously initiates it, it is most likely not yet mastered. True mastery emerges when the child is able to initiate the skill confidently and spontaneously in a variety of settings.

Identifying the child's mastered and emerging skills often requires clinical judgment; in other words, you must evaluate a number of factors and rely on your knowledge of the child and prior experience to make an accurate judgment call. If you are not sure if the skill is mastered, err on the side of emerging and create more opportunities for the child to solidify the skill in session.

MASTERED SKILLS	EMERGING SKILLS
○ Used frequently (2+ instances for gestures, 3+ types for play acts on the SPACE)	○ Used sparingly
○ Able to be spontaneously initiated	○ Not used spontaneously (only imitated or in response to prompts)
○ Easy, consistent, and flexible	○ Rigid and repetitive
○ Integrated with other skills (e.g., paired with eye contact)	○ Difficulty using the skill
○ Used across multiple contexts, (e.g., different activities, people, and situations)	○ Unclear skills (word approximations, partially formed gestures)

FIGURE 4.1. Mastered versus emerging skills.

4.2.2 Why Not Target Higher Skills?

JASPER targets skills within the child's *zone of proximal development* (Vygotsky, 1978). In other words, we target skills within one step of the child's mastered level, not too low or too high. This ensures that the target is realistic and achievable. If the child is starting at the lowest developmental level (A) and we want the child to be at the highest developmental level (Z), we must make sure the child learns all of the small and important steps in between (B through Y). By targeting skills within the child's developmental range, we keep the demands reasonable and "bite-sized," so that we do not overload the child with too many difficult expectations at once. If we jump to the highest skills, the child may have more difficulty engaging in a high-quality interaction and may be more likely to interact in limited (even scripted) ways.

4.3 Targets by Domain

In the sections below, we provide information and practice for setting targets in each domain, represented in Form 3.1 (SPACE Data Collection and Targets). Within each domain, the order of the skills reflects the typical developmental sequence from the earliest and simplest skills to later developing and more complex skills, as outlined in Chapter 2. In general, you will first identify the child's mastered skill in each domain and then set the child's targets one step higher, following the order of skills listed in Form 3.1. Keep the child's age in mind as you work toward your goals. The highest goals in each domain may not be appropriate, depending on the child's chronological age. For example, we would not expect an infant to be in a state of coordinated joint engagement for much time or to play symbolically, since these are unreasonable goals at that age.

4.3.1 Engagement and Regulation Targets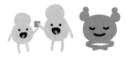

Set the target one step higher than the time point you circled. For example, if the child only has *fleeting moments* (e.g., 3–5 seconds) of regulation, the target is *sustained intervals* (e.g., 15–30 seconds) of regulation. Once you identify the child's target, work toward incrementally longer periods of joint engagement and regulation.

4.3.2 Gesture Targets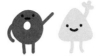

Set the target gesture one step higher than the child's mastered gestures on the SPACE. For example, if the child has mastered the JA show, target a JA point. The gesture is likely mastered if the child uses it clearly and spontaneously two or more times on the SPACE. If the gesture is unclear or partially formed, then it is likely emerging. Here are some examples of unclear gestures:

- *Unclear point.* Points with loose hand or with different finger instead of clear, index finger.
- *Unclear show.* Turns object inward toward self or does not clearly direct object toward another person.
- *Unclear give.* Sets object in front of person but does not attempt to place in hand.
- *Unclear reach.* Reaching for object without clear social requesting intent.

In most cases, you can follow the order of Form 3.1 (SPACE Data Collection and Targets) to set targets; however, in some cases, it may be more logical to choose the target gesture based on the child's emerging skills. For example, if the child demonstrates an emerging skill that is out of sequence (e.g., the child is starting to use a JA give but has not shown JA points or JA shows), you can target a JA give first. We are flexible in the order we target gestures since gestures emerge in overlapping order or very closely together in typical development.

If you choose to target respond to JA, JA look, or look to request, you should also choose a gesture target (e.g., show, point, or give). If the child is using language and gestures separately, target combining these skills, so the child can use them concurrently (e.g., using a JA show to hold out a yellow block while saying, "Yellow!"). Practice identifying the child's mastered and target gestures in Exercise 4.1.

EXERCISE 4.1. Mastered and Target Gestures

Identify the child's mastered and target skills based on the information provided.

REQUESTING TARGETS

1. The child looked at you a few times to gain access to toy and reached once for the windup.

Mastered requesting skill:	Eye contact	Reach	Give	Point	Coordinate skills
Target requesting skill:	Eye contact	Reach	Give	Point	Coordinate skills

2. The child looked at you several times, reached for several objects, pointed several times to gain access to the toys on the shelf, and gave the windup once to ask for it to be activated again.

Mastered requesting skill:	Eye contact	Reach	Give	Point	Coordinate skills
Target requesting skill:	Eye contact	Reach	Give	Point	Coordinate skills

3. The child did not look at you. He reached once toward the balloon.

Mastered requesting skill:	Eye contact	Reach	Give	Point	Coordinate skills
Target requesting skill:	Eye contact	Reach	Give	Point	Coordinate skills

JOINT ATTENTION TARGETS

4. The child pointed several times to share and raised several toys toward herself as if to show the toy.

Mastered JA skill:	Respond to point	Look	Show	Point	Give	Coordinate skills
Target JA skill:	Respond to point	Look	Show	Point	Give	Coordinate skills

5. The child pointed several times and shared a figure with the assessor using one JA give.

Mastered JA skill:	Respond to point	Look	Show	Point	Give	Coordinate skills
Target JA skill:	Respond to point	Look	Show	Point	Give	Coordinate skills

---

4.3.3 Language Target

To identify the child's language target, first determine the child's length of utterance (as defined in Chapter 3) and then set targets for diversity and complexity. The immediate goal is to increase the diversity of the child's current language level, and the long-term goal is to increase the complexity by targeting one step higher. Thus, if the child primarily uses one-word utterances during the assessment, the targets are *one-word utterances* (diversity) and *two-word combinations* (complexity).

EXERCISE 4.2. **Mastered and Target Length of Utterance**

Circle the child's mastered and target length of utterance and write in targets for diversity and complexity based on the information provided. Note: Vocalizations are marked with V.

1. Horse, cat, dog, truck, circle, it crashed, Old MacDonald, cookie

   Mastered MLU: No words/partial words   1 word   2 words   Phrases   Sentences

   Diversity target: _____

   Complexity target: _____

2. More shapes, truck, go, sleep time, block on, eat cookies, eat more cookies

   Mastered MLU: No words/partial words   1 word   2 words   Phrases   Sentences

   Diversity target: _____

   Complexity target: _____

4.3.4 Play Target

To identify the child's play target, determine the child's mastered play level and set the target one play level higher. The child's mastered play level is typically the highest level at which the child shows three or more different spontaneous play acts. It is *not* the highest play level the child demonstrates. If the child's play level is presentation combination, then target general combination. If the mastered play level is general combination, target pretend self, and so on. Note that while indiscriminate is the first level of play, it is never a target in JASPER. If the child does not show any play acts or primarily shows indiscriminate acts, we begin to work on discriminate acts. As you set targets, keep in mind that play targets are not always linear and the order of development may vary with each child. We address some additional considerations below.

Consider the Context of the Play Act

You may not always know the play level based upon the actions alone and may need to consider the broader context and other indicators. The same play act can demonstrate different levels of ability depending on the child. For one child, the act of putting food into the bowl is simply a general combination of putting things together in different ways. For another child, this act could be symbolic. For example, the child says he is "making soup" and describes the ingredients he is putting in, demonstrating the more symbolic idea of cooking.

Be Aware of Splintered Play Skills

Sometimes, children with ASD learn play skills out of order. When there is a big jump from the lower play levels to higher play levels, with skills missing in between, we call these *splintered skills*. For example, the child primarily shows combination play actions but has a few emerging symbolic actions. Situations like these can be confusing at first, because it appears as though the child's developmental level is higher than it is. Yet there are typically indictors that these higher-level symbolic actions are not fully flexible and natural. In these cases, you should continue to follow the developmental sequence of skills on Form 3.1 (SPACE Data Collection and Targets), targeting the first skill that the child has not yet mastered. In the example above, you would focus on mastering combination play actions and then moving onto presymbolic.

Remain Flexible within the Presymbolic Levels

Even though you will set a mastered and target level, you must be flexible in how you teach the presymbolic skills. You may recall from Chapter 2 that there is often variability in how the presymbolic skills emerge (see examples of three potential pathways in Figure 4.2). Some children learn the presymbolic combination acts first, others learn the presymbolic acts with agents first, and others learn both at the same time. Therefore, we often teach the presymbolic skills simultaneously in play. Based on the nature of the play, opportunities may arise during the routine where you can work on a different play skill within the presymbolic level. For instance, if the child chooses to play with blocks, that might be a good opportunity to work on physical combination and child as agent play levels. If the child moves on to a food routine during the same session, you can work on conventional combination, pretend-self, and child-as-agent acts.

Practice identifying the child's mastered and target play levels in Exercise 4.3.

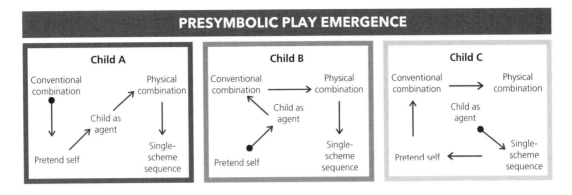

FIGURE 4.2. Presymbolic skills are flexible in the order that they emerge.

EXERCISE 4.3. Mastered and Target Play Skills

Circle the child's highest mastered and target play levels based on the information provided.

1. The child demonstrated three types of discriminate acts, three types of take-apart, one type of presentation combination, one type of general combination, and one pretend-self action.

   Mastered play level: Discriminate acts   Take-apart

                               Presentation combination   General combination

                               Pretend self   Physical combination

   Target play level: Presentation combination   General combination

                               Pretend self   Physical combination

                               Child as agent   Conventional combination

2. The child demonstrated three types of general combination acts, one type of physical combination act, three types of child-as-agent acts, and one doll-as-agent act.

   Mastered play level: Presentation combination   General combination

                               Pretend self   Physical combination

                               Child as agent   Conventional combination

   Target play level: Pretend self   Physical combination

                               Child as agent   Conventional combination

                               Single scheme   Doll as agent

4.4 Practice Setting Intervention Targets

Before you administer the SPACE for the first time, practice scoring an assessment and setting targets using the case example below. Reference the following for assistance:

- Form 3.1, SPACE Data Collection and Targets
- Section 3.6.1, Recording Skills on the SPACE Data Collection and Targets Form
- Sections 4.2–4.3, instructions for setting targets
- Figure 4.3, SPACE Data Collection and Targets Form for Jackie

After the case example, we will introduce some common questions that may have come up as you practice.

4.4.1 Case Example

Below is a description of a child's performance on the SPACE:

Jackie is a 6-year-old girl with autism who is considered minimally verbal. The SPACE was administered in the classroom by her teacher. During the assessment, Jackie showed very few play skills and required a lot of support to regulate. She banged a few toys on the table and used a lot of eye contact to request and share with her teacher. She was drawn to the doors on the barn and spent much of the time opening and closing them. Jackie enjoyed the bubbles and frequently shared excitement with her teacher using coordinated looks. When her teacher pointed to pictures on the wall, Jackie sometimes responded by shifting her gaze. She reached for the bubbles several times. Jackie used minimal language to request during the interaction (e.g., "More"; "Go").

Jackie showed a few simple play skills and some combination skills, such as placing two cookies on the tray and stacking up three blocks. There were also a few moments during the assessment when she showed presymbolic skills, such as putting a spoon and a cookie to her mouth (pretend self). Jackie had difficulty staying engaged throughout the assessment. As she became dysregulated, she rocked back and forth in her seat and made loud vocalizations. Her teacher used sensory squeezes and brief songs at several points to help her regulate. Her teacher also commented on Jackie's play, but Jackie did not seem to notice.

We filled out Jackie's SPACE Data Collection and Targets Form in Figure 4.3. Using the information provided, circle the child's targets.

4.4.2 Explanation of Intervention Targets

In this section, we provide answers and rationale for the intervention target choices within each domain.

Joint engagement goal: Sustained intervals
- Jackie is only engaged for fleeting moments (e.g., 3–5 seconds) during the SPACE, so her target is sustained intervals (e.g., 15–30 seconds). Jackie's engagement is often disrupted by moments of dysregulation, so we want to increase the time she is in higher states of engagement and facilitate longer moments of joint engagement.

SPACE Data Collection and Targets Form

Child: _J. M._   Adult: _C. S._   Date: _July 02_

Instructions:
- Record the overall quality of joint engagement and regulation and then set targets for each state.
- Tally and circle communication skills and then set targets for these skills.
- Use page 2 to record the child's play skills and targets.
- Record only *spontaneous initiations* of skills (*not* imitated or prompted responses).

DATA COLLECTION				
Joint engagement	**Regulation**	**Joint attention skills**	**Requesting skills**	**Language (MLU)**
None	None	RESPOND to JA points *Not yet 1 2 3*	LOOK to request *Not yet 1 2+*	No words
Fleeting moments	Fleeting moments	LOOK to share *Not yet 1 2+*	REACH to request *Not yet 1 2+*	Partial/ approximations
Sustained intervals	Sustained intervals	SHOW to share *Not yet 1 2+*	GIVE to request *Not yet 1 2+*	*1 word*
1–2 minutes	1–2 minutes	POINT to share *Not yet 1 2+*	POINT to request *Not yet 1 2+*	2-word combinations
Several minutes	Several minutes	GIVE to share *Not yet 1 2+*	LANGUAGE to request *Not yet Yes*	Phrases
Most of the interaction	Most of the interaction	LANGUAGE to share *Not yet Yes*	COMBINES eye contact, gesture, and language *Not yet Request Joint attention*	Sentences

JOINT ENGAGEMENT AND REGULATION TARGETS					
Joint engagement:	Fleeting moments	Sustained intervals	1–2 minutes	Several minutes	Most of the interaction
Regulation:	Fleeting moments	Sustained intervals	1–2 minutes	Several minutes	Most of the interaction

COMMUNICATION TARGETS					
Joint attention:	Respond*	Look*	Show	Point	Give	Coordinate skills
Requesting:		Look*	Reach	Give	Point	Coordinate skills
Language:	Diversity: _____		Complexity: _____		

*If chosen, also choose a *gesture* target (show, point, or give).   (continued)

FIGURE 4.3. Example of filled-out SPACE Data Collection and Targets Form.

SPACE Data Collection and Targets Form *(p. 2 of 2)*

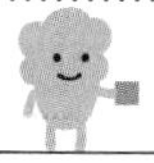

DATA COLLECTION OF PLAY SKILLS		

	Indiscriminate *None* *1–2 types* *3+ types*	Discriminate *Not yet* *1–2 types* *3+ types*	Take-apart *Not yet* *1–2 types* *3+ types*
Simple	Bang toys on table	Push truck Open/close barn doors	Take blocks out Take cookies off Dump cookies

	Presentation combination *Not yet* *1–2 types* *3+ types*		General combination *Not yet* *1–2 types* *3+ types*	
Combination	Puzzle piece in Cookie on tray Shape in sorter		Stack blocks	

	Pretend self *Not yet* *1–2 types* *3+ types*	Physical combination *Not yet* *1–2 types* *3+ types*	Child as agent *Not yet* *1–2 types* *3+ types*
Presymbolic	Cookie to mouth Spoon to mouth		
	Conventional combinations *Not yet* *1–2 types* *3+ types*	Single-scheme sequence *Not yet* *1–2 types* *3+ types*	

	Substitution with object *Not yet* *1–2 types* *3+ types*	Substitution without object *Not yet* *1–2 types* *3+ types*	Doll as agent *Not yet* *1–2 types* *3+ types*
Symbolic			
	Multi-scheme sequence *Not yet* *1–2 types* *3+ types*	Sociodramatic *Not yet* *1–2 types* *3+ types*	Thematic *Not yet* *1–2 types* *3+ types*

PLAY TARGETS

Mastered play level: _____   Target play level: _____

Remember to increase the quality of the skills too!

Diversity   Flexibility   Creativity

Notes: Communication:
         Req. lang.: "more" "go"
         Partial give for bubbles (emerging)
         Need: SGD, table/chair support

         Regulation: bouncing in seat, vocal stims
         (easily dysregulated)

         First read:
         Mostly unengaged, some object

FIGURE 4.3 *(continued)*

Regulation goal: Sustained intervals

- Jackie needs help with regulation. She is only regulated for fleeting moments during the SPACE, so her target is sustained intervals. The interventionist will need to implement strategies to address this (e.g., environmental support, supporting engagement), understanding that being regulated for sustained intervals of time is a reasonable target for this child.

Play target: General combination

- Jackie's mastered play level is presentation combination. She showed several discriminate acts and presentation combinations and one general combination. Although she demonstrated a couple of emerging presymbolic acts, Jackie did not show many skills in between simple and presymbolic. In order to build up these missing skills, we will target general combination first. Since Jackie's combination and presymbolic skills are emerging concurrently, we can use toys that promote both combination and some presymbolic actions during the JASPER session.

Requesting gesture target: Give

- Jackie was able to use a reach with eye contact to request several times. We will target the next missing skill, the give to request.

JA gesture target: Show

- Jackie responded to two of the teacher's points and used looked to share, so we will target the next developmental skill, a JA show.

Language target: One word

- Jackie has not yet mastered one-word utterances. She used a couple of words to request and is not yet using language to share. Since she has partial and single words, we will set one word as the target for both diversity and complexity (as we do not target partial words and two-word combinations would be too high).

4.4.3 Common Questions

In the section below, we address some common questions on choosing targets.

What if the child did not use a skill that I know he has?

If the child did not use a skill you believe he already knows, there may be a few reasons:

- The child knows how to use the skill only to respond, not to initiate.
- The child may not be fully comfortable using the skill, because it is not yet mastered.
- The child is simply having an "off" day. This might be a sign that the child is not completely comfortable in this new setting.
- The child was not provided with clear opportunities to demonstrate the skill.
- The skill is so far below the child's mastered level that it is no longer interesting to the child.

Set your targets based on the skills you saw during the SPACE. If it is clear later during intervention that the child has fully developed a skill, you can adjust your targets accordingly.

Can I target the same gesture for JA and requesting?

You may notice that some of the gestures are overlapping between requesting and joint attention. Although joint attention and requesting are two different functions of communication, the physical form of the gesture can be the same. For example, a child may point to socially share (joint attention) or to get a need or want met (requesting). When a child is first learning to use gestures to communicate, you may choose joint attention and requesting gesture targets that differ in form. Choosing gestures that are different in their visual and physical form may help the child to link each distinct gesture to a different communicative function. For example, you may choose a show for joint attention and a point for requesting, rather than choosing a point target for both joint attention and requesting.

4.5   Conclusion

This chapter explained how to identify the child's mastered and emerging skills and to choose intervention targets for the core JASPER domains. You will rely heavily on this information throughout the intervention as you work toward the child's targets. As the child progresses, you should see improvement in the child's play and communication skills and engagement and regulation states. Continue updating the child's targets accordingly as you identify new skills and after each SPACE assessment. This concludes Part II. Part III introduces the first set of core strategies of JASPER, starting with an introduction to JASPER play routines.

PREPARING FOR SESSION

In this section, you will learn how to strategically set up the learning environment and plan play routines.

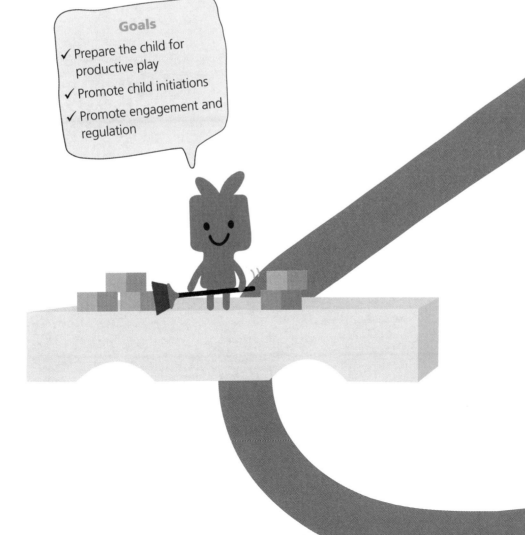

Goals

✓ Prepare the child for productive play

✓ Promote child initiations

✓ Promote engagement and regulation

Introduction to JASPER Routines

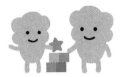

5.1 Introduction

In this chapter, we will begin discussing the core strategies of JASPER, starting with play routines. Play routines are the context in which all the core domains of the intervention come together—play, communication, engagement, and regulation. JASPER play routines help support our goals by providing both the structure necessary to help the child engage and the flexibility and fun of typical play interactions. In this chapter, we will define routines, explain the components and qualities of routines, and then describe your role within the routine.

5.2 Description of Play Routines

The idea of a "routine" is common throughout many interventions and activities. In JASPER, we define *play routines* as toy-based interactions that include developmentally appropriate toys, two active players, repeated practice, and a mixture of familiar and flexible steps that build toward a central purpose or theme. Rather than having a clear beginning, middle, and end to the routine, JASPER routines are ongoing. They can unfold in many different ways, start over, and end at any time. Routines include clear opportunities for communicating and learning, while also maintaining the fun, natural, and flexible qualities found in typical play interactions. Figure 5.1 shows how all these features come together within a routine.

5.3 Components of a Play Routine

The basic structure of the routine includes a *base* (i.e., a starting point), several *expansions* (i.e., novel additions), and opportunities to *restart* (i.e., additional practice), as illustrated in Figure 5.2. These steps are repeated with small changes over time to provide both familiarity and flexibility.

In order to have a successful routine, you must first establish a strong foundation of play steps at the base and then either restart or expand the routine. Together, these steps extend engagement and keep the interaction moving forward. Here is an example of how the components of the routine work together:

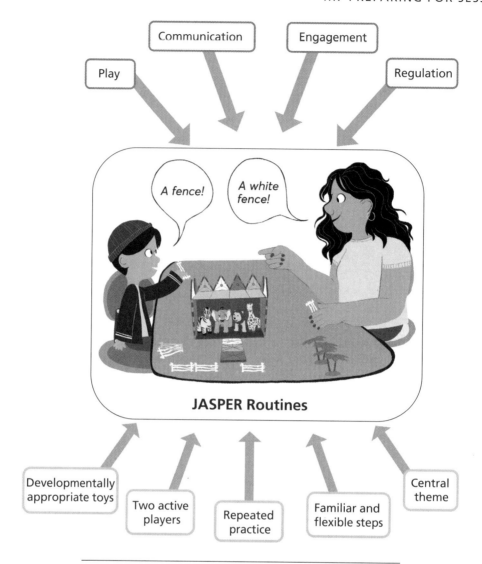

FIGURE 5.1. Play routines support each of the JASPER goals.

The adult and child stack blocks until they build a zoo (base); they knock the zoo down and start building it up again (restart after the base); they build another zoo (base); they add animals to the zoo (expansion); they knock the zoo down together and start building again (restart after the expansion).

The components of the routine are most apparent when children are first learning to play. For children with ASD, it may take some time and effort to establish the base and expand the routine, and you may need to restart more often to establish these steps. As children learn more play skills at higher play levels, routines become more flexible and complex. While the components of the base, restart, and expansion are still present, they may be less apparent and often emerge more naturally.

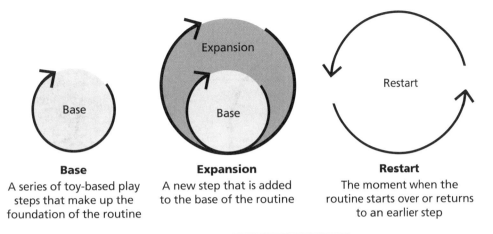

Base
A series of toy-based play steps that make up the foundation of the routine

Expansion
A new step that is added to the base of the routine

Restart
The moment when the routine starts over or returns to an earlier step

FIGURE 5.2. Components of a routine.

5.3.1 Base

Every routine starts with a base. This is a single play step or a short sequence of play steps. These steps should be at the child's mastered play level. (Refer to Chapter 4, Section 4.2.1, for indicators of mastered play). The purpose of the base is to establish a series of play acts that the child can comfortably sustain, add to, and return to throughout the life of the routine. We restart to repeat the base until the child is familiar with these initial steps. This creates a foundation for more skills, such as language, gestures, and eventually new play acts. In Figure 5.3, the base involves attaching frosting to the cookies and then placing cookies on the tray.

The number of base steps can vary depending on the child. For example, the cookie routine could have a one-step base (e.g., put the cookies on the tray), or it could have a multistep base (e.g., put frosting pieces on cookies, put cookies on tray, pretend to eat cookies), as illustrated in Figure 5.4. The number of base steps should be determined by the child's need for immediate repetition, the child's comfort adding new steps, and the familiarity of a specific routine. The base steps should be comfortable and easy for the child to sustain and repeat several times, with the

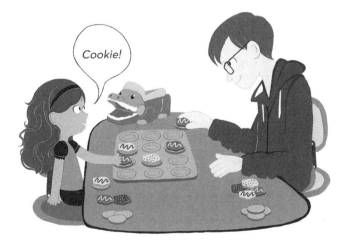

FIGURE 5.3. The adult and child add cookies to establish the base of the routine.

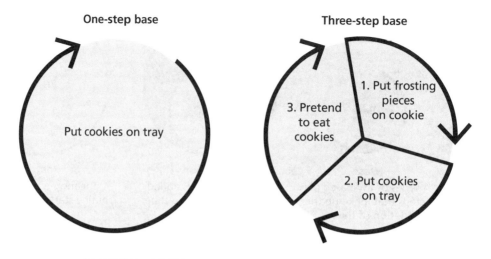

One-step base

Put cookies on tray

Three-step base

1. Put frosting pieces on cookie

2. Put cookies on tray

3. Pretend to eat cookies

FIGURE 5.4. The base can include one step or several steps.

child primarily initiating and you following along. We will explain how to choose toys for the base in Chapter 6 and discuss the details of establishing the base in Chapter 10.

5.3.2 Expansion

Once the child is comfortable with the base steps, you can expand the routine by adding one new step. For example, in Figure 5.5, the child expands the routine by feeding the cookies to the alligator toy. Where the base is predictable and repeatable, expansions help the routine grow to be flexible, diverse, and creative over time. They also make the routine more fun and more like natural play!

As you expand the routine, there are various options for which direction the routine can go, depending on the child's play level and available materials. For example, in Figure 5.5, the child initiates feeding the alligator (child as agent), but other expansions could have been to stack the cookies on top of each other (general combination) or put the cookies onto a plate (conventional

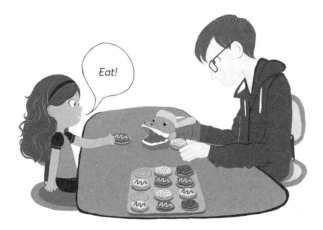

Eat!

FIGURE 5.5. The child expands the routine by putting the cookie in the alligator.

combination). We keep a number of toy choices available for every routine to support the many ways the routine could evolve.

Expansions can be more or less complex depending on the child's ability. Some children have routines that expand to include just a couple new steps, whereas other children have routines that develop numerous expansions across a longer story line. Some children will be able to expand more quickly; other children will need more time and repetition to establish the base before they expand. You should always be thinking about how you can use these steps to grow the routine and help it become more flexible and diverse. This is how we work toward our play targets and eventually increase the child's play level, extend engagement, and increase opportunities for communication and initiations. We will explain how to choose toys for expansions in Chapter 6 and discuss the details of expanding in Chapter 11.

5.3.3 Restart

You can also restart the routine to transition back to an earlier step. To do this, you simply crash or reset the materials to return to a previous part in the routine. You can restart at any time throughout the routine; however, the most natural moments are after the base steps, after expanding, during a moment of decreased engagement (to reengage the child), or simply when a fun opportunity arises (e.g., a monster comes and crashes the tower you were building). See Figure 11.11 for signs that it is time to restart.

Restarting after the Base

In JASPER, we repeat the base until the child is familiar with these initial steps. For example, in the cookie routine from Figure 5.5, you could restart the routine by taking the frosting off the cookies and the cookies off the tray. This gives the child another chance to become accustomed to the base steps before you add an expansion. A child who is just learning to play might restart the base several times before demonstrating a strong foundation of engagement, while another child might be ready to expand immediately. We will discuss the details of restarting after the base in Chapter 10.

Restarting after an Expansion

You can also restart after an expansion. In Figure 5.6, the adult dumps the cookies out of the alligator's mouth. After restarting, you can return to the base and try adding the same expansion once again. Or you can return to an earlier step in the routine and add a new expansion. Restarting helps the child practice the new expansion step as part of the routine. We will discuss the details of restarting after an expansion in Chapter 11.

Restarting to Maintain Engagement

Restarting is a useful tool to support the child's engagement. If the routine gets too complex or the child begins to lose engagement, you can choose to restart the routine partway through. This allows the child to practice the easier, more familiar steps of the base and to reestablish engagement. See Chapter 15 for more information on how to use the routine to maintain the child's engagement.

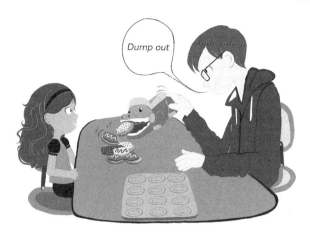

FIGURE 5.6. The adult dumps out the cookies to restart the routine.

Restarting When Natural Opportunities Arise

You do not have to wait until the child completes a certain number of steps to restart the routine. You can also restart during natural moments in the routine, such as if the tower you are building falls apart. This reflects typical play, with flexible steps and just a bit of added structure.

5.3.4 Transitioning to a New Routine

At some point, the child will lose interest in the routine. When this happens, you can move on to something else. While it is okay to try to extend the child's engagement in the routine for a while, you should not fight the child to stay in the routine beyond a reasonable point, nor require the child to "finish" the activity. It is natural and expected for children to lose interest with a specific toy or routine eventually. See Chapter 11 for more information on transitioning to a new routine.

5.3.5 Common Questions

We address some common questions about the components of the routine in the section below. In many cases, there is not a definitive answer that applies to all children; rather, you should think about the bigger picture and the particular needs of the child in front of you.

How many steps are in a routine?

Routines do not have a predefined number of steps. The steps can change within each routine, across routines, and over time. You may have more steps or fewer, depending on the child's play level, level of regulation, and the quality and duration of engagement. However, the number of steps in a routine should increase over time as different routines become more comfortable and the child builds new play skills.

Can I return to a previous routine during the same session?

Yes! The child can return to a previously used toy or routine during the same session. As long as the child is able to engage with the toys and you, there is benefit in repeating the same routines.

This is common of typically developing children as well, who often return to favorite play steps or activities. However, if the child seems overly interested in a routine and begins to play rigidly or repetitively, you may choose not to return to these particular steps.

How many routines should the child have total?

Over time, you and the child will begin to develop a collection of routines that you can use across sessions. The number of routines depends on the child and the length of intervention. You will start out with a few routines, make changes to those routines, add more routines over time, and perhaps set some routines aside for a time. In general, we are not concerned with number of routines or the number of play acts within a routine. Rather, the purpose is to create varied contexts for the child to practice different play acts, diverse communication, and rich social interaction.

Before we move on to the next section, take a moment to complete Exercise 5.1 on the components of a routine.

EXERCISE 5.1. **Components of a Routine**

Indicate whether each statement is true or false according to JASPER guidelines.

1. A routine can have multiple steps that make up the base.	True	False
2. There must be at least two expansions in every routine.	True	False
3. Restarting should happen only after an expansion.	True	False
4. A routine should be repeated as long as the child is still interested and the routine remains flexible.	True	False
5. If the child is ready for a new routine, you should have the child complete the current sequence of steps before you move on.	True	False

---

5.4 Qualities of a Play Routine

The best way to understand the "feel" of a routine is to watch several JASPER sessions with children who have different interests, characteristics, and developmental levels. While the structure of the session and the routine are the same, the look and feel of the session is adapted to the needs, motivation, and interests of each child. In reality, no two sessions or routines look exactly the same. In the sections below, we discuss the qualities of JASPER routines.

5.4.1 Routines Are a Natural, Playful Context

For children, a natural learning environment is one that is playful and fun! It should be motivating and enjoyable for the child and have a feeling of openness, curiosity, and exploration. When you place too much focus on "teaching" instead of "playing," you lose the natural context that we aim to create. The challenge is in finding the appropriate balance between providing support for learning and maintaining a motivating experience.

Support a Purposeful Direction

A routine is not a series of random actions taken in sequence. It must have a purposeful direction that is connected by a story or theme that makes sense *to the child*. Consider the following steps: The child puts a figure in a house, gives a stuffed animal a bite of food, and then puts a block on a tower. This is not a routine because it lacks cohesion between the steps. Instead, the play steps should come together in a meaningful way, as if you and the child are creating a story together. When you engage in a string of disconnected acts, you are unable to build the momentum in the routine, expansions no longer make sense, and there is no central topic for the conversation. A purposeful direction is essential for promoting longer periods of engagement and regulation and the development of play, cognition, and communication skills.

Avoid Drilling Particular Words or Play Acts

Routines are not teaching trials. The child does not have to say specific words or learn specific play acts that you predefine ahead of time. Rather, there are many teaching opportunities that can be naturally incorporated within play routines. To truly learn how to play and communicate, children need more than the discrete skills. They need to learn how to connect these skills together into flexible reciprocal interactions and to do so without frequent prompts from the adult.

Do Not Treat the Routine Like a Task

A routine is not a task to be completed. We do not expect the child to accomplish a defined sequence or a specific number of steps before moving on to something else. For example, if we give the child a ring stacker, the routine is not over when the rings are stacked. Instead of ending the routine at that standard step, we can continue the routine by restarting (e.g., taking the rings off of the stacker) or adding creative expansions (e.g., adding another type of rings to the stacker).

5.4.2 Routines Are Tailored to the Child

Tailor the routines to the interests and experiences of each child.

Follow the Child's Interests

Follow the child's play ideas as much as possible and allow the child to make decisions that direct the course of the routine. Notice the child's attentional focus and follow the child's choices. (This is how we work toward a state of coordinated joint engagement.) With that said, we are also careful when following the child's choice of activity. If the child's play acts become rigid, repetitive, or far below his developmental level, we do not follow the child's steps; instead, we provide toy choices that lead to more productive actions and joint engagement.

Consider the Child's Experience

As you build routines, think about the experience of the child in front of you. You can get quite creative and even tailor the routine to the child's daily experiences, as long as you stay within the child's developmental level. For example, if the child frequently rides the metro and is learning to play at a symbolic level, you could build a routine that involves figures buying a metro pass, scanning the tickets, boarding the train, and pretending to get off at a familiar stop. This incorporates the child's experience in a fun and playful way. If the child has not had the particular experience you are trying to re-create in the routine, then he will be unlikely to initiate new steps, share ideas, or communicate about what is happening. As children become more comfortable with symbolic play steps and ideas, you can begin to add more abstract topics (e.g., novel experiences or fantasy) to help encourage their creativity and symbolism.

5.4.3 Routines Match the Child's Developmental Level

Routines consist of steps at the child's developmental level. There should be some steps at the mastered level to establish the base, new steps at this same level to build play diversity, and other steps at the child's target level to build play complexity. This balance of familiarity and novelty helps maintain engagement, while building new skills. Routines can look very different depending on the play level. We describe some of these differences below.

Routines at Lower Play Levels

Routines at lower play levels may look more "structured" with a clear base, restart, and expansion. These routines typically have more repetition and are less thematic. For example, nest boxes (base), stack the boxes (expansion), put other shapes inside the boxes (expansion), and take each box off to nest them again (restart); cut toy food (base), put food on a plate (base), give the food to a tummy stuffer (expansion), and have the tummy stuffer pretend to sneeze as you dump all of the food out (restart).

Routines at Higher Play Levels

Routines at higher play levels are often made up of several actions that connect to a broader theme, for example, baking a cake or taking dolls to an amusement park. These routines look less like a repeated sequence and more like a story that evolves. For example, the child might pretend that the dolls are getting ready to go to the zoo, getting in the car, petting the different animals, and so on. The dolls might then get ready to go to a new location. While the components of the routine are still present at higher levels, they may be less apparent. There may be a greater number of unique steps, and the components of the routine may be more flexible. At the very highest levels of play, you may not have a traditional restart at all; rather, the routine may continue to grow and change, with a variety of steps across numerous levels.

Examples

Here are some examples of routines at different levels:

> **Simple play routine:** *The adult and child roll a ball back and forth to each other, take turns dropping balls down a ramp structure, and then take the balls out of the structure one at a time before doing it all again.*

> **Combination routine:** *The adult and child put shapes in a shape sorter. They dump out the pieces, stack the pieces, put the shapes into the container again, stack nesting boxes on top*

of the container, and then crash the structure. They then stack the nesting boxes, put each shape piece into a nesting box, stack smaller blocks on top of the boxes, and then reintegrate the shape sorter by placing the blocks and shapes back into the container.

Combination and presymbolic routine: *The adult and child assemble a birthday cake, putting the slices together one by one. They both add toppings and candles and then cut the slices with a toy knife and put them on plates. After they pretend to eat the cake, they reassemble the cake to begin the routine again.*

Presymbolic and symbolic routine: *The adult and child dress up dolls together. They place different pieces of clothing on the dolls and then build a "school bus" out of blocks. They walk each doll into the bus and then push the block structure across the room, pretending to drive the dolls to school. The adult and child build a school out of magnetic tiles and walk the dolls out of the bus into the structures.*

Symbolic routine: *The adult and child pretend to be firefighters. They pretend that the tower in their pretend city is up in flames. They use buckets and pretend to toss water on the flames and rescue all the people from the burning building. They return to the firehouse and pretend to wait for another fire.*

As you can see, the components of the routine are often more salient in lower-play-level routines where children have simpler steps and are just learning to play. In higher-level routines, the components may be less apparent, and the steps often have more variability. Over time, we help the child progress from more linear and repetitive play to increasingly flexible and creative stories. It might not look and feel seamless at first, but the goal is to start at the child's level and to increase the quality and complexity of the interaction over time.

5.4.4 Routines Are Flexible

Use the base, restart, and expansion flexibly throughout the routine. While you may have some idea of how the routine will progress, the various steps and components should play out naturally. The child might initiate different steps than you predicted, or she might carry them out in a different order than planned. She might restart early or expand before you reach the end of the base steps. As long as the routine continues to make sense (rather than being a set of random actions), this level of flexibility is encouraged.

Evolve Routines over Time

Routines should also grow and change flexibly over time. This helps the child learn many ways to play with the toys. Here are some aspects that might change:

- The expansions change and progress across sessions.
- The base includes more steps as the expansions become more comfortable and familiar.
- You choose not to repeat certain steps of the routine. For example, the base might involve

building a road; instead of rebuilding the road every time you restart, you might leave the road intact and restart by building something new, such as houses along the road.

- The base may change entirely. For example, in one session, the base routine might involve cutting food, but in the next session, the child might begin the routine by putting food into a pot.

This level of flexibility and change in routines is encouraged! It shows that the child can play flexibly with the same toy, while maintaining the story of the routine. This is another example of how routines should reflect typical play. When the routine evolves, it typically means that the child is learning new skills and playing in more natural and dynamic ways. (See Chapters 11 and 17 for more examples.)

Complete Exercise 5.2 below to test your knowledge of the qualities of a play routine.

EXERCISE 5.2. **Qualities of a Play Routine**

Indicate whether each statement is true or false according to JASPER guidelines.

1. You should decide the steps of the routine ahead of time and teach the child to follow that specific order.	True	False
2. You should expect the child to complete specific play acts in each routine.	True	False
3. You should have several routine options for each session.	True	False
4. The sequence of play steps can be flexible. They do not have to be completed in the same order or the same way every time.	True	False
5. You should follow all of the child's ideas even if they are repetitive or interfering.	True	False

---

5.5 Be an Equal and Active Partner in the Routine

Now that you understand the components and qualities of the routine, it is time to discuss your role in the interaction. The child cannot be in a state of joint engagement without you, so it is imperative for you to be engaged. In every routine, you should perform the role of an *equal and active play partner*. Being an equal and active play partner involves playing and communicating alongside the child, as shown in Figure 5.7. It means that you play a balanced role in the routine and provide support without taking over the interaction. It also means that you are actively engaged and attentive to the child. You and the child should both have opportunities to generate and share new ideas. Distinct from being compliant as a responder, the child should have the opportunity to be an active participant in the shared experience. The goal is to support the child's role, so that the routine is led by the child's motivations and initiations as much as possible.

Sometimes, it can be difficult to find the balance in your role. Some common mistakes are discussed in the text and in Figure 5.8.

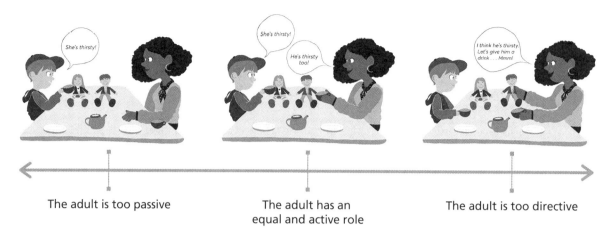

The adult is too passive   The adult has an   The adult is too directive
                                equal and active role

FIGURE 5.7. The adult's role can range from too passive to too directive. The adult should take an equal and active role as she plays along with the child.

5.5.1 Do Not Be Passive

Be an active, rather than passive, play partner. Sometimes adults end up sitting back and watching the child play, rather than actively joining in the routine. In the first picture in Figure 5.7, the child takes all the play actions as the adult watches. This is a passive role that does not contribute to the child's learning. Another form of passivity is to "narrate" the child's actions and offer praise without taking any active play turns. For example, the adult says, "You're having a tea party with the dolls . . . Oh, are you giving them a drink? That's a good idea!" It may sound as though the adult is participating in the interaction, but narrating is not a play turn.

5.5.2 Do Not Be Directive

Another mistake is to be overly directive by playing or talking too much. While it is important to be supportive, you should not be overly directive. A directive adult and compliant child are not in a state of joint engagement (as you may recall from Box 2.1), nor in equal and active roles. The most common ways adults make this mistake is by telling children how to play, asking many questions,

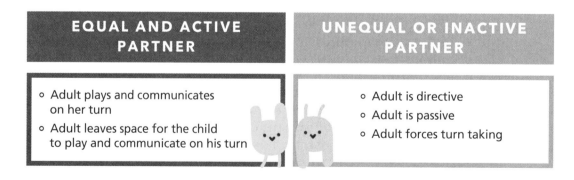

EQUAL AND ACTIVE PARTNER	UNEQUAL OR INACTIVE PARTNER
○ Adult plays and communicates on her turn ○ Adult leaves space for the child to play and communicate on his turn	○ Adult is directive ○ Adult is passive ○ Adult forces turn taking

FIGURE 5.8. Equal and active partner versus unequal or inactive partner.

or providing too many ideas of their own. In the last picture in Figure 5.7, the adult takes most of the play and communication turns, such that the child is only able to respond. The interaction can also feel too directive when the adult does not give the child enough time to initiate or respond (e.g., the adult jumps in with a model too soon rather than waiting).

When you make all the decisions and direct the play, you end up dominating the interaction. This play routine is less enjoyable for the child, and the child becomes more reliant on prompts from the adult. This leaves the child with minimal opportunity to initiate communication and play acts of her own.

5.5.3 Avoid Forced Turn Taking

Being an equal and active play partner means that you get to take play turns too; however, it does not mean that you must take exactly the same number of play turns. Turn taking should be fluid and support the routine. For example, the adult may need to take two quick turns to the child's one turn in order to keep the routine going. It is not the turn taking that maintains the interaction; rather, it is what you do on your turn that provides the necessary support. When we force turn taking, play quickly becomes unnatural instead of flexible and fun. For example, the adult's dialogue might sound like this: "My turn. Okay, your turn. Wait, wait! It's *my* turn [*grabs toy away from the child*]. Okay, *now* it's your turn [*hands child a toy*]." Instead of following the child, the adult ends up leading a rigid interaction. We recommend avoiding the following:

- Avoid counting the number of turns or enforcing equality.
- Avoid taking toys away or blocking the child's turn.
- Avoid labeling turns (e.g., "my turn," "your turn").
- Avoid telling the child to wait for you to take a turn.
- Avoid recruiting the child's attention to your turn.

5.5.4 Find a Balanced Role

A routine should have balanced roles for both you and the child. Neither of you should be responsible for making all the decisions in the interaction. Instead, you should prioritize following the child's ideas, only supporting in select moments when necessary. To support balanced roles, we must often create more room in the interaction for the child to share ideas; therefore, we do not talk or take actions on the child's turn. Instead, we wait quietly during this time and watch to see what the child will do. As you watch and wait, you should not attempt to recruit the child's attention or provide prompts of any kind. This is the child's opportunity to demonstrate ideas of her own. Once she does, you can *then* use your turn to reinforce the child's actions (or to provide support if necessary). Another aspect of your role is to manage the environment and support engagement and regulation. Figure 5.9 provides an overview of your role, and we will explain the details of these strategies in Chapters 9–12.

Use Exercise 5.3 to practice identifying the balance in the adult's role.

CHILD'S TURN	YOUR TURN	THROUGHOUT THE ROUTINE
○ Leave room for the child to initiate ○ Do not talk or take play actions ○ Watch for play and communication	○ Respond to the child's initiations ○ Imitate and model play ○ Use language and joint attention gestures	○ Manage the environment ○ Support engagement and regulation

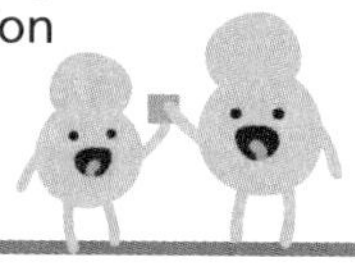

FIGURE 5.9. Overview of roles.

EXERCISE 5.3. Equal and Active Roles

Identify whether the adult is too passive, is too directive, or has an equal and active role in the interaction.

1. The child stacks a block. You move more pieces into the immediate environment. The child stacks another block, and you say, "Good stacking!" while passing the child another block.   Passive   Directive   Equal and active

2. The child puts a spoon to the doll's mouth and says, "Eat." You put a spoon to the doll's mouth and say, "Eat food!"   Passive   Directive   Equal and active

3. You and the child are playing with Velcro food. The child pretends to eat a piece of food. You say, "Not yet. Let's cut!" as you continue to cut the food.   Passive   Directive   Equal and active

4. You and the child are assembling cupcakes. The child puts the frosting on a cupcake. You put frosting on another cupcake and say, "On." The child puts a cupcake in the tray. You put a cupcake in the tray and say, "Cake."   Passive   Directive   Equal and active

5. You and the child are putting figures in a bus. The child puts a figure in, and you say, "Let's drive to school." Child says, "Okay, let's go!" and pushes the bus. You say, "We're here. Everybody off the bus!" You both take figures off the bus, and then you ask the child, "Do you want to be the teacher or the student?" The child says, "I want to be the teacher!"   Passive   Directive   Equal and active

5.6 Conclusion

JASPER routines provide a structure that allows the child to access the many benefits of play. The routine strips away distractions and allows the child to focus on the learning opportunities most relevant to his targets and goals. Once you begin a routine, you will continue to restart and expand until the child is ready to move on to something new. This process of establishing the routine, expanding the routine, and transitioning to a new routine is repeated until the end of the session. Review the strategies and information regarding the routine in Figure 5.10. In the chapters to come, we will look closer at each step of the routine, troubleshoot common challenges, and begin layering on the child's learning targets.

Chapter 5 Summary

LEARN THE **COMPONENTS** OF A PLAY ROUTINE	LEARN THE **QUALITIES** OF A PLAY ROUTINE	LEARN TO PLAY AN **EQUAL AND ACTIVE** ROLE
Build a solid base routine o Start at the child's mastered play level **Expand** o Add new steps to the base routine **Restart** o Return to a previous step in the routine o Restart after the base or an expansion step	o Create a natural and playful context o Tailor the routine to the child's interests and experiences o Match the child's developmental level o Stay flexible	o Take a clear role in the play o Allow the child space to initiate play and communication o Let play turns be natural o Balance your role

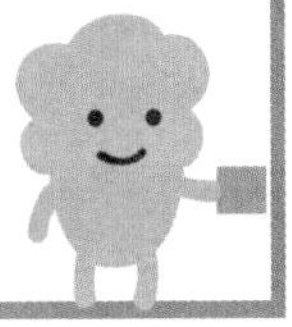

FIGURE 5.10. Chapter 5 summary.

Assembling JASPER Routines

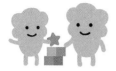

6.1 Introduction

In this chapter, you will prepare the toys, actions, and communication for several play routines. We will start with instructions for the toys and actions, and then introduce some basic guidelines for communication. Next, you will use this information to fill out Form 6.1 (Assembling Play Routines, p. 113) to compile routine options that are tailored toward the child. In this process, remember that the toys and actions are contingent on the child and your choices should support the child's goals and targets of the intervention. Though you will put a significant amount of effort in choosing and preparing toys, you must be flexible in the moment, depending on what the child decides to do.

6.2 Choose Toys and Actions

In JASPER, we do not have a standardized set of toys. In fact, we often use toys from the child's school or home, because these are the toys that the child will most likely play with outside of intervention. The toys you choose do not have to be high tech or made by a particular brand. You can improvise with homemade toys, for example, using cardboard boxes for building materials or plastic utensils, cups, or plates for food routines. You can also substitute objects, for example, using a book as a ramp for vehicles. More important than type of toy is the developmental appropriateness of the actions. Use the guidelines in Figure 6.1 to compile a list of toy choices for the first session.

6.2.1 Choose Developmentally Appropriate Toys and Actions

Choose toys and actions that are within the child's developmentally appropriate range, illustrated in Figure 6.2. The majority of the toys and actions should be at the child's mastered play level. You will also need to support steps at the child's target play level for times when the base is established and the child is ready to expand, as well as toys a step below the child's mastered level for

---

GUIDELINES FOR TOYS AND ACTIONS ☑

☐ Select toys and actions within the child's developmentally appropriate range

☐ Include toys that are motivating, are productive, and foster social connection

☐ Include actions that are creative and make sense to the child

---

FIGURE 6.1. Guidelines for choosing toys and actions.

moments when the child needs an easier step to increase engagement or after a moment of dysregulation (see Box 6.1; Chapter 15, Section 15.3.2; and Chapter 16, Section 16.3.2). When play acts are too far above the child's mastered play level (i.e., too challenging), the child will have difficulty maintaining engagement, will not be able to initiate play or communication, and may grow frustrated. When play acts are too far below the child's mastered play level (i.e., too easy), this is suboptimal for engagement as well, as the child may become bored and look for another activity.

It is generally not the toy itself that determines the play level; it is what you do with the toy that makes it developmentally appropriate or not for a particular child. For example, a toy pizza can be used for a variety of play levels. You can stick toppings on the pizza (presentation combination), place slices of pizza on plates (conventional combination), pretend to eat the pizza (pretend self), pretend to feed the pizza to a doll (child as agent), have the doll serve pizza to another doll (doll as agent), and so on (see more on play levels in Chapter 2). That said, some toys lend themselves better to certain play levels than others. For example, a shape sorter is perfect for presentation combination, but it is typically not appropriate for higher play levels. A doll and hairbrush are appropriate for presymbolic or symbolic play, but are less appropriate for earlier play levels.

In Exercise 6.1, we provide examples of four children with different mastered play levels. Take a moment to match the different profiles with their developmentally appropriate toy options. Keep in mind that the toys below represent just a few options and may or may not be right for your child, even if he is at the same level.

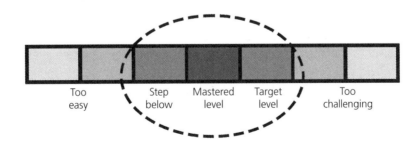

FIGURE 6.2. Choose toys within the child's developmentally appropriate range of play levels.

EXERCISE 6.1. Choosing Toys

Match the description of the child with the most developmentally appropriate toy options.

Description of child	Toy options
1. The child mouths most toys and occasionally bangs a toy on the table.	A. Figures, several structures, puppets, food, a doctor set
2. The child puts shapes in the shape sorter but performs no other play acts.	B. Shape sorter, nesting boxes, magnetic building tiles
3. The child puts all the shapes in the shape sorter and completes the puzzle, puts together food and place settings, fills the dump truck with blocks, and pretends to eat a piece of food.	C. Pop-up, drum, ring stacker
4. The child builds a structure out of magnetic tiles, assembles the food, has the doll hold the comb and brush her hair, has the doll walk to the house and sit on furniture, and then has the doll walk to the barn to sit down.	D. Blocks, food, magnetic building tiles, figures

6.2.2 Choose Motivating Toys and Actions

As you choose toys, consider the child's interests. It is much easier to sustain periods of joint engagement when your child is playing with motivating toys. For example, if the child is interested in animals, you can incorporate these toys in developmentally appropriate ways by choosing toys that feature animals, such as putting sea animal pieces in puzzles (presentation combination), placing animals into a truck (child as agent), or having farm animals snore while they sleep in bed (doll as agent), depending on the child's play level. Be aware that some toys may be so distracting that they lead to *interfering* rather than *productive* actions, as described below.

6.2.3 Choose Toys That Lead to Productive Play

We want the child to play with toys in ways that are productive toward our goals. *Productive play* is developmentally appropriate, flexible, diverse, and creative and allows the child to remain jointly engaged. Avoid toys that lead to *interfering actions,* such as electronic toys with lights and sounds (or remove the batteries), toys that are particularly distracting, and those that lead to dysregulation, object engagement, rigid and repetitive behaviors, or restricted interests. See Figure 6.3 for signs to help you determine if the child's play is productive or interfering. If a toy is particularly distracting for the child, you may choose to exclude it from the session for a time. Once you have successfully built some routines with the child, you can help incorporate the toy in more productive ways.

SIGNS THE CHILD'S PLAY IS PRODUCTIVE	SIGNS THE CHILD'S PLAY IS INTERFERING
o Play acts are at the child's developmental level o Play acts are flexible, diverse, and creative o Child demonstrates increased joint engagement o Child's affect is appropriate to the routine o Child is more likely to initiate play and communication o Child is more likely to share enjoyment with you (e.g., smiling, laughing, looking at you)	o Child is unable to use the toy in developmentally appropriate ways o Child shows an increase in rigid and repetitive behaviors o Child will not let you play with the toy o The toy leads to periods of lower engagement o The toy leads to periods of overly high positive affect (e.g., clapping, uncontrolled laughter) o The toy leads to periods of negative affect (e.g., throwing toys, banging)

FIGURE 6.3. Signs of productive and interfering play.

6.2.4 Promote Creativity

Be creative! Children and adults often think about play in different ways. Adults tend to follow more standard ways of playing, whereas children tend to be more creative. In order to increase the flexibility and diversity of the child's skills, you may need to set aside your traditional ways of thinking. This is especially important as you learn to expand the routine. You can mix toys from different toy sets, combine routines together, and use toys in new ways. For example, rather than building with only wooden blocks, you can use both wooden and plastic blocks together. Remember, you should also follow the child's creative ideas, even if it deviates from the routine you had planned. For example, a child may pretend that the box for a toy is a bathtub and use it to wash a doll. This is a creative, productive play act that you should imitate and encourage. Aside from considerations of developmental appropriateness and productive actions, there is no "right" or "wrong" way to play.

6.3 Choose Communication

Next, brainstorm communication you could use in your routines. Similar to play, we choose language that is developmentally appropriate, motivating, flexible, and creative. We also model joint attention gestures. See Chapters 12 and 13 for additional communication strategies. Use the guidelines in Figure 6.4 to choose appropriate communication for the first session. (For children who use augmentative and alternative communication [AAC], prepare the words you expect to use during the routine and follow the guidelines in Chapter 14.)

6.3.1 Match the Child's Mean Length of Utterance

The typical pace, vocabulary, and language level of adults is often too complex for the child to produce. Instead of talking as you normally would, stay within one word of the child's mean length of utterance (MLU). As you may recall from Chapter 3, this is the approximate number of

```
┌─────────────────────────────────────────────────────────────────┐
│              GUIDELINES FOR COMMUNICATION  ☑                       │
│   ☐  Choose words that match the child's language level            │
│   ☐  Choose words that are related to the play routine             │
│   ☐  Use commenting language that fosters social connection        │
│   ☐  Use joint attention gestures throughout the routine           │
│   ☐  Prepare symbols for users of speech-generating devices (see Chapter 14) │
└─────────────────────────────────────────────────────────────────┘
```

FIGURE 6.4. Guidelines for choosing communication.

words the child says in each utterance, as shown in Table 6.1. Remember, this is measured by the approximate number of words the child can use spontaneously and independently, not the number of words the child can imitate. This means that, for most early language learners, you must significantly cut back on how much you speak and that your language models could be reproduced independently by the child.

Use Exercise 6.2 to practice choosing the appropriate language level.

TABLE 6.1. Match the Child's Length of Utterance

Child's spontaneous length of utterance		Adult's length of utterance
Uses vocalizations, word approximations, or no language	➜	Uses one-word comments
Uses one-word utterances	➜	Uses one- to two-word comments
Uses two- to three-word utterances	➜	Uses two- to four-word comments
Uses short sentences	➜	Uses short sentences
Uses long sentences	➜	Uses long sentences

EXERCISE 6.2. Adult Language Level

Match the child's length of utterance to the most appropriate language for the adult to use in a bath routine.

Child's MLU	Adult's language
1. Approximations (e.g., "Buh")	A. "Baby."
2. One word	B. "Baby takes a bubble bath."
3. Two to three words	C. "I put shampoo in baby's dirty hair."
4. Short sentences	D. "More soap on."
5. Long sentences	E. "Wash."

6.3.2 Use Commenting Language

Use simple *commenting* language that is related to the toys and actions in the routine. For example, you could say what the object is ("Car"; "Baby"), what is currently happening or just happened in the routine ("Crash!"; "We're driving"), or highlight something interesting about the toys or events ("The tower fell down!").

Avoid directive language that seeks to change the child's behavior or produce a certain response during play (e.g., "Put the square in"; "Find the orange animal"). You should also limit language that recruits the child's attention, asks questions, or tests the child's knowledge (e.g., "Look!"; "Can you push the car?"; "What color is this?"). See Figure 6.5 for examples of commenting language compared to directive language.

Many of our children are already accustomed to responding but do not know how to play or share ideas of their own; therefore, it is important to model language that the child could use. If the child is dysregulated or in need of behavioral direction, this might be an appropriate time to use directive language (see Chapters 8 and 16).

6.3.3 Be Flexible and Natural in the Way You Communicate

Children with ASD sometimes learn rote or repetitive speech patterns. Our goal is to help the child to develop more flexible and natural ways to communicate. For this reason, we try to be flexible and natural ourselves in the way we speak.

Use a Variety of Words

Use a variety of words during the routine. For example, if you are modeling language in a picnic routine, do not say "Eat" on every turn as you give the figures a bite. This is too repetitive and only exposes the child to one new word. On the other hand, if you use a different word on every turn (e.g., "burger," "bun," "cheese," "ketchup," "eat," "more"), there might not be enough predictability for the child to learn the language. Try to find a natural balance.

JA LANGUAGE TO USE	LANGUAGE TO LIMIT
o "Red ball." o "Crash!" o "Scary dinosaur." o "Building the blocks!" o "The baby is sleepy." o "We're feeding the babies!"	o "What color is it?" o "Now crash it." o "What kind of dinosaur is it?" o "You should put the block on." o "Can you put the baby to sleep?" o "Find the boy baby."

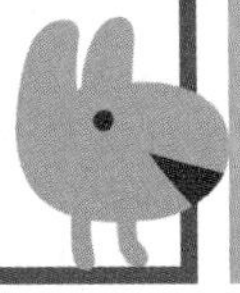

FIGURE 6.5. JA language to use and language to limit.

Be Natural in Intonation and Speech

The child will imitate all aspects of your speech, from the words you say to the intonation you use. When some people use positive affect, they raise the pitch of their voice at the end of the utterance, making the comment sound more like a question: "Build *blocks*?" As a result, the child's language also starts to sound like this, with every utterance also sounding like a question. Try to remain natural. You should not be monotonous or robotic, nor should you overemphasize syllables, draw out words, use a melodic cadence, or speak in third person.

6.3.4 Adjust Based on the Child's Length of Utterance

You should also be flexible and natural based on the child's length of utterance.

Build on Word Approximations

If the child is using word approximations, build on the sounds the child is already using and choose words that match those sounds, so long as they make sense within the context of the routine. For example, if the child can make the *b* sound but has a difficult time with *s,* you might model the word *build,* rather than *stack*.

Adjust for One to Two Words

If the child has a language level of one to two words, it can be difficult to keep your language flexible and natural. In this case, you can add another word intermittently to keep your models from feeling rote or awkward. For example, if you typically model *stack,* mix it up every few turns by saying, "Stack blocks." If you typically say, "In," as you put figures into a bus, then occasionally say, "In the bus."

Be Creative with Phrases and Sentences

You can be a lot more creative and natural with children who have more language, especially those who speak in sentences. If the child speaks in long phrases or sentences, you can exercise more flexibility, with comments that sound more conversational. For example, if the child says, "I'm the teacher. It's time to start the lesson!" you can say, "Okay, I'm the student. I'll get out my books." You may also be able to work on other language functions that arise as children become more conversant, such as playful (rather than directive) requests and question asking that is related to the routine. For example, if the child says, "I'll have the corn dog," the adult could respond, "I'll have pizza. What would you like to drink with that?"

6.3.5 Use Joint Attention Gestures

In addition to communicating with words, you will also model joint attention gestures on your play turn. These models are valuable for all children, regardless of their language level. We place some priority on the child's target gestures and make sure to model these frequently; however, you can also model the gesture that makes the most sense in the moment, given the context of the routine. We will explain the details of modeling gestures in Chapter 12, Section 12.4.3.

6.4 Assemble Play Routines

Once you choose developmentally appropriate toys, actions, and communication, use Form 6.1 (Assembling Play Routines, p. 113), as well as the following guidelines, to compile a list of materials for the first session.

Steps for Assembling Play Routines

- Create a list of motivating toys at the child's developmental level.
- Prepare for eight or more routines.
- Choose toys for the base and expansions.
- Choose actions for the base and expansions.
- Select the words and gestures at the child's level for each routine.

6.4.1 Fill Out the Master List of Toys, Actions, and Communication

At the top of the form, record the child's mastered and target play levels, target requesting and joint attention gestures, and length of utterance. These should be informed by the SPACE assessment in Chapter 3.

Routines

Choose at least eight different routines and write a brief title or description of the routine. Try to get a sense of your child's needs during the SPACE to guide this process. You may need more or fewer routines, depending on how quickly the child goes through the materials. At this stage, it is better to be overprepared than to scramble when you do not have what you need, so plan for more toys than you might think you need at first. As you build routines, try to think of steps that are developmentally appropriate and go naturally together. For simple and combination levels, routines are often made up of two to three play levels. As the child enters presymbolic and symbolic play, it is natural for routines to incorporate more levels as the child builds more skills. This is common in typical development as well. For example, a symbolic play routine might include a lower play level of putting food toys in an oven (conventional combination) as part of a larger idea of pretending to have a restaurant. Prepare a routine to support engagement and regulation as well (see Box 6.1).

BOX 6.1. Prepare a Routine to Support Engagement and Regulation

You should prepare a routine that is well mastered or a step below the child's play level, in the event the child needs extra support to regulate and engage. Choose something comfortable and motivating that you think the child will likely enjoy. This is especially helpful when the child is new to JASPER. Later in the intervention, once the child has more routines, a very familiar routine at the child's mastered level serves the same purpose. We will discuss this more in Chapter 15.

Toys and Actions for the Base

Write down toys and actions you could use to establish the base. Remember, the base is the foundation of the routine, so the toys should facilitate steps at your child's mastered play level. For presymbolic and symbolic play, some mastered base steps are often best supported by other play levels. For example, you may find it easier to build momentum with a physical combination step, compared to a single-scheme step, since the larger number of pieces allows you to establish more consistent back-and-forth turn taking; therefore, you might first build a tree out of Lego blocks before placing each toy squirrel in the tree. See Table 6.2 for a list of base steps at various play levels.

Toys and Actions for Expansions

Choose several toys to facilitate new steps at the child's mastered or target level. Make sure the actions are logically connected to the base and build on your current routine. See Table 6.3 for expansions at various play levels. See Chapter 11 for more information about choosing toys for expansions.

Gestures and Words

Preplan gestures and words that you can use to comment while taking your turn. Think of ways to include the target gestures you chose for your child in Chapters 3 and 4. Choose a variety of words or phrases that match the child's language level. Cycle through a few content words or phrases (rather than repeating the same word on every turn) to help the child become familiar with them.

TABLE 6.2. Examples of Toys and Actions for the Base

Play level	Developmentally appropriate toy		Potential base steps
Discriminate	Pop-up	→	Push buttons
Take-apart	Ring stacker	→	Take rings off of stacker
Presentation combination	Coin Pig	→	Put coins into pig
General combination	Blocks	→	Stack blocks
Pretend self	Cookies and utensils	→	Put cookie on tray; pretend to eat cookie
Physical combination	Foam blocks	→	Build "submarine" with blocks
Child as agent	Figures, house, and furniture	→	Put figures on furniture
Conventional combination	Figures, house, and furniture	→	Set furniture in house
Single-scheme	Babies, food, bottles	→	Put food together; extend food to each baby
Substitution	Tiles, figures, pizza	→	Put blocks on pizza as "toppings"
Substitution without object	Tiles, figures, pizza	→	Cook pizza in oven; blow on "hot" pizza
Doll as agent	Playground structure, figures	→	Dolls climb up structure
Multi-scheme	Playground structure, figures	→	Dolls play tag and then climb up structure
Sociodramatic	Doctor costume, animals	→	Veterinarians suit up for surgery
Thematic	Superhero cape, blocks	→	Drive *Batmobile* to a crime

TABLE 6.3. Examples of Possible Expansion Steps

Play level	Base step		Possible expansion step
Discriminate	Bang drum with a stick	→	Bang xylophone with a stick
Take-apart	Take apart nesting boxes	→	Nest boxes together
Presentation combination	Put cookies into cookie jar	→	Put cookies on a tray
General combination	Build a structure out of blocks	→	Place figures on the structure
Pretend self	Pretend to drink from a cup	→	Extend the cup to a doll
Physical combination	Build a "zoo" out of blocks	→	Place animals in the zoo
Child as agent	Put figures on chairs	→	Have figures eat ice cream
Conventional combination	Blanket on bed	→	Pillow on bed
Single-scheme	Set two dolls on a bed	→	Add blankets to the dolls
Substitution	Build "road" out of tiles	→	Drive car on road
Substitution without object	Mix "cake" in bowl	→	Pour "cake" into muffin tins
Doll as agent	Pretend the doll is drinking tea	→	Pretend to add sugar into tea
Multi-scheme	Doll walks to car; doll drives car	→	Build "school" for dolls
Sociodramatic	Pretend to be a doctor checking heartbeat	→	Offer patient medicine
Thematic	Fly on magic carpet	→	Arrive at home and feed a tiger

You can use a mixture of nouns, verbs, prepositions, and adjectives as long as they are linked to your actions and at the child's level.

6.4.2 Prepare Enough Toys to Share

In JASPER, you get to play too! Therefore, you should prepare enough pieces for both the child and you to actively participate together. If the child has a car, you should also have a car. If the child stirs with a spoon, you should also have a utensil so you can stir. This does not mean you must play with the exact same *type* of toy as the child or that you cannot mix items or share but rather means you should have all the materials necessary to play together. When it comes to larger items (like an oven, car ramp, or barn), you and the child can play with the same toy together. You do not need to have your own. There should also be enough toys to maintain a shared play interaction for about 7 to 12 turns before you have to start over. For example, if you are putting pegs on a pegboard, there should be enough pegs for you and the child to build together. It is difficult to build momentum in the routine if you keep running out of pieces.

6.4.3 Update Toys over Time

Review your list of toys after each session and write down changes you would like to make for the next session. Some children may be able to play with the same routines across several sessions; other children will need new routines to keep the session motivating. Consider removing or adding support around toys that were distracting and interfering, and plan to build routines around toys that were motivating in productive ways. Over time, you should build a collection of routines you can use to accomplish the goals and targets of the session.

Give Popular Toys a Break

After many sessions, you may find that a toy or a routine that was once exciting may become less motivating. If you have already added many expansions and the child is starting to lose interest, it could be time to give familiar toys a break for a few sessions. This can make a big difference in the child's motivation. When you reintroduce the toy after a short break, children are often excited to see the toy and are better able to engage for longer periods of time once again.

6.4.4 Case Example

In Figure 6.6, we provide an example of a completed Form 6.1 (Assembling Play Routines). This includes several routines for a child who has a length of utterance of one word and who plays at a simple play level with some emerging presentation combination skills. Additional examples of routines are provided in Appendix C.

6.5 Common Challenges Assembling Routines

Choosing toys is a process of trial and error. The child may not like the toys you have chosen, struggle to play productively, or fly through all the options, leaving you wondering what to do next. It takes time and experience to learn what toys the child finds motivating and distracting. We will address some common questions first and then provide a few case examples. If you get stuck at any point, go to the ACT framework from Chapter 8 to troubleshoot.

6.5.1 Common Questions

In the section below, we address some common questions that may arise as you choose toys.

What if I do not have the "right" toys for JASPER?

Toys may not be abundant in some cases, such as with teachers or families in low-resourced communities. In this case, you can be creative and make toys with the materials you have available. Here are some examples:

- Use shoeboxes in place of blocks.
- Use household items such as bowls, spoons, and toothbrushes.
- Use baskets for baby baths or cradles.
- Repurpose old clothes or rags into clothes and blankets for figures.
- Cut a hole in the lid of a jar or plastic container to fill with coins.
- Save cereal boxes and food wrappers for food-theme routines.
- Shape cardboard into symbolic play props (e.g., deep-sea diving costumes).

What if the child will only play with something for a few seconds?

Make sure that toys are at the appropriate play level so they are not too easy or too difficult, and keep the child's development in mind. If you are playing with a child who is only 15 months old, it is normal for him to take a couple of turns with one toy and then move around the room to

Assembling Play Routines

Child: __J. M.__

Adult: __C. S.__

Date: __July 06__

Mastered play level: __Presentation combination__

Target play level: __General combination__

Target requesting gesture: __Give__

Target joint attention gesture: __Show__

Target language level: __1–2 words__

ROUTINES			
Assemble eight different play routines.			
Routines	**Toys**	**Actions**	**Gestures and Words**
Routine 1: Peg board	Base: pegs, peg board	Base: put pegs into each hole in the pegboard, stack pegs up into a tower	peg, up, stack, in, out, ring, on, off, box, more / JA point, JA show, give to request
	Expansion: rings and ring-stacker, nesting boxes	Expansion: put rings onto the pegs, put pegs into nesting boxes, stack boxes, stack rings on boxes	
Routine 2: Ice cream	Base: ice cream, ice cream jar	Base: stack up ice cream pieces, put ice cream in jar, dump ice cream	ice cream, stack, on, off, colors, cookie, tray, stick, more, eat / JA show
	Expansion: ice cream scoop, tummy stuffer, cookies on tray	Expansion: scoop ice cream, place ice cream on cookies, feed ice cream and cookies to tummy stuffer	
Routine 3: Shape sorter	Base: shapes, shape sorter	Base: put shapes in, dump out pieces	in, out, shapes, dump, stack, truck, drive, go, box, build / JA show, give to request
	Expansion: dump truck, interlocking road pieces, nesting boxes	Expansion: stack shapes up, put shapes in dump truck, put together road, drive truck, stack up boxes, put shapes into boxes	
Routine 4: Cake	Base: cake pieces, toppings	Base: put together cake slices, add toppings to cake, stack cake pieces	cake, on, off, make, stack, toppings, candles, eat, more / JA point, JA show, give to request
	Expansion: candles, plastic nesting cakes, ice cream, tummy stuffer	Expansion: add candles to cake, sing "happy birthday," stack nesting cakes, stack ice creams on cake, feed cake slices to tummy stuffer	

FIGURE 6.6. A completed example of Form 6.1 (Assembling Play Routines).

explore other toys. The child may need some time to increase his capacity for engagement. It is also okay to give the child time to explore. The child might not have access to the same toys at home, and some are probably novel. If the child has not seen the toys before, you might have to show him how a toy works by modeling (see Chapter 9). Just because the child did not seem interested at first does not mean a lack of interest in those toys at all.

What if the child is not motivated by the toys?

Think about what the child enjoys and try to find ways to incorporate that interest. For example, if the child is very interested in butterflies, you could incorporate butterfly figures into a child as agent level play routine (as long as she is able to play productively with them). Notice which toys the child will play with, even if for only one or two turns, and which toys are being completely ignored. See if the child is more motivated by novel toys or familiar toys. Update your toys regularly to accommodate for the child's preferences, and try circling back to the unsuccessful toys another time.

Should there be only two to three play levels represented in every routine?

Not necessarily. At lower play levels, this may be developmentally appropriate. But as play becomes increasingly presymbolic, it is often natural for your routines to incorporate more play levels. A symbolic "airport" routine, for example, may start with physical combinations, such as building an airport and an airplane, even though this step is lower than the child's current mastered level. This is developmentally appropriate and mirrors typically developing play. The goal is simply to choose toys that facilitate natural routines that are sustainable for the child, while also targeting higher skills. Recall, as well, that you choose from a few appropriate presymbolic targets, depending on the child's motivation, as presymbolic skills often develop concurrently in typical development (see Chapter 4, Section 4.3.4 and Figure 4.2).

6.5.2 Case Examples

The following case examples illustrate the troubleshooting process. They are formatted in the style of advice columns and will appear throughout the remaining chapters under the heading "Case Examples" to illustrate the strategies discussed. These are fictional examples but highlight common scenarios we have encountered over the years.

Just Trying to Get Started

Dear JASPER,

I just finished my third session with a little boy who is emerging in his general combination skills. He has a little bit of language and is quite interested in toys. Our biggest problem is that it takes us a long time to actually get going in a routine. I bring different toys to every session hoping that something will spark a great routine! I've tried changing the play environment, using a visual schedule, and increasing my affect when he takes the first play act with a toy, but nothing seems to work. He still goes from toy to toy for almost 10 minutes before we start making progress. What am I doing wrong?

Thanks,

Just Trying to Get Started

Dear *Just Trying to Get Started,*

We are glad that you are using a variety of strategies to interest the child. From your story, it sounds as if he might benefit from more consistency of materials. While variety is great, changing the toys every session might be too much novelty for this particular child and may be one reason he is spending so much time exploring. Try providing more consistent toy choices, so he can quickly find a familiar place to begin. Then, as soon as the child chooses a toy, move the other toys off to the side to help him attend to his chosen routine.

Best,

JASPER

Stuck on Repeat

Dear JASPER,

I completed the SPACE and set my child's mastered play level at pretend self and her target play level at child as agent. When I started planning routines, I could only think of things like combs, toothbrushes, and food toys. Then, when I started thinking of base steps and expansion steps, I got stuck! How am I supposed to come up with eight different routines made up of actions the child can extend only to herself or to another doll? I'm worried our play won't be very fun, and it will feel more like adaptive skills training. What should I do?

Help me make this fun!

Stuck on Repeat

Dear *Stuck on Repeat,*

You are right that your routines will not feel very natural or fun if you rigidly stick to actions at pretend self and child as agent. In play routines, you will often incorporate several play levels in order to create steps and a story that go together. Instead of limiting yourself to these two play levels, you can add in steps at other similar play levels. For example, you could add in combination steps to a food routine, such as putting the food together, cutting the food, and putting the food on plates or into an oven, in addition to steps like pretending to eat or drink or extending food or drinks to the figures. You could also include different themes for the base (e.g., building with blocks) to incorporate physical combinations, and then add in child as agent or pretend self steps as expansions to keep your actions diverse and interesting.

Keep up the hard work!

JASPER

6.6 Conclusion

Once you fill out Form 6.1, you will have a list of appropriate and motivating toys, actions, gestures, and words for your routines. Although you are planning ahead, remember that you are not predetermining the steps of the routine. The child might choose different toys than you antici-pated or start with a different set of base steps. This could lead to a new routine with a different set of words for you to follow along. Continue to update your toys across sessions to keep the toys motivating and responsive to the child's targets. As you continue to develop routines, you should see progress toward the child's goals over time. You should have a better sense of the toys and actions that are motivating to the child, and it should get easier for the child to initiate ideas and build on actions from previous routines. In Figure 6.7, review the strategies for assembling routines. In the next chapter, we will explain how to prepare the play environment, including how to set up the routines.

Chapter 6 Summary

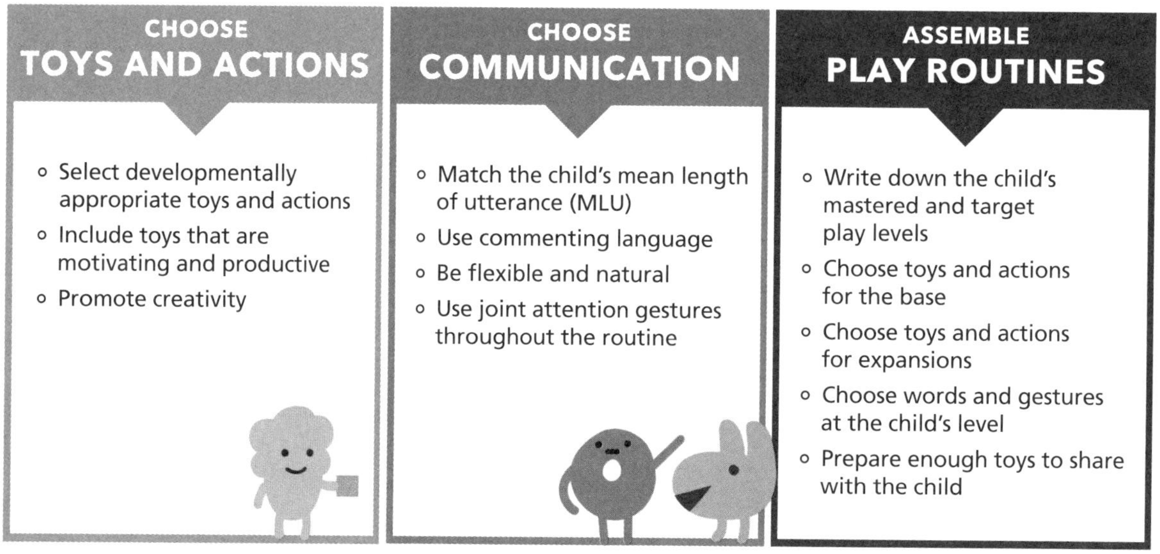

CHOOSE **TOYS AND ACTIONS**	CHOOSE **COMMUNICATION**	ASSEMBLE **PLAY ROUTINES**
○ Select developmentally appropriate toys and actions ○ Include toys that are motivating and productive ○ Promote creativity	○ Match the child's mean length of utterance (MLU) ○ Use commenting language ○ Be flexible and natural ○ Use joint attention gestures throughout the routine	○ Write down the child's mastered and target play levels ○ Choose toys and actions for the base ○ Choose toys and actions for expansions ○ Choose words and gestures at the child's level ○ Prepare enough toys to share with the child

FIGURE 6.7. Chapter 6 summary.

FORM 6.1. **Assembling Play Routines**

Child: _____

Adult: _____

Date: _____

Mastered play level: _____

Target play level: _____

Target requesting gesture: _____

Target joint attention gesture: _____

Target language level: _____

ROUTINES Assemble eight different play routines.			
Routines	**Toys**	**Actions**	**Gestures and Words**
Routine 1:	Base: Expansion:	Base: Expansion:	
Routine 2:	Base: Expansion:	Base: Expansion:	
Routine 3:	Base: Expansion:	Base: Expansion:	
Routine 4:	Base: Expansion:	Base: Expansion:	

(*continued*)

Routines	Toys	Actions	Gestures and Words
Routine 5:	Base: Expansion:	Base: Expansion:	
Routine 6:	Base: Expansion:	Base: Expansion:	
Routine 7:	Base: Expansion:	Base: Expansion:	
Routine 8:	Base: Expansion:	Base: Expansion:	

Notes:

Preparing a JASPER Environment

7.1 Introduction

This chapter explains how to set up and maintain the environment for a session. When we discuss the environment, we are referring to all aspects of the physical space, including the setup of the room, the placement of the toys, and your position related to the child. In JASPER, we do not have one recommended layout for all children. Instead, we tailor the environment to the child and arrange the toys—and ourselves—to maximize play and engagement. We will begin this chapter by explaining some of the goals and features of a JASPER environment. Then we will explain how to set up the environment, including preparing the play area, setting up routines, and managing your position and materials throughout the routine. Finally, we will end with some common challenges and case examples.

7.2 Use the Environment to Support the Child's Goals

Before explaining how to prepare the environment, we will outline the features of a JASPER environment and discuss how we use this strategy to support our goals. An ideal JASPER environment should create a setting in which the child can actually *play* (as described in Chapter 5). We are talking about more than mere actions taken with toys but the natural learning process that takes place through creative, spontaneous exploration of activities the child finds motivating and fun. The environment is an essential tool that can be used to support children's engagement and regulation and set the stage for the child to initiate the play steps. When you set up the environment, you are giving the child visual cues that serve as subtle indicators of where the child should sit and what the child should do. This increases the child's ability to initiate and reduces the need to use frequent models and more directive prompts. In order to support this kind of interaction, we need to ensure that the environment provides an appropriate amount of structure to help the child engage and an appropriate number of toy choices to support the child's ideas and initiations. In Figure 7.1, we provide three examples of different environmental arrangements ranging from too many choices and distractions to too much structure and support, with the JASPER environment in between.

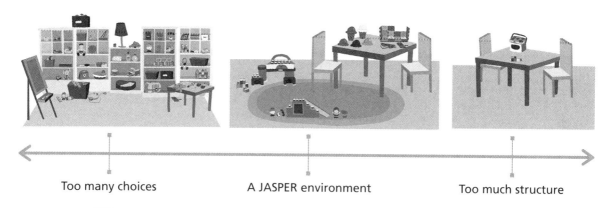

Too many choices   A JASPER environment   Too much structure

FIGURE 7.1. A JASPER environment balances structure and opportunity for choice.

7.2.1 Provide Structure to Support Engagement and Regulation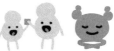

The structure of the environment can either support or hinder engagement and regulation. If the environment is not properly prepared, it can be a source of dysregulation and distraction. Clutter and disorganization, for example, can be overwhelming. If the environment is too distracting like the first image in Figure 7.1 with too many choices, the child might walk around the room, touching toys but not playing with them; she might jump from toy to toy, never settling into an activity, or she might play with the toy in rigid or repetitive ways. Yet if the environment is too restricted, like the third image in Figure 7.1 with too much structure, it is no longer motivating, fun, or conducive to play. Although the child may know where to sit and what to do, she is less likely to make choices, pursue interests, or initiate ideas of her own. Thus, in JASPER, we try to organize the environment so that the child can see a clear and easy way to participate. We limit distractions, provide a clear place for the child to sit, and provide toy options for the child to engage, as shown in the second image of Figure 7.1.

7.2.2 Prepare to Follow the Child's Lead

The environment is prepared with productive and motivating toys to support the child's initiations and help the child take the lead. All materials available in the play space are considered fair game and available for the child's use. A JASPER environment always provides toy choices, including several choices of different routines, as well as options for actions within each routine that are matched to the child's mastered and target play levels. The environment also includes several pieces of each toy. This allows the child to choose the toys he wants to play with and make choices about the steps within the routines and also allows the adult to follow the child's idea.

7.2.3 Tailor the Environment to the Child

The environment should always be tailored to the child. Some children need more physical structure to engage comfortably in the room, while others need more freedom to move around and make choices. You will likely need to make changes to your environmental setup across sessions as you get to know the child's needs. Over time, you should be able to fade environmental structure to prepare the child to play in a more natural environment (e.g., a preschool classroom).

7.3   Prepare the Play Area

Before each session, you will prepare the play area for the child. We typically look for a small area with enough room for the adult and child to sit comfortably facing each other, with toys and objects in between, at either a table or on the floor. We often start with an area that is roughly 5 feet by 5 feet in a clear and uncluttered corner of a room, and we adjust depending on the child's needs (see Figure 7.2).

If you are working in a home or school, you may need to rearrange the room to create the area that works best for the child. You can create a smaller designated area by using furniture or dividers to section off the room, as shown in Figure 7.3. You can use a couch, chairs, or a shelf to create the same effect in the home.

Whenever possible, face the child away from distractions. If you are at a school and the child becomes distracted by other people going in and out of the room, set up the play area in a quiet corner of the room to reduce distractions within the child's immediate line of sight.

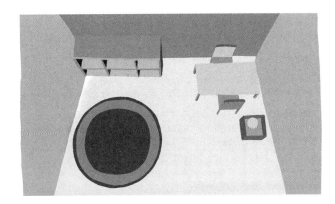

FIGURE 7.2. A clear, uncluttered play space.

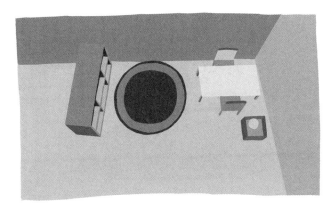

FIGURE 7.3. Partitions provide a smaller designated play area.

7.3.1 Choose the Table, Floor, or Both

JASPER sessions typically take place on the floor, at a small table, or at a combination of the two. One is not necessarily better than the other, and you can change the amount of structure throughout the session or across sessions. What matters is that you select the layout that best supports the child's ability to engage.

Choosing the Table

For some children, it is easier to play and stay engaged at a table. The table offers physical support, as well as more organization for the toys, as illustrated in Figure 7.4. It is a familiar place for school-age children and provides a clear visual cue of where to sit or stand. The surface of the table also provides a designated area where you can set up clear choices and control the number of toys available. Some signs that you might try a table include the following:

- The child is very active, moves around, or frequently wanders.
- The child has low tone or has difficulty sitting up without assistance.
- The child transitions quickly between toys.
- The child is more engaged with more structure.

Consider the height and shape of the table. If possible, avoid large or wide tables that make it difficult to reach the toys and each other. The child should be able to rest her arms on the table and her feet on the floor.

Choosing the Floor

For some children, the floor is a more suitable environment. The floor is less restrictive and provides more room for the child to move (see Figure 7.5). The added space makes it easier to have

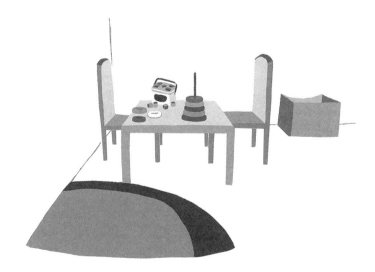

FIGURE 7.4. Routines set up at the table.

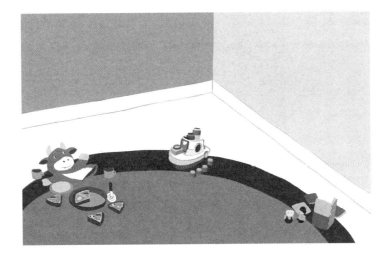

FIGURE 7.5. Routines set up on the floor.

numerous toy choices, as well as routines that require more materials or a larger layout. Some signs that you might try the floor include the following:

- The child is more comfortable having several choices presented at the same time.
- The child has routines that require a larger layout or numerous materials.
- The child finds sitting at the table constricting, aversive, or dysregulating.
- The child is more engaged with more freedom to move around.

If you are setting up on the floor, create a clearly defined place for the child to sit, such as a flat seat, a small rug or mat, or an area defined by colored tape. This visual cue helps the child know where to be within the space and can support the transition into the room.

Choosing a Combination

Often, the best option is to have a combination of the table and floor, as shown in Figure 7.6. This allows you to provide as much support as the child needs at any given time. Signs that you might try a combination include the following:

- The child can engage on the floor most of the time but has moments where he needs help to reengage (e.g., becomes distracted, fixated, or dysregulated).
- The child does not need as much support at the end of the session as he does at the beginning, or vice versa.

Some children may need to start at a table to ease into the session but can later transition to the floor, or vice versa. If you are unsure which environment is right for your child, start with a combination. If you do not end up needing the table, it is easy to move it to the side. Take a moment to complete Exercise 7.1. See if you can determine which environment best matches the profile of the child.

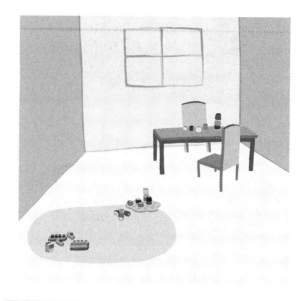

FIGURE 7.6. Routines set up on the table and the floor.

EXERCISE 7.1. **Choosing the Environment**

Match the description of the child with the most appropriate environmental layout.

Child profile	Appropriate environment
1. The child tends to wander around the room, has difficulty staying in one place, and often gets dysregulated.	A. Mostly floor
2. The child easily stays in the same place, can support his body while sitting, and is not often distracted by other objects in sight.	B. Mostly table
3. The child has moments of dysregulation and wandering but can sustain periods of time in the same spot and can play with several objects in sight.	C. Combination of floor and table

---

7.3.2 Provide Environmental Modifications

Within the play areas described above, you can further adjust the level of support to meet the child's needs. The goal is to reduce any barriers that may take energy away from the child's ability to play. Use any of the following modifications (or others not listed so long as they increase the child's engagement). Avoid modifications that are overly restrictive, controlling, or otherwise dysregulating to the child. The goal is to consider the strengths and needs of the individual, so you can set up the environment for a positive, fruitful, and fun interaction, where the child has appropriate support to comfortably play and engage.

Table Modifications

Here are some examples of modifications you can make to the table arrangement:

- Allow the child to stand instead of sit at the table.
- Use furniture, the wall, or other boundaries next to the child to help define the space.
- Use a chair with a back and/or arms (e.g., a cube chair) to support the child in sitting up.
- Sit adjacent to the child (orient face-to-face with the toys directly in between you and the child), as shown in Figure 7.7.
- Seat the child in the corner of the room and move the table forward to create boundaries on either side of the child, as shown in Figure 7.8.

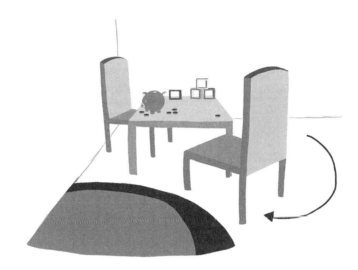

FIGURE 7.7. Adjacent seating arrangement.

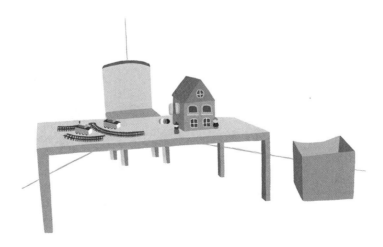

FIGURE 7.8. Table in corner.

Floor Modifications

Here are some examples of modifications you can make to the floor:

- Seat the child with his back against a wall or in the corner of the room to support the child's body.
- Use a legless chair for back support, as shown in Figure 7.9.
- Prop up the toys to increase accessibility and reduce the need for the child to lean forward, as shown in Figure 7.9.
- Use your own body to create a smaller space by sitting with your legs in a *V* shape.

7.3.3 Reduce Distractions

Make sure the room is tidy and your play area is free of clutter. There are often distractions in the environment that you may not immediately notice. A good general rule is to keep the floor and surrounding area clear of objects that are not a part of the intervention. Everything placed within the child's sight and reach is "fair game." This means that if the child can easily access an item, it should be appropriate for the session. If an item distracts from the child's engagement during the session (e.g., items to climb, electronics, developmentally inappropriate toys), then consider removing these items.

7.4 Set Up Routines

Once you have arranged the play area, you can set up the routines you prepared in Chapter 6. You will not set out all the toys you prepared; rather, you will provide a few clear options for the child to choose between. The goal is for the child to see the options available, make a choice, and begin playing. This creates opportunities for the child to initiate and supports the child's engagement in the routine. Figure 7.10 shows an example of a JASPER environment for a child with mastered general combination play and a target of presymbolic skills.

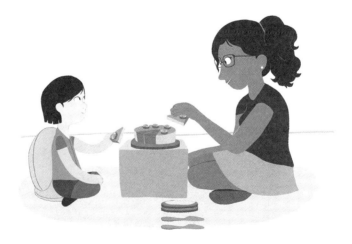

FIGURE 7.9. The adult provides a legless chair and a small platform for the toys..

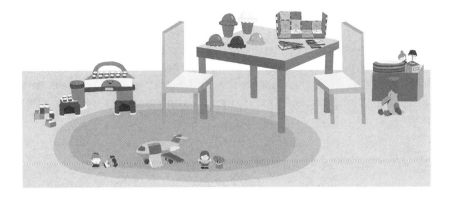

FIGURE 7.10. Routines set up for mastered general combination and target presymbolic levels.

7.4.1 Provide Clear Choices

Set up the initial routine choices within reach of where you want the child to sit, whether on the table, the floor, or both. Group the toys together by routine, while maintaining some space in between the different routines to create a clear distinction. This helps the child notice the different choices available and supports the first steps of the routine. For example, in Figure 7.10, we provided four routine options: a combination barn structure with blocks, an airplane with figures, ice cream stackers, and magnetic tiles with some of the structure prebuilt. Each of these routine options has a few starting pieces for the base, and we also have a box of expansion options nearby. This is one example of how you might set up the environment for a particular child.

Partially Assemble the Toys

When you set up each routine, put some of the pieces together to provide a visual cue of how to play with the toy. In Figure 7.10, for example, you could have a pile of magnetic tiles with several tiles prebuilt into part of a structure or a couple of ice cream scoops already stacked on a cone. This gives the child some ideas of how to start playing with the toy without modeling or prompting the first step. (The child is not required to play with the toy in this way; this is simply a way to spark action.)

Provide Enough Pieces to Establish the Base

You do not have to fully set up all the toys for each routine. This would be too distracting and take up too much space. Instead, provide just enough pieces to begin the routine, and perhaps an expansion option or two. For example, if you have set up the room like the example in Figure 7.10, you can provide a few ice cream pieces on the table. If the child chooses the ice cream routine, you will then add more pieces to the table so you can each continue taking turns and keep the routine going.

Keep Extra Toys and Expansions Organized and Within Reach

Extra materials should be organized and easily accessible at all times so you can quickly access what you need. Use clear, zip-top bags; small boxes, baskets, or bins; tubs with lids; or other organizational containers. Keep the extra toys behind you, next to you, or on a nearby shelf so they are easily accessible but out of the child's reach. In Figure 7.10, there are additional materials close at hand for each of these routines. (Note that these additional materials are not always captured in our illustrations. See Box 7.1.) If you move from the table to the floor, bring the toys with you. In order to keep engagement with the child, you will not have time to get up from the routine, search for particular toys, or fumble with containers that are difficult to open, so it is important to plan ahead.

7.4.2 Set Up Stations for Higher-Level Players

Children at higher play levels eventually bridge separate routines together to create one larger routine. You can use toys to help the child make these connections. For example, in Figure 7.11, we use the road pieces to facilitate the connection between the furniture and people and the animals and boxes. This keeps the routines flexible, helps the routine flow naturally, and encourages the child to play in creative ways.

7.5 Maintain the Environment throughout the Routine

We have extensively explained the way that you set up the environment *before* the session. Another aspect of this set of strategies is the way that you manage the environment *within* the session.

7.5.1 Stay Face-to-Face

You are also part of the environment. Therefore, it is essential to make sure you are in the best position to engage the child. Sit directly across from the child with toys in between. See Figure 7.12 for seating at a table and Figure 7.13 for seating on the floor. In most cases, you should avoid sitting next to the child, behind the child, or with the child in your lap, as these positions require the child to turn his head or body in order to see you.

Try to remain near the child's eye level. Ideally, the child should not have to move his body at all in order to see your face. In some cases, you may need to lower your body closer to the table or floor to make it easier for the child to glance at you. You can lean forward or slightly recline on

---

BOX 7.1. A Note on Illustrations

We have provided many illustrations throughout the book. Note that these illustrations are simplified examples intended to highlight particular strategies or behaviors. They do not always represent the complexity of a JASPER environment. For example, the illustrations provide very clean- and clear-looking environments. This is important to maintain for the child; however, in the background, a typical JASPER environment includes additional expansion options within reach, organizational bins for the clinician, and other routine options close at hand. Some children may also do well with more toys in the environment than is feasible to illustrate while highlighting specific strategies.

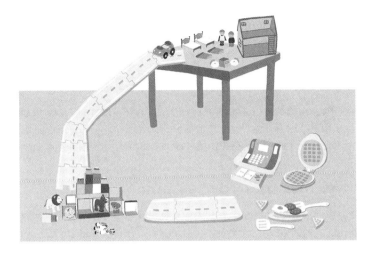

FIGURE 7.11. The road creates a visual cue that connects three distinct routines.

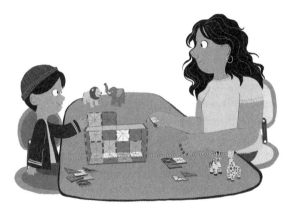

FIGURE 7.12. The adult and child sit in the optimal position at the table with the toys in between them.

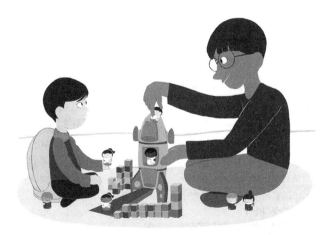

FIGURE 7.13. The adult and child sit in the optimal position on the floor with the toys in between them.

the floor; however, try to remain natural. You do not need to get close to the child or seek out eye contact directly. Keep a comfortable, natural distance.

Adjust Your Position as the Child Moves Around

Over time as the child moves and you begin different routines, your position and the toys can shift. If you notice that you are no longer in front of the child, move *your* body or subtly shift the toys between you to get face-to-face instead of prompting the child to move to you.

7.5.2 Orient the Toys toward the Child

As you play, notice the orientation of the toys. If a toy is physically too high, too low, or off to the side, make an adjustment so it is in a better position for the child. For example, you can turn the piggy bank so the slot faces the child, move the cuttable food so it is positioned correctly for the child's knife, or tilt the shape sorter so it is easier for the child to insert the shapes. If the toy has a clear front and back, like the rocket ship in Figure 7.13, make sure the front is oriented toward the child. This means you will have to reach around the back of the toy in order to take your turn. If one person has to use more effort to participate in the routine, it should be you, not the child.

7.5.3 Continue to Take an Equal and Active Role

Be purposeful as you rearrange the environment. Throughout the session, you will need to replenish the environment with new options as the child plays. Effective environmental arrangement should support the child's engagement and regulation and help the child initiate new play and communication ideas. You can use the environmental arrangement in moments when the child might have a new idea (e.g., adding new toys to expand the routine) or needs more support to reach joint engagement (e.g., removing the clutter of extra pieces to reduce distraction). See Figure 7.14 for qualities of environmental arrangement that you should strive for.

Remember to Take Your Turn as You Arrange the Environment

Good environmental arrangement is subtle, not overt. It should not take the place of your turn, interrupt the routine, or be distracting to the child. Take your turn with one hand, as you get out

ENVIRONMENTAL ARRANGEMENT SHOULD	ENVIRONMENTAL ARRANGEMENT SHOULD NOT
○ Provide the child with choices ○ Be subtle, discrete, and timely ○ Support next steps in play ○ Support the child's motor abilities ○ Provide opportunities for the child to initiate a new idea	○ Take the place of your play turn ○ Be overcontrolling ○ Interrupt the routine ○ Be noticeable and distracting to the child ○ Create downtime where the child is waiting for materials

FIGURE 7.14. Qualities of environmental arrangement.

more pieces for the child with the other hand, while keeping your focus on the child at all times. You should not be spending time looking for toys, turning away from the child, organizing, or setting up.

Avoid Overcontrolling Materials

As you monitor the materials, be careful not to be overcontrolling. Do not give the child one piece at a time or continually prompt the child to ask for more. When you overly control the materials, you end up controlling the play steps, the pace, and the entire direction of the routine as well. You make the play interaction feel more like a discrete trial or a task rather than a spontaneous and fun interaction.

7.5.4   Use the Environment to Support New Skills

You can also use the environment to establish the base, expand the routine, and create specific opportunities to practice communication (i.e., programming in Chapter 13). We also use the environment as a subtle, suggestive prompt to help the child build new skills without depending on more intrusive prompting. More information on each of these strategies is in subsequent chapters, signaled by the environment character.

7.6   Common Challenges with the Environment

When challenges arise in the session, begin by reassessing the environment. Ensure that the play area is set up clearly, that toys choices are available, and that you are in an optimal position to engage. You might consider adjusting the number of toys present or move from the table to the floor (or vice versa). In the following sections, we will answer some common challenges you may have and provide a few case examples to highlight the troubleshooting process.

7.6.1   Common Questions

In the section below, we address common questions that may arise as you prepare the environment for a JASPER session.

How many toys should I provide in the environment at any given time?

The amount of toys in an environment at a given time varies from child to child. This is determined by the child's engagement and regulation. Take note from the child's SPACE and your early sessions to try to find a balance between too few and too many toy choices. If there are too many toys present, the child might swipe toys off the table, throw toys, become unengaged, or have difficulty remaining regulated. However, if there are too few choices, the child might become frustrated and bored.

Signs Your Child May Need FEWER Toys

- Routines have fewer steps.
- Child gets overwhelmed by multiple options (or many pieces).

- Child plays at a slower pace.
- You anticipate staying at the base for a longer period of time.
- Rigid or repetitive behaviors increase when there are many items available.

Signs Your Child May Need More Toys

- Routines have numerous steps.
- Child quickly gets bored with the toys.
- Child plays at a higher play level.
- Child plays at a faster pace.
- You anticipate incorporating more expansions.

How do I set up in an environment where I have less control?

When working with children in settings like school or at home, you may not be able to perfectly arrange the environment. In these settings, you can use materials creatively to shape your space, for example, moving a couch toward the corner of the room or turning around a bookcase to limit distractions. Before arriving at the session, organize your toys by theme and routine using containers or bags so you can quickly set up your session and so the toys are easily accessible. Bring a blanket or sheet to cover materials that you want to set up but introduce later in your session. You may need to engage the child with a motivating toy or activity for a few minutes as you set up the routines for session. In this case, be sure to choose an activity that will help the child engage but not be so interesting that it causes dysregulation when you are ready to begin session.

What if the child does not want to sit in front of me?

Some children may want to sit on your lap while others may want to play on their own and away from you. In either case, you should adjust the environment to help them stay face-to-face with you so you can better respond to any social bids. Here are some suggestions: Move the toys away from the edges of the room so the child cannot face the wall; add structures such as chairs or dividers into the space; or set materials on a small box or stool to lift them up off of the floor.

How do I prevent the child from sliding under the table?

Check that the child fits comfortably in the table and chair you have provided. The child may need a shorter chair so his feet can rest on the floor, a smaller table so he can properly reach the toys, or a setup with more structure, such as a cube chair and attached table. The child may also slide underneath the table to avoid or escape the demand of play. In this case, use your environment to provide more structure, such as moving yourself to sit at the corner of the table or placing a box underneath the table to block the child's escape. You could also try starting the session on the floor.

What if the child is moving so fast that I do not have time to clean up my environment?

There is a lot to manage in the session, and the room can quickly become cluttered and overwhelming for both you and the child. When this begins to happen, it is sometimes necessary to take a quick break to reorganize or clean up materials. After the child has engaged in a high-quality routine, you may need to take 1 to 2 minutes to tidy up, assess the room and materials, and prepare choices for your next routine. Consider also the pace of the child's play. If the child is a fast-paced player, you may need to modulate the pace of the routine as described in Chapter 10.

7.6.2 Case Examples

Bouncing Off the Walls

Dear JASPER,

I am working with a child who is quite active and plays at the combination level. His mother says he loves to jump and run around, and I can definitely see this during our sessions! He is constantly moving from toy to toy, walking around the room, and bouncing around during our session. I decided to move him from playing on the floor to standing at a table, since he seems to engage more when he is able to wiggle a bit while standing. For the most part, this has been an improvement, but sometimes this results in him wanting to leave the table to run around even more. I'm not sure what to do. How can I help him stay connected and play for longer?

Thanks,
Bouncing Off the Walls

Dear *Bouncing Off the Walls,*

Great job adjusting your environment to meet this child's needs. You are definitely taking a step in the right direction by giving him the opportunity to stand and play. Another way to help extend time playing is to incorporate movement within or between routines. You can try setting up stations around the room so he has opportunities to get his wiggles out when moving from one routine to another. You can try adding toys that facilitate more gross motor movements, such as large blocks or shoeboxes where he needs to bend down to pick up blocks and stand up to stack them. You might also check into how long the child has been seated prior to your session (e.g., seated in transit, long day in school). You can help the child get the wiggles out prior the session by giving him time outside (if you're lucky to be close to a playground or open safe space) or creating a quick gross motor routine (jumps, scooters, etc.) so the child enters the session ready to engage.

Happy playing!
JASPER

Eager to Get Engaged

Dear JASPER,

I am working with a 6-year-old girl who loves to wander around the room and explore all the toys in the play space. She's quite active, and it's hard to get her attention. However, I recently had some luck in getting her engaged with a base routine where we put coins into a piggy bank. Sometimes she starts the routine, and sometimes I model the first steps. We can put all 10 coins into the pig, which feels like a huge win! When we run out of pieces, I typically look to my toy shelf to see what other objects might fit into the pig so that I can expand. Even though it only takes me a couple seconds to find an expansion or another toy option, she is wandering around the room by the time I turn around again. It's super overwhelming when this happens, because it feels like a lot of work to get her interested in a toy again! How can I help her stay engaged with me?

Thanks for the help,
Eager to Get Engaged

Dear *Eager to Get Engaged,*

It is great that you have had success in getting this little one engaged in a presentation combination base routine! It sounds as if you may need to quicken your pace during moments when you add more steps to the routine. Plan some expansions ahead of time and keep them easily accessible so you are ready before the child has finished putting in the last coin. This way, you will not need to turn away or shuffle through materials during a key moment when the child needs support to stay engaged. For example, if you plan to add cookies to the coin bank as an expansion, you can prepare the cookies in an open container nearby (e.g., under the table, on a shelf, next to your chair, in your lap). As the child begins to put the final coin into the pig, move a couple of the cookies onto the table into the child's reach. This way, the child will have access to materials for the next step immediately and can continue the routine, rather than getting up and wandering off.

Great job!
JASPER

7.7   Conclusion

Although it is impossible to avoid all distractions, you should enter every session mindful of the environment, minimizing distractions when and where you can. Once you find a layout that works well for the child, you can keep many aspects of the environment consistent from session to session to create a sense of familiarity. Take a moment to review the strategies from this chapter in Figure 7.15. As you use these strategies, you should see improvements toward your goals. The child should improve in her ability to choose toys and initiate play and communication within the routine. The tailored environmental structure should help the child play for longer amounts of time with fewer interruptions, breaks, and periods of dysregulation. With this structure in place, you should see more productive play and fewer interfering behaviors, and you may be able to reduce environmental support over time. In the upcoming chapters, we will explain how you can use environmental arrangement to support the specific stage of the session, strategy, or step of the routine.

Chapter 7 Summary

PREPARE THE PLAY AREA	PREPARE PLAY ROUTINES	MANAGE THE ENVIRONMENT
o Choose the table, floor, or both o Adjust the amount of structure to meet the child's needs o Reduce any distractions	o Set up 2–3 routine choices o Partially assemble the toys to provide a visual cue o Keep extra toys organized and within reach	o Stay face-to-face o Orient toys toward the child o Be quick and purposeful while arranging toys o Continue to take your turn o Adjust structure to support engagement and regulation

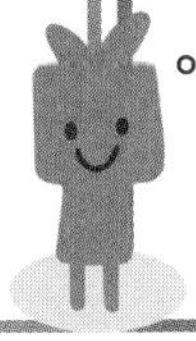

FIGURE 7.15. Chapter 7 summary.

Setting the Foundation for Engagement and Regulation

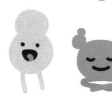

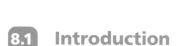

8.1 Introduction

The purpose of this chapter is to begin laying a foundation for engagement and regulation. As you begin, it is helpful to remember the child is entering a new situation. For some children, this may be their first exposure to intervention (or even a teaching context). And even those familiar with intervention may not know what is expected, who will be there, how long they are supposed to stay, and so on. For children who have minimal communication, anxiety around change, or rigidity in routine, this can add an extra layer of challenge. Thus, it is necessary to create a plan to support the child.

In this chapter, we provide a variety of strategies that may help children understand the expectations and participate more successfully in the session, such as visual supports, a plan for transitions, and positive reinforcement. We will also introduce a prompting hierarchy that can be used in select cases to help children follow through with demands, and a troubleshooting framework to evaluate challenges that may arise. With these strategies in place, our goal is to set a positive tone from the beginning of the interaction and to lay a foundation for regulation and engagement. You will continue to build on this foundation with other strategies, as many of the environmental strategies (from Chapters 6 and 7) and the play and communication strategies (from Chapters 9–14) support engagement and regulation as well. In Chapters 15 and 16, we will address challenges with engagement and regulation and provide additional explanation of how to use your full toolbox of strategies to respond.

8.2 Incorporate Visual Schedules and Supports

Many children benefit from visual supports. Like a clearly arranged environment, visual supports provide clear visual cues to help children understand the directions and expectations of a session in a way that is more efficient and effective for them. This extra layer of input can help children relax, be successful, and hopefully have fun! There are many types of visuals available for children of all ages and abilities. If a child uses a system at home or school, you can tailor the visual to the needs of the JASPER session. You can also create a visual from scratch to match your session needs. We have provided a list of supports that are helpful to have on hand before the session begins.

8.2.1 Prepare Supports Ahead of Time

Use your early impressions from the SPACE assessment and first few sessions to include supports to help the child regulate and engage. Children who have shorter periods of engagement and regulation, significant or reoccurring periods of dysregulation, or challenging behaviors may need more support. Others may not need visual support at all. (See Chapters 15 and 16 for indicators the child may need more support.) We will introduce some common types of visual supports below.

Visual Schedule

A visual schedule is a simple visual representation of a sequence of steps that can be used to clarify your statements and the expectations of the session. Visual schedules can vary in complexity, so you should choose a system that is simple, clear, and easy for the child to follow. A simple type of visual schedule includes a "first, then" statement—for example: "First sit, then play," or "First play, then all done" (see Figure 8.1). More complex schedules can include other steps and instructions as well (e.g., sit down, play with toys, all done playing, and go home; see Figure 8.2). If you use a visual schedule, keep the schedule consistent between sessions to help the child understand your expectations and facilitate transitions.

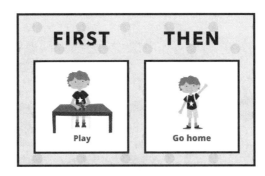

FIGURE 8.1. A simple first, then schedule can help the child understand what comes next.

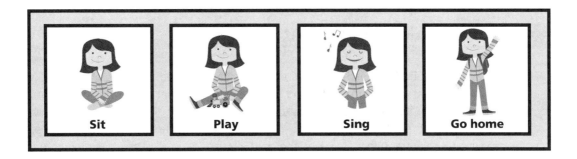

FIGURE 8.2. A multistep schedule can clarify expectations for the session.

All-Done Bin

Some children, especially those in preschool programs, may be familiar with a visual cue to clean up, such as an all-done bin. Incorporating this in your session can be a helpful way to transition the child out of session and onto their next activity for the day.

Social Story

For some children, it is helpful to practice a particular social skill or expectation using a simple narrative. For example, if a child has a difficult time with the expectation of playing with a partner, you could create a short story around the concept of sharing ideas and then read the story together before starting session. This story, often written from the child's perspective, provides a reminder about what will happen (e.g., "I will have a turn to play and then my friend will have a turn") and how the child might feel or behave (e.g., "Sometimes I do not want my friend to move the dinosaurs, and then I might feel frustrated"). Next, you can add a strategy the child can use (e.g., "I will take a deep breath and count to 3") and a positive statement about what happens when we do this (e.g., "We'll have so much fun playing together when we take turns!"). This preview can help increase regulation and understanding of expectations, and even give the child an opportunity to practice new regulation strategies at the beginning of the session.

Timers

A visual timer can help the child understand expectations about timing. You can pair the timer with the visual schedule or an all-done bin to show the child how much time is left until the end of session.

8.2.2 Use Supports to Clarify Expectations

Use the visual supports as necessary throughout the session to help the child understand your expectations and to clarify directions. For example, you can use these supports to help the child transition in and out of the session, to sit down, or to redirect the child back to play after a period of dysregulation or unengagement. Incorporating visual supports allows you to limit verbal input (which can add to dysregulation during challenging moments) while still helping the child follow through with expectations.

8.3 Transitioning In and Out of Session

Children with ASD often need support during transitions. Therefore, it is helpful to have a plan that you can repeat at the beginning and end of every session so that the child knows what to expect. This plan should be consistent enough to create expectations the child can rely on, yet flexible enough to meet the child's changing needs. The following sections provide examples of how you can support each transition. However, the child may not need all of these strategies, and you can often fade the level of support over time.

8.3.1 Support the Beginning of the Session

While some children may transition joyfully into session, others may have a difficult time. You may notice some challenging behaviors when the child first enters the room, such as crying, clinging to a caregiver, resisting sitting down, or attempting to escape the room. Your approach in these moments is vital to supporting the child through this stage. Here is an example of how we typically begin a JASPER session.

1. ***Greet the adult and child.*** Share your goals for the session and the approximate length you expect it to be. Fulfill any needs the child may have before you begin (e.g., give the child a drink of water, take her to the bathroom). Put aside items that have come along with the child (e.g., special toys, electronics, snacks, outerwear). During therapist-mediated JASPER, it is most common for the caregiver to wait outside of the play area unless the child is very young or there is another reason for the adult to be present (see Section 8.8.1 for more information). If this is distressing for the child, you can assist in having her successfully separate from the caregiver across the first few sessions. For example, begin the first session with the caregiver sitting next to the child as you play, and in subsequent sessions you can have the caregiver move farther away from the child until the child no longer relies on the caregiver being in the room.

2. ***Transition into the play space.*** As you transition into the play space, the goal is to help the child settle into the environment and begin playing. Do not linger in this transition window. Slow, hesitant transitions can create space for worry, anxiety, and upset. Instead, the transition should be quick and fun! The play area and toys should be set up already to provide visual cues of where to sit and what toy options are available, as described in Chapter 7. This makes it easier for the child to understand that it is time to play and to make a choice. If needed, you can show the child the visual schedule you prepared to explain what he will do next (e.g., "Sit down then play").

3. ***Help the child take a seat in front of the toys.*** If the child does not sit down on her own, help her to take a seat in front of the toys you have prepared. Make sure the child has clear choices immediately within sight and reach. Ideally, the child will pick a toy that is motivating and initiate the first steps, as illustrated in Figure 8.3.

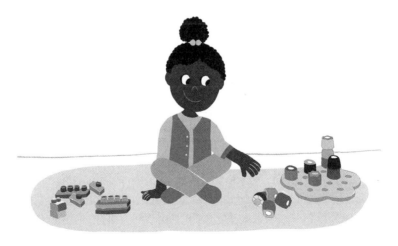

FIGURE 8.3. The room setup allows for the child to make a choice.

If the child does not immediately start playing, invite the child to do so by saying something like, "It's time to play!" or "Let's play!" Then pause and look expectantly at the child. Watch carefully to see if the child shows any signs of interest in any of the toys. For example, she might look at a toy, pick it up, or carry it around the room.

4. *Support the first steps of play.* If the child shows interest in a toy but still does not start playing, model an action. For example, if the child in Figure 8.3 picks up a peg, you could model by putting the peg in the pegboard. If the child has not indicated an interest in the toys, you could hold up a toy in each hand and offer a choice (e.g., say "Pegs or blocks?" and then wait a few seconds for the child to select one). The child might indicate a choice through words, gestures (e.g., a reach or point), gaze, or even a slight turn of the body. Once she has indicated interest in something, you can support the first steps of play by handing her a piece to get started or modeling a first play step. If the child is having a hard time settling into the room or choosing toys, you could use the visual schedule to help her understand what to do or use a short social activity to help her get more connected with you before you start playing. See Box 8.1.

5. *Establish the base of the routine.* Once the child begins playing productively with the toys, the goal is to establish the base of the routine. Use the environmental strategies in Chapter 7 to get situated to play. For example, if the child chooses the pegboard in Figure 8.3, put the board between you and her, make sure she has pegs within reach, and move the other routine options to the side, so they are not a distraction. You should also make sure you have expansion toys for the pegboard within your reach (e.g., blocks, figures, and flags that could be stacked along with the pegs). To support the child's first steps, use the strategies of imitating, modeling, and restarting, which will be covered in Chapters 9 and 10. The fictional case examples in Table 8.1 demonstrate how you might use the strategies in this section to start a session.

BOX 8.1. **Use a Quick Transition to Toys**

Sometimes children need a "warm-up" activity to transition into the higher demands of play. This can take on many forms. It could be an easier base step, a well-mastered routine, or a routine one step below the child's mastered play level (see Chapter 6, Box 6.1). You could also use a moment of person engagement, for example, singing "Old MacDonald" and then transitioning to toys by putting animals in a barn. For children with significant episodes of dysregulation, you could try an alternative activity, such as reading a book. For example, you could read *The Very Hungry Caterpillar* with the child and then transition into a play routine once the child is regulated and engaged by putting play food inside a stuffed caterpillar (see Box 16.1 for more on alternative activities). The goal is for the child to connect with you first and then the activity, so you can then quickly build momentum in a routine. During these transition activities, you should still model the same appropriate language and gestures you would use and target in your JASPER play routines. For more information on using transition activities to promote the child's engagement, see Chapter 15, Section 15.3.2.`

TABLE 8.1. Starting the Session

Javier (age 4)	Spence (age 2)	Erika (age 5)
Setting: Clinic	*Setting*: Child's home	*Setting*: Child's classroom
Engagement and regulation targets: Several minutes	*Engagement and regulation targets*: Sustained intervals	*Engagement and regulation targets*: Most of the interaction
Notes from SPACE: Shy, enjoyed playing once he warmed up. Did not use any language or gestures. Mastered combination play.	*Notes from SPACE*: Cried and wandered for the first half and repeated, "All done." Mastered simple play.	*Notes from SPACE*: Hard time leaving toys. Used some gestures and language. Mastered presymbolic play.
Javier and his mother arrived at the clinic for his first JASPER session. The interventionist *greeted* them, *shared the plan for session,* and invited Javier to play. Javier had never been in a session before and began to look around in distress. The interventionist used a *first, then schedule* to help him understand the expectations. She pointed to the visual: "First sit, then play." The interventionist had two routines on the table in front of Javier. She *watched attentively* as he looked at the toys. He picked up a block and stacked it on top of another block. The interventionist *imitated* Javier's play act while saying, "Build!" and quickly moved the other option off to the side.	The interventionist arrived at Spence's house with her toys organized and a small quilt to sit on to add some *structure to the environment* to play. She remembered Spence loved to read with his mom, so she brought one book for him to look through while she quickly set up and another for them to read together to use as a *quick transition activity.* She set out *toy choices* to begin building a routine and waited for Spence to choose. He picked up a plastic coin and began rolling it on the ground. The interventionist *modeled* putting the coin into a piggy bank and moved the piggy bank toward Spence. He imitated her action, and she quickly added more coins in front of him to begin building a routine.	Because Erika had a hard time leaving arts and crafts in her classroom to go to session, her interventionist *prepared an "all-done" bin and visual schedule* to support the transition. She showed Erika the schedule ("Walk, Play, Clean up, Art") so that Erika knew she was coming back to continue her art project. Erika put her project in the "all-done" bin, and they walked to the session together. The interventionist had three routines set up and *paused* as Erika chose the Velcro cupcakes. The interventionist *imitated* putting cupcakes in the oven. After a couple of turns, Erika said "Art!" and ran to the door. The interventionist *calmly showed her the visual schedule* and *helped her take a seat.* They began building a routine with the cupcakes.

In each of these examples, the interventionist proactively supported the child's engagement and regulation. They were prepared with a variety of supports and made use of those that were needed to help each child start the session on a positive note. When they noticed hesitation and early signs of dysregulation, they quickly stepped in to prevent future challenges. They also provided each child with room to make decisions and were not too quick to provide support during the moments when the children were regulated so that they had opportunities to engage with the toys.

8.3.2 Support the End of the Session

Children often need support near the end of the session as well. The child may grow tired as energy, engagement, and regulation begin to wane, or the child may be enjoying himself so much that he does not want to leave. JASPER sessions typically last between 45 and 60 minutes. The goal is to end on a positive note when the child is regulated and engaged, rather than a moment when the child is dysregulated or trying to leave. This reinforces positive behavior and helps the child build endurance over time. Use the strategies below to support the end of the session.

1. *Give a transition warning.* Tell the child how much time is left and what is going to happen next—for example: "Two more minutes, then all done with toys." This signal should be provided prior to, rather than in response to, dysregulation. The amount of time you choose depends on the child. Some children need more warning, while others do better with less. You can also provide a couple of transition warnings, for example, when there is 5 minutes left, and another when there is 1 minute left. You may also include this step with a visual schedule. Once the approximate amount of allotted time has passed, help the child transition from playing to leaving.

2. *Create an appropriate stopping point.* After the time has elapsed, have a consistent plan that you repeat at the end of every session to signal that it is time to leave. A simple and quiet activity, such as a goodbye song, can help the child transition smoothly. The activity should be interesting so the child wants to participate, but not so motivating that the child would have difficulty ending. This could be a routine that the child has successfully engaged in, a simple cleanup activity (see Box 8.2), or a brief song.

- Choose only *one* activity.
- Choose an activity that is enjoyable or neutral, rather than unpleasant.
- Choose an activity that is familiar and easy for the child to do (e.g., if the child follows a particular sequence at school, you can do the same).

If a moment of dysregulation occurs during this activity, maintain the expectation, help the child regulate (use strategies from Chapter 16), and end on a positive note. If you place a demand such as cleaning up, you need to be clear that you are setting a demand and then help the child follow through; however, you do not have to set a demand for all children. The crucial part of this step is to signal the end of the session. It is okay for the child to watch while you put a few toys away or listen while you sing.

3. *Say goodbye.* If you have successfully completed the transition and the child is regulated, say goodbye! In Table 8.2, we continue our fictional case examples from Table 8.1 to see how the interventionists end each JASPER session.

In each of these examples, the interventionists provide the right amount of support for each child. Some children will need less support, while others will need more. If you find that these steps are not enough support and the child continues to have difficulty, you may need to adjust the environment (Chapter 7), address engagement (Chapter 15), or address dysregulation (Chapter 16).

Use Exercise 8.1 to practice matching the appropriate level of support to different child profiles.

BOX 8.2. **A Note on Cleaning Up**

Cleaning up is a common transition activity and one way you can create a clear end-of-session routine. If you do choose to clean up, *do not make the child pick up all of the toys*. This is a big request at the end of a long session! Choose a small number of toys and help the child by also putting toys away.

TABLE 8.2. Ending the Session

Javier (age 4)	Spence (age 2)	Erika (age 5)
The interventionist noticed they had about 3 minutes left in their session. Javier was happily playing and regulated in that moment; however, his mom had warned that he typically has a hard time transitioning away from toys. The interventionist decided that a *brief song would help him transition* since his mother had reported that he loves singing songs with her. Since they were playing with a boat toward the end of the session, she began singing "Row Your Boat." Javier ran away from the table and reached for the door handle. Joyce *showed Javier the visual schedule,* pointed to it, and said, "First song, then all done." When they finished singing the song, she said, "All done playing!" and walked Javier to meet his mom in the hallway.	After 30 minutes, the interventionist decided to *finish session on a positive note* since Spence was so engaged in their routine. She gave Spence a *warning of "2 more minutes."* As soon as he heard the warning, Spence dropped his toys and began running around the room. The interventionist decided to show Spence a *visual timer* with 2 minutes and repeated the expectation: "2 more minutes of play." She *helped Spence sit down* and *handed him a piece* to continue the routine. When the timer went off, the interventionist said, "All done. Awesome playing!" with a big smile and walks Spence to the kitchen to find his mom.	As they reached the end of session, the interventionist *gave Erika a warning* that they had "1 more minute." About a minute later, the interventionist decided they would reach an *appropriate stopping point* after they expanded the routine. The interventionist *showed Erika the schedule* saying, "We played, now time to clean up, and then go back to art." Erika and the interventionist *cleaned up a few toys* and then the interventionist *walked Erika back to her classroom.* They checked in with Erika's teacher, who then helped Erika continue her art project.

EXERCISE 8.1. Support Transitions

Match the scenario of each child with an appropriate amount of support to transition.

1. The child is used to spending all day with his dad and cries when his dad leaves at the beginning of the session.

2. After asking the child to clean up, the child throws all the toys on the floor and begins crying.

3. The child is 5 years old and enjoys his preschool routine of waving goodbye to his mom, hanging up his backpack, and going into his classroom.

4. As you finish session and tell the child you are all done, he stubs his toe and begins crying.

A. Greet the child cheerfully, quickly transition into the room, direct the child to the seat, and start the routine.

B. Use a "first, then" visual schedule to show the child that he will see his parent after you play together.

C. Help the child calm down by singing a favorite song and then leave the session on a positive note.

D. Use a visual support such as an all-done bin and help the child follow through with the expectation you have set.

8.4 Use Natural Reinforcement

Throughout the session, we primarily use intrinsic rewards that are socially motivated (such as responding with communication, imitating play acts, and using positive affect), more so than extrinsic rewards (such as frequent verbal praise and external reinforcers). By providing a fun, calm, engaging environment for the child to learn, the goal is to help the child find the *interaction itself* to be rewarding, thus eliminating the need for external incentives.

8.4.1 Use Your Turn in the Routine to Reinforce the Child's Actions

Use naturalistic play-based responses with *commenting* language (see Chapter 6, Section 6.3.2) on your own play turn as your primary mode of reinforcement. By noticing and responding to the child's appropriate behaviors, you encourage these behaviors to happen more frequently. Reinforcement is especially crucial after the child uses a new skill or after moments of dysregulation and low engagement have resolved. For example, if the child shows you a toy, you can respond naturally with positive affect, and say, "A purple car!"; or if the child puts a figure on the bus after a period of dysregulation, you can respond by putting another figure on the bus and saying, "On the bus!" with a cheerful tone. By imitating the child's actions and commenting with excitement, you are conveying a pleasant message while also modeling a phrase that the child can use within the play interaction. In most cases, this is rewarding enough to reinforce the behavior.

Limit Verbal Praise

In general, we avoid (or significantly limit) verbal praise, such as "Good playing," "I hear you," "I like your talking," or "Thank you for using your words." Verbal praise may unintentionally imply that there are specific play actions the child is expected to take. Additionally, when the adult constantly uses verbal praise, the child has less time and space to initiate communication and hears fewer language models to possibly imitate.

Avoid Extrinsic Rewards

In general, we avoid (or significantly limit) the use of external rewards, such as tangible reinforcers, special toys (e.g., bubbles), food, and long breaks from the session. Tangible reinforcers are viewed as supplementary to JASPER and should not be the default for most children. When you add external reinforcers such as highly motivating sensory toys, it can lead to object engagement and make it very difficult to expand the routine. Thus, these are only incorporated for a brief period of time if a child has a particular need for this level of extra support and then is quickly faded out once the child has built up other skills.

Avoid Punishments

Avoid strategies that lend themselves to a negative social environment, such as punishments, reprimands, and time-outs. These are often incompatible with play and having fun. In general, using positive reinforcement is a more effective and appropriate approach to helping children learn new skills and behaviors.

8.4.2 Use Positive Affect

Every JASPER session should have a warm and positive social atmosphere. One of the best ways to create an inviting social environment is to use positive affect in a way that is motivating to the child. *Positive affect* refers to the way that a person experiences and communicates their positive feelings. There are many ways to use positive affect, such as by smiling, using a cheerful tone of voice, and demonstrating interest in the child's activities. Make sure your voice is natural when you use positive affect, so that it sounds appropriate if the child imitates you. You should infuse this attitude throughout your interaction with the child, so that the child begins to understand that engaging with you is fun! Here are some additional tips for using positive affect.

Learn the Child's Affective Style

All children have different levels of affective expression and response to positive affect. Some children respond well when you are upbeat, positive, and enthusiastic, while others need a calm, quieter approach to stay regulated and engaged. In general, we model positive affect within the child's natural range. Get to know the child and try to create an atmosphere that works best for him. You can also adjust your affect based on what is happening in the moment. For example, if the child is quiet and concentrating on a particular play act, then it may be more appropriate to demonstrate support or encouragement in a soft volume, whereas a moment of excitement or discovery might warrant higher affect.

Modulate Affect

Sometimes children demonstrate affect that does not appropriately match the social context. Extremes in affect (e.g., being overexcited) can create challenges in building joint engagement. In these cases, you can use your own affect to model a balanced and appropriate state for the child. For example, the child might get very silly, laugh a lot, and want to repeat funny words or actions over and over again. While this may seem like a good exchange, it can lead toward lowered engagement (or possibly an attention-seeking behavior). If the child is overly excited, you can use a more neutral tone and facial expression to help the child settle down. On the other hand, the child's affect might seem lower than expected, and it may appear as though he is not motivated at all by even the most exciting aspects of the interaction. For example, you feed a silly puppet while making eating noises; however, the child may only glance at you briefly or he might not have any reaction at all. If the child has flat affect, you can increase your positive affect to help the child find motivation in the interaction.

8.5 Understanding the Prompting Hierarchy

There may be instances where you need to add more support by providing additional prompts. Prompts can be used to teach new skills and to help the child follow through with the expectations of the session. In JASPER, we are very intentional in how we define and use this strategy.

8.5.1 Consider Engagement and Regulation while Using Prompts

Before we discuss the details of prompting, it is critical to consider how this strategy can either support or derail engagement and regulation. Remember from Chapter 5 that achieving a state of joint engagement requires an *equal and active* role from the adult. Your role is not to direct the child through prompts. Using prompts can feel rewarding as you see the child succeed in new skills. However, when the adult becomes overly directive, the child may be less motivated to participate, and the interaction begins to feel like a task rather than a social activity. This can also lead to fewer initiations and more episodes of dysregulation. Thus, it is important to keep the child's big pictures goals in mind.

8.5.2 Follow a Least to Most Prompting Hierarchy

In JASPER, we follow a least-to-most prompting hierarchy, which includes the following prompts: environmental, modeling, gestural, verbal, and physical prompts (see Figure 8.4).

- *Environmental prompts.* Rearrange the environment to provide a visual cue of what is expected (e.g., move one toy forward, hand the child a toy, hold up two choices, show the child a visual support).
- *Modeling.* Show the child an action (e.g., model a productive play action or a gesture).
- *Gestural prompt.* Support the child by gesturing toward the desired action or object (e.g., extend your hand with your palm facing up to encourage the child to give you an object).
- *General verbal prompt.* Ask the child an open-ended question (e.g., "What happened?" or "What do you want?").
- *Specific verbal prompt.* Instruct the child to use the target skill (e.g., "Show me") or provide the child with words he can use (e.g., "Say, 'Want train' ").
- *Partial physical prompt.* Gently touch the child's arm or hand (e.g., tap the child's elbow to remind the child to point).
- *Full physical prompt.* Help the child take the action (e.g., gently form the child's hand into the target gesture).

Suggestive and Directive Prompts

Environmental prompts and modeling are what we call *suggestive prompts,* meaning they provide the child with a possible "next step," but without an explicit expectation. For example, you move the toys forward with the hope that the child will choose one, and you model an action as a prompt for what the child could potentially do next. These prompts should be subtle and unobtrusive and should not include additional verbal or physical cues. In JASPER, the child does not *have* to follow through with your ideas after an environmental prompt or modeling; rather, these strategies are used to encourage the child to take an appropriate action.

Gestural, verbal, and physical prompts are considered *directive prompts*. With directive prompts, there is a clear demand, a target response for the child, and an expectation that the child follows through. We are careful not to become overly reliant on directive prompts to meet our goals. As you can see in Figure 8.4, suggestive prompts are part of the *core* strategies of JASPER. They are frequently used to provide the child with opportunities. Directive prompts are *conditional*

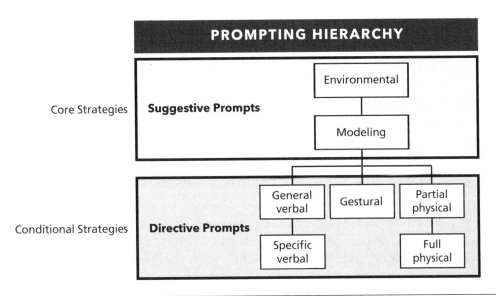

FIGURE 8.4. The prompting hierarchy begins with suggestive prompts and moves into directive prompts.

strategies. They are used much less frequently, and only after troubleshooting. (See Chapter 1, Section 1.6.1, for more information on when to use core strategies versus conditional strategies.)

8.5.3 Guidelines for Prompting

Follow the guidelines below to provide successful prompts.

- ***Pause after prompting.*** Give the child enough space to respond to the prompt. For example, if you choose a verbal prompt, do not say, "What do you want . . . Joey? What do you want?" Instead, make sure the child is paying attention, say the prompt once, and pause for him to respond. If the child does not respond to the prompt, move to a higher level prompt before he loses engagement.
- ***Move through the prompt hierarchy.*** Increase the level of prompt to help the child be successful. For example, if you start with a general verbal prompt (e.g., "What do you want?"), you can move on to a specific verbal prompt ("Do you want the blocks or the cars?").
- ***Help the child follow through with directive prompts.*** Use clear directions and visual supports as necessary to help the child understand and follow through. By using a directive prompt, you are setting an explicit demand. This is not something we do often in JASPER, but when you do, you must carry it out. This helps the child understand the expectations and makes it more likely that the child will respond to your prompts in the future.

8.5.4 Avoid Prompt Dependence

Children can easily become prompt dependent, meaning they will rely on prompts, instead of learning to use the skill on their own. Therefore, use prompts sparingly and quickly fade support so that the child begins using the skills with less input from the adult. Here are some strategies we use to avoid prompt dependence.

- *Use core strategies whenever possible.* Before using a directive prompt, evaluate your use of core strategies and suggestive prompts.

- *Start with the least explicit prompt.* Start with the least explicit prompt that you suspect will be successful. In other words, do not use the most intrusive form of prompt if a less intrusive prompt might produce the skill. (In most cases, this means relying on suggestive prompts over directive prompts.)

- *Fade prompts quickly.* The child should not be dependent on prompts for long (particularly directive prompts). Once you prompt at one level, consider prompting at a lower level next time. Eventually, the goal is for the child to use the target skill spontaneously.

In order to avoid prompt dependence, we often have to push the child's level of comfort a little bit each time, so the child is eventually able to use the skill on his own. Be optimistic about the child's ability to learn from that moment. You should expect the child to be a little closer to using the skill with a little less support in the next attempt. It may not always work out, but it is important to keep your expectations high for the child. Use Exercise 8.2 to test your understanding of using prompts in JASPER.

EXERCISE 8.2. Using Prompts in JASPER

Indicate whether each statement is true or false according to JASPER guidelines.

1. Start with the least intrusive prompt that allows the child to be successful.	True	False
2. Continue to repeat the same prompt until the child produces a skill.	True	False
3. You must follow through after providing a suggestive prompt.	True	False
4. Fade prompts as quickly as possible.	True	False
5. Verbal prompts and gestural prompts are core strategies of JASPER.	True	False

---

8.6 Set Clear Expectations

In some cases, you may need to set some expectations in order to accomplish the long-term goals of the session. For example, if the child wanders around the room, you must help the child stay in front of the toys and you. This is particularly important when you are establishing expectations early in the intervention and when you encounter challenging behaviors. These expectations should be clear, so the child understands what you are asking, and developmentally appropriate, so the child is able to follow through.

8.6.1 Choose One Clear Direction

When you instruct the child, make sure the direction is specific and achievable. Rather than asking a question the child can say no to, such as "Will you come sit down?" you should offer one clear direction, such as "It's time to sit" or "Sit down." Say the direction *once* and wait for the child to respond. If he does not follow your instructions, help him meet the demand. For example, move his chair closer, point to his chair, or physically help him to sit down. Follow a consistent plan across sessions to help establish the expectation (e.g., use consistent, developmentally appropriate words so the child becomes familiar with what he needs to do).

8.6.2 Be Consistent

Once you use a give the child a direction, help the child carry out the expectation. Your response teaches the child what type of communication is most successful, whether it is whining when he wants something or more productive communication that will help him in future interactions. While these moments can be challenging, remain calm and consistent in your expectations to prepare the child for future successes.

8.6.3 Maintain Confidence

Maintain confidence throughout the session. You should stay calm and in control of your own expressive state. Use appropriate affect and tone, take action during difficult moments, provide support appropriate to the moment, and follow through on prompts and demands. Try not to show signs of anxiety, frustration, or distress, even if the child has a meltdown or the session feels like it is falling apart. Find a balance in your role and avoid being too timid or domineering:

Signs You Are Being Too Timid

- Talking too softly or quietly
- Appearing anxious or hesitant
- Asking the child for permission
- Giving in to the child's demands
- Abandoning a prompt or demand
- Freezing or panicking

Signs You Are Being Domineering

- Using a brusque or overly harsh tone of voice
- Being too directive
- Placing demands without providing necessary support
- Overlooking the child's experience and the broader context

Before moving on, identify in Exercise 8.3 whether a clear expectation has been set.

EXERCISE 8.3. Setting Expectations

Identify whether the scenarios provide clear expectations for the child. Circle "Yes" if the adult follows JASPER guidelines, and circle "No" if not.

1. You realize the session time has elapsed and tell the child, "It's time to clean up and put your shoes on." The child starts to get upset, so you continue the routine for a few more turns and plan to try again. You instruct the child, "Clean up. Do you want to go? Come on, let's pick up!" The child does not clean up, so you continue to repeat the directions.   Yes   No

2. After the child crawls under the table, you tell her to sit on the chair. She does not respond, so you help her move her body onto the chair.   Yes   No

3. When the child is slow to come into the room or choose a toy you ask, "Do you want to play?" The child stays still and does not answer, so you say, "Come on, let's go play. Don't you want to play with me?"   Yes   No

8.7 ACT Troubleshooting Framework

Despite your best efforts, you will encounter challenges as you implement the intervention. Ultimately, it is your responsibility to help the child through these difficult steps. In JASPER, we provide a three-step process for troubleshooting: Assess the situation, Create a plan, and Test for success (ACT framework). The ACT framework is a systematic and iterative process where we assess the child's actions and our own actions, develop a strategy plan based on an informed hypothesis, and then test the plan until we find solutions that improve the child's overall engagement, regulation, social communication, and play. As you troubleshoot, ask yourself the following questions:

- *Assess the situation.* What happened? What challenges occurred in the routine or in the child's behavior?
- *Create a plan.* What can I do to help? How can I use core and conditional strategies to produce change?
- *Test for success.* Did my plan have the intended effects? Is there anything I can improve?

We apply this structure throughout the upcoming chapters to troubleshoot challenges that may arise. This is a continual process that happens both in the moment when challenges occur and in reflection after the session. When patterns of challenging behaviors are particularly perplexing or difficult to address, we recommend filling out Form 8.1 (ACT: Assess the Situation, Create a Plan, and Test for Success, p. 152) after the session to look closer at the situation and brainstorm solutions. Filling out the form will help you be more thorough and creative as you investigate the situation and brainstorm solutions. This process is described below.

8.7.1 Assess the Situation

Assess the current situation. When something goes awry, you will likely see evidence in the quality of the routine and the child's behavior. Try to be specific about what you see, including the change itself and the surrounding context.

Check the Routine

You may encounter trouble starting the routine, maintaining the routine, adding new steps to the routine, and adding flexibility to the routine over time. You may also notice other changes in the overall quality of the routine, such as a having too much adult direction. The challenge may also occur during the transition between routines.

Check the Child's Behavior

Look for signs in the child's behavior. In this case, we mean all signals from the child, including actions, communication, affect, pace, regulation, and engagement. The child might look around the room, fiddle with the toys, get stuck on particular play acts, push toys off the table, cry, and so on. Look for signs of diminishing engagement (see Chapter 15), dysregulation (see Chapter 16), or rigid and repetitive behaviors (see Chapter 17). When challenges occur repeatedly or at a high level of intensity, it may be necessary to evaluate the *function of the behavior,* that is, the message the child's behavior is sending (see Chapter 16).

Assess the Impact

Consider the impact of the current challenge on the session, ranging from mildly interfering (e.g., child always initiates the same expansion step) to significantly interfering (e.g., child wanders the room crying and throwing toys). The level of impact will influence the strategy you choose as well as the amount of support you provide to get the session back on track. If the behavior is only mildly interfering, you may need to make a minor adjustment using a core strategy, compared to a moderately or significantly interfering behavior that may require a more targeted approach. See Chapters 15–17.

8.7.2 Create a Plan

Once you have assessed the challenge, the next step is to create a plan to address it. You will use the strategies in Chapters 6–16 to make changes to the environment, improve your own actions, and respond to the function of the child's behavior.

Change the Environment

Set up the environment to support the child. If something goes awry, you can adjust the level of environmental support to help the child play, regulate, and engage.

Change Your Actions

You may also need to change your own actions to better support the child. Remember that you play a role in challenges as well. It is often the case that something you are doing (or not doing) contributes to a change in the child's behavior or the routine. Sometimes challenges arise when we are too inflexible, have the wrong balance of strategies, push the child too hard, or keep expectations too low. Be aware of the role you play in the challenges that arise.

Respond to the Function of the Child's Behavior

Use the core and conditional strategies to respond to the function of the child's behavior, as explained in Chapter 16. This function helps you understand why the behavior might be occurring so you can create an appropriate response, particularly in the case of dysregulation when behaviors may not always be clear.

Prioritize Core Strategies over Conditional Strategies

Adjust your level of support to the needs of the situation, generally beginning with the least amount of support the child needs to be successful and increasing support as needed. Prioritize core strategies. If the child needs more support to resolve the challenge, you may need to use the conditional strategies. The core and conditional levels of support are introduced in Chapter 1, Section 1.6, and the guidelines for these strategies are further discussed in Chapters 15–17.

8.7.3 Test for Success

The last step is to test your plan for success. Did your plan work, or do you need to continue troubleshooting? Be aware that sometimes it gets worse before it gets better. The child might not understand the expectation and might resist the change by increasing the old patterns of behavior. It may take several attempts to find a solution that works. And once you find the solution, it may require some persistence to produce change.

Note What Worked

Begin by noticing which aspects of your plan worked. Use this knowledge to set yourself up for success in the next session. For example, if you planned to increase environmental structure by moving to the table partway through session, start your next session with these strategies in place.

Plan for the Future

Use the information you gathered through the ACT framework to be proactive and prevent challenges in the future. Get to know the child's early signs of diminished engagement or dysregulation so you can respond before the situation interferes with the routine. Notice also how the child responds to your actions. Avoid reinforcing behaviors you do not want to see repeated (see more in Chapter 16). Begin considering how you can fade support and encourage the child's independence and initiations.

8.8   Common Challenges Supporting Engagement and Regulation

In the sections below, we answer some common questions and provide a few case examples of specific challenges.

8.8.1   Common Questions

In this section, we address common questions that may arise as you create a plan to support the child.

What if the child is consistently dysregulated when entering the room?

If the child is dysregulated during the transition into the playroom, you may need to increase the amount of support you use during the transition. You can start by giving the child a clear warning of when it will be time to enter the session. For example, if the child is playing in a waiting room of the clinic or participating in an activity in class, you should let him know how long he has to wrap up the activity. For some children, you may need to pair the verbal transition warning with a visual schedule to show the child exactly what is going to happen. Once you deliver this expectation, it is important to follow through. You may also need to assess the function of the child's behavior and address dysregulation using the strategies in Chapter 16.

What if the child wants the caregiver in session?

Sometimes the child will want the caregiver to come into session but have a hard time engaging with you when the caregiver is there. We often work with caregivers to determine how best to support the child. Many caregivers choose not to be present, as they recognize that they may be a source of distraction. For some children, especially those who are very young, it can be more developmentally appropriate and regulating to have the caregiver in the session. However, for other children, this may be more distracting and can even encourage silly or challenging behaviors. (This book covers interventionist-mediated JASPER. In caregiver-mediated JASPER, the caregiver will be a full participant.) In these cases, it is best to practice separating from the caregiver using transition strategies. For example, you could include a visual schedule, give kind and clear verbal directions of the expectations, and welcome the child into an environment with interesting and motivating toy choices.

8.8.2   Case Example

So Many Cars!

Dear JASPER,

I have a little girl who always brings something special with her to our sessions. She loves all vehicles. Sometimes she comes with tiny cars in her pockets or a big stuffed airplane. We've tried including these favorite toys in our sessions, but she loves them *so much* that it's very hard for me to even touch the toys or add them into our routines in new ways.

I know it's hard for her mom to get her in the car to come to our session without them, so I don't think leaving them at home is an option. I have tried to take the toy when she arrives, but she gets very upset and keeps asking until I finally give them back. How can I deal with these vehicles?

Sincerely,

So Many Cars!

Dear *So Many Cars,*

This sounds like a tough transition into your session. We love that you have tried to use these favorite toys, but it sounds as if it is very challenging for the child to play with these items in flexible ways, and this is hampering the progress in your routines and the child's engagement. Perhaps you can create a plan to help her put the vehicles aside before starting your session. One strategy is to set up a cubby or safe place for the child to store her things. Just as at school, she could hang up her jacket, place her backpack on the hook, and then put her vehicles in a special safe spot in the cubby. You might consider pairing a "first, then" or visual schedule with the introduction of the cubby to help her understand that the cars are put in her cubby where they stay safe until she finishes the session.

Good luck!

JASPER

8.9 Conclusion

Using Figure 8.5, take a moment to review the strategies you learned in this chapter. As you become more familiar with the child over time, you will learn to make better choices to support the session. We cannot always perfectly predict how a child will act and how best to respond. The measure of your success is defined not by whether you encounter challenges (you will and should expect to!) but rather by how often these behaviors arise, how long they last, and whether they decrease in severity over time. If you notice that challenges are emerging less often, are briefer in duration, and are less interfering, then you are making progress toward you goals and providing a stronger foundation for the session.

This chapter concludes Part III. You will return to these strategies often to keep the physical and emotional environment responsive to the child's needs, to advance the child's goals, and to troubleshoot when challenges arise. In Part IV, we will explain how to build routines within this environment you have carefully prepared.

Chapter 8 Summary

PREPARE **VISUAL SUPPORTS**	FACILITATE **TRANSITIONS**
o Prepare supports for the child (e.g., visual schedule, timer) o Use supports to clarify expectations	o Create a transition routine o Make transitions quick and fun o End session on a positive note

CREATE A SUPPORTIVE **LEARNING ENVIRONMENT**	TROUBLESHOOT WITH THE **ACT FRAMEWORK**
o Use natural reinforcement (e.g., use positive affect, imitate productive play and communication) o Use the least-to-most prompting hierarchy o Plan to fade prompts o Set clear expectations and follow through	**Assess the situation** o Check the routine o Check the child's behavior **Create a plan** o Change the environment o Change your own actions o Respond to the function of the behavior **Test for success** o Note what worked o Plan for the future

FIGURE 8.5. Chapter 8 summary.

ACT: ASSESS THE SITUATION, **C**REATE A PLAN, AND **T**EST FOR SUCCESS

Child: _____   Adult: _____   Date: _____

Assess the situation: What happened? What challenges occurred in the routine or in the child's behavior?

Check the routine	Check the child's behavior

Try using the "Check the Child's Behavior" Form!

Create a plan: What can I do to help? How can I use core strategies and conditional strategies to produce change?

Change the environment	Change your own actions	Respond to the function of the child's behavior

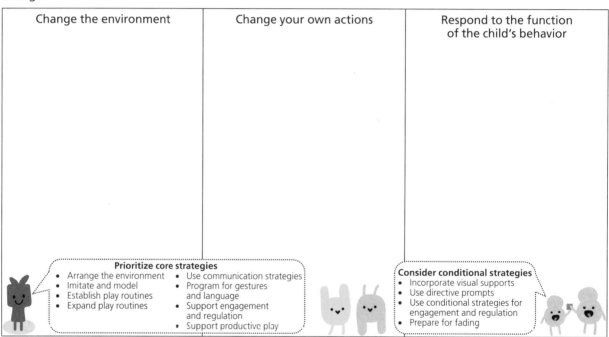

Prioritize core strategies
- Arrange the environment
- Imitate and model
- Establish play routines
- Expand play routines
- Use communication strategies
- Program for gestures and language
- Support engagement and regulation
- Support productive play

Consider conditional strategies
- Incorporate visual supports
- Use directive prompts
- Use conditional strategies for engagement and regulation
- Prepare for fading

Test for success: Did my plan have the intended effect? Is there anything I can improve in the future?

Note what worked	Plan for the future

Prepare to fade support!

PART IV

PLAY

In this section, you will learn how to
build dynamic play routines through
imitating and modeling, establishing
the base, and expanding.

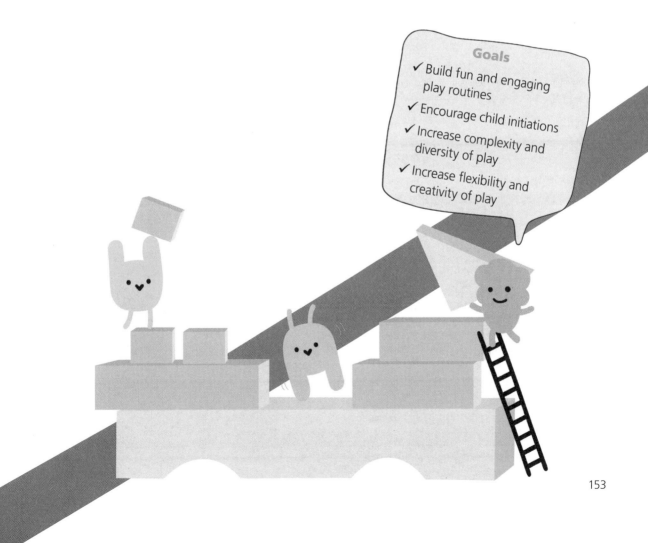

Goals

✓ Build fun and engaging
play routines

✓ Encourage child initiations

✓ Increase complexity and
diversity of play

✓ Increase flexibility and
creativity of play

Imitating and Modeling Play

9.1 Introduction

Now that you have the tools necessary to prepare the environment, it is time to introduce the strategies for play. In this chapter, we discuss the guidelines for imitating and modeling play acts. As you may recall from Chapter 1, *imitation* is the process of repeating and reinforcing the child's actions, and *modeling* is the process of demonstrating a developmentally appropriate play act. Together, these strategies support the child's goals for engagement, productive play, and initiations. These strategies also make up a large part of your role as an equal and active play partner. Once you understand how and when to imitate and model, you will use them to establish, maintain, and expand routines, as described in Chapters 10 and 11.

9.2 Imitate and Model in Response to the Child

In every JASPER session, you will imitate and model play acts in response to the child's actions. If the child takes a productive play act, you can *imitate* to reinforce the child's action; if the child does not play or needs help to do so appropriately, you can *model* to provide support. It is imperative to notice what the child is doing in the moment to determine which strategy to use and how best to respond.

9.3 Guidelines for Imitating

Your primary role is to imitate the child's play acts (see Figure 9.1). When the child takes an action, you should have an immediate responding action with a similar toy (see Figure 9.2). For example, if the child puts a shape in the shape sorter, you can imitate by also putting a shape in the shape sorter. If the child pretends to drink out of a cup, you can pretend to take a drink out of a cup too. Imitation is one of the primary ways we reinforce the child's actions. Rather than using verbal praise or an external reinforcer, we imitate as a more natural form of reinforcement to show the child that we like his ideas. This strategy also supports the continuation of the routine and your role as an equal and active play partner.

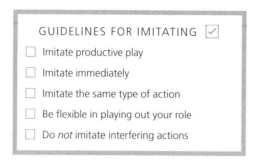

FIGURE 9.1. Guidelines for imitating.

9.3.1 Imitate Productive Play Acts

In JASPER, we do not imitate every single action the child takes. Instead, we only imitate the child's *productive* play acts. Remember, productive play acts are developmentally appropriate, are flexible, and support our goal of being jointly engaged (see Chapter 6, Section 6.2.3). Sometimes children surprise us with creative ideas and unique ways of using toys that we had not considered. As long as the action is productive, you should imitate. Here are some additional guidelines to make the most out of your imitation.

Imitate Immediately

Imitate immediately after the child's play act, so it is clear you are following the child's ideas. Children often move quickly, so you must act fast. You may only have a second or two to complete your action before the child takes another turn.

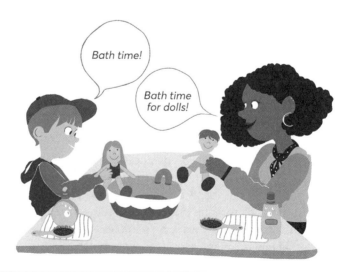

FIGURE 9.2. The adult imitates the child's productive play act by placing another doll in the bath.

Imitate the Same Type of Action

This does not mean you must take the *exact same action* as the child or imitate in the *exact same way* that the child does. For example, if the child puts a circle in the shape sorter, you can put any other shape in the shape sorter too; you do not need to put in the exact same color or shape.

Play Out Your Role

In presymbolic and symbolic play routines, it may be more appropriate to *play out your role* in the interaction, rather than to imitate the role the child is playing. For example, if the child pretends a figure is the teacher, and says, "Okay, class, time to sit down," you can play along by pretending to be a student: "Okay, teacher, I'll sit here." It would be unnatural to pretend to be the teacher as well and repeat the exact same actions.

9.3.2 Do Not Imitate Actions That Interfere with Engagement

Sometimes children with ASD use toys in ways that are not playful and do not contribute to the purpose of the routine. We refer to these as *interfering* actions in Chapter 6. For example, in Figure 9.3, the child is visually inspecting the soap bottle instead of using it for the purpose of play within the routine. These actions may be rigid or repetitive, they may serve as sensory exploration, or they may be far below the child's play level. They are often a sign of diminishing engagement and may occur in isolated instances or as an early sign of dysregulation. If the child's actions do not seem productive or do not serve the purpose of play, you should not imitate. This takes time away from social play and limits the amount of time the child spends learning.

Here are some additional examples of actions we typically do not imitate:

- Spinning objects
- Opening and closing doors
- Lining up or sequencing toys
- Repeatedly knocking down toys
- Repeatedly pushing buttons
- Visually inspecting
- Banging, throwing, or mouthing toys
- Flapping hands

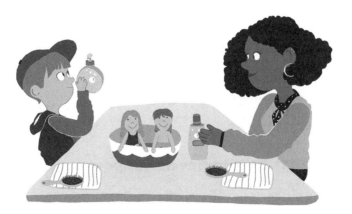

FIGURE 9.3. The adult refrains from imitating when the child visually inspects the soap bottle.

Before you move on, take a moment to complete Exercise 9.1 to check your understanding of this strategy.

EXERCISE 9.1. **Appropriate Use of Imitation**

Identify whether the adult imitates according to JASPER guidelines. Circle "Yes" if the adult provides an appropriate response and "No" if the adult does not.

1. You and the child are playing with a puzzle. The child taps the puzzle pieces two times before placing each piece in the puzzle. You tap the pieces twice before placing them in the puzzle as well.   Yes   No

2. You and the child are putting figures in stacking boxes. The child says, "It's a car" and pretends to drive the box. You say, "I have a car too!" and pretend to drive a figure in another box.   Yes   No

3. You and the child are putting toppings on a pizza. The child puts a pepperoni on the pizza. You put a mushroom on the pizza.   Yes   No

4. The child picks up an airplane and throws it across the room. You say, "It's flying!" and throw another airplane across the room.   Yes   No

5. The child pretends that she is the chef and you are the customer. The child says, "I'm the chef! Here's your order!" You give a hamburger back to the child and say, "I'm the chef! Here's your order too!"   Yes   No

---

9.4   Guidelines for Modeling

There will also be moments when the child needs help to play and engage, in which case you can model (see Figure 9.4). Modeling allows you to provide support and continue the interaction without taking over or physically prompting the child. Modeling can also encourage productive play actions and introduce new ideas into the routine. While it may seem like a good idea to model frequently to show the child new ideas, we want to remember to prioritize the child's own ideas and initiations. We always look for opportunities to imitate the child first; then if we cannot, we model.

9.4.1   Model When the Child Needs Support

If the child stops playing or needs support, model a productive play action to show the child what to do.

GUIDELINES FOR MODELING ☑

☐ Model when the child needs support

☐ Model one action at a time

☐ Model at the child's developmental level

☐ Model with the child's toy choice

☐ Ensure the child has materials and time to respond

FIGURE 9.4. Guidelines for modeling.

Model to Increase Engagement

If the child does not know what to do with the toys, model to show the child a step he could take. For example, if the child is looking at a puzzle but is not playing, you can put a piece in the puzzle. If the child was playing but stops, you could model another action to help him continue the routine. Try to model *before* the child loses engagement. Do not wait until the child stops playing entirely or becomes upset. By this point, it will be difficult to reengage the child in the routine.

Model after Interfering Behaviors

If the child's actions interfere with the routine, you can model to show the child something more productive he can do with the toy. In Figure 9.5, the child becomes object engaged with the soap bottle, shaking and visually inspecting it, and is no longer playing productively in the routine, thus the adult models putting soap in the bath to show the child something else to do. This helps the child learn a more productive action and a new way to play.

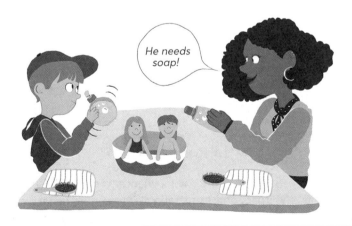

FIGURE 9.5. When the soap bottle becomes interfering, the adult models a productive play act by adding soap to the bath.

9.4.2 Model an Action the Child Is Likely to Imitate

Model actions that are developmentally appropriate, motivating, and reasonable for the child to repeat. When you model, the goal is for the child to imitate. If the step is too easy, too difficult, or poorly timed, the child is less likely to imitate. Here are some guidelines to make your models most effective.

Model One Action at a Time

Model only *one* action at a time. An appropriate one-step model might be placing a piece of play food in a bowl, whereas a two-step model would be placing a piece of play food in a bowl and stirring it. When you model too many actions at one time, it is difficult for the child to process the action and imitate.

Model a Developmentally Appropriate Action

Models are most likely to be successful at the child's developmental play level. If you are trying to establish a routine, you should model at the child's mastered play level (or possibly an earlier step). If the child is getting bored or you are trying to expand the routine, you can model an action at either the child's mastered or the child's target play level (see Chapter 11).

Model with the Child's Toy Choice

Follow the child's interests. If the child shows interest in a particular toy, try modeling a step with the same *type* of toy first. For example, if you have a routine that involves a train, tracks, cargo, and people figures, and the child begins tapping the piece of cargo on the table, you should model with the cargo rather than the figures or the trains. If the child is not holding or looking at any of the toys, you can pick an action you think might be motivating.

Provide Materials for the Child to Take His Turn

The child should have materials to respond to your model. For example, if you put a figure in a school bus, make sure there is at least one other figure within the child's reach. If you model cutting a cake, make sure there is another toy knife within the child's reach. These toys should be visible and easily accessible. If the child does not have access to the toys or cannot easily find them, he cannot respond even if he wants to, so it is important to be prepared.

9.4.3 Give the Child Time to Respond

After you model, *pause* to give the child a chance to respond. During this time, you should look at the child with eagerness and expectation. Do not talk or take any other actions to evoke a response, such as rapidly pointing at or shaking the toys. Do not provide further prompting or direction. Simply wait a couple seconds. The child may need a moment to process the action and decide what to do next. Now that we have introduced the guidelines for modeling, complete Exercise 9.2 to practice the proper use of this strategy.

EXERCISE 9.2. Appropriate Use of Modeling

Identify whether the adult models according to JASPER guidelines. Circle "Yes" if the adult provides an appropriate response and "No" if the adult does not.

1.	The child is looking at a puzzle with sea animals but is not playing. You pick up the starfish and "walk" it to the puzzle board.	Yes	No
2.	The child is lining up cars. You place a car into the garage.	Yes	No
3.	At the beginning of the session, you prepare the environment with two choices of toys: cupcakes and sandwiches. The child looks at the sandwich pieces but does not start playing. You put frosting onto a cupcake.	Yes	No
4.	The child sits down in front of a jungle routine with trees and clip-on monkeys. The child looks at the monkeys but does not start playing. You clip a few monkeys together and connect them to the tree.	Yes	No
5.	At the beginning of the session, you provide the child with a choice of two toys: a train set and magnetic tiles. The child picks up a magnetic tile but does not start playing. You stack one tile on top of another.	Yes	No

9.5 Notice the Child's Response to Your Model

After you model, the goal is for the child to imitate or demonstrate another developmentally appropriate play act. You can respond to the child's action, by either imitating or modeling with more support.

9.5.1 Reinforce the Child's Response

If the child imitates your model, imitate to reinforce the new action. Your model might also spark a new idea, and the child may respond by trying something new. For example, while building a routine at the simple play level, you might model shaking a tambourine, and the child could respond by patting the tambourine like a drum (both *discriminate acts*). You should imitate in this case as well.

9.5.2 Increase the Clarity of the Model

In some cases, children may need more support to understand and follow your models. If the child is consistently struggling to follow your models, you should first evaluate the clarity of the action you modeled, ensuring it is developmentally appropriate, appropriately timed, and within the child's lines of sight. If your model is clear, you can consider increasing the level of support. Try to provide the least amount of support necessary to help the child respond. Table 9.1 shows a list of appropriate responses based on the child's action.

TABLE 9.1. Increase the Clarity of Your Model

Child's action		Your response
Child did not notice the action.	➜	Model the same action again.
Child noticed the action but was not interested.	➜	Try modeling a different action.
Child did not like the action or became dysregulated.	➜	Try modeling a different action.
Child noticed and understood the action but needs additional support to try it out.	➜	Model the same action and push a toy forward or hand the child a toy.
Child initiates a different productive play act.	➜	Stop trying to model and instead imitate the child.
Child lost engagement.	➜	Stop trying to model and instead reengage the child (see Chapter 15).

9.6 Balance Imitation and Modeling

Like any strategy, imitation and modeling are only effective when used at the right time for the right purpose. We think of imitation and modeling as a dynamic duo. They play different roles during the routine, and each is important for sustaining the interaction. When the child initiates a productive action, we imitate. When the child needs more support, we model. Like a steady drumbeat, imitation and modeling are essential for maintaining the pace and rhythm of the session. Finding an appropriate balance often requires an understanding of the child and the context of the routine. We have provided Figure 9.6 and some additional tips to help you find this balance.

9.6.1 Err on the Side of Imitation

If you are unsure whether you should imitate or model, err on the side of imitating. This may not be intuitive at first. Modeling feels productive, especially if the child is responding. However, if you continue modeling, you create a dynamic where you do all the leading and initiating, and the child does all the imitating and responding. This quickly starts to feel like a trial or a task. Instead, use imitation to put the child back into the position of the leader. Remember, imitating the child is our way of reinforcing the child's productive play and keeping the routine going. (You will have opportunities later to work toward new skills as well. Once the base of the routine is established and the child is comfortable with play, you will introduce new toys in the environment and new play steps through expansions. This ensures that the child's play does not become too repetitive and that the child has a chance to learn new skills.)

9.6.2 Consider the Context before You Model

Whereas we are quick to imitate, we are more cautious in how quickly and frequently we model. A routine should not be entirely dependent on your models. The child should be initiating some of the time. If you feel you are consistently modeling play acts in an attempt to maintain the interaction, this is a sign that something else is going wrong in the routine or that the child needs a different form of support. Evaluate the environment, the toys, or the play level. Before you model, consider the following questions.

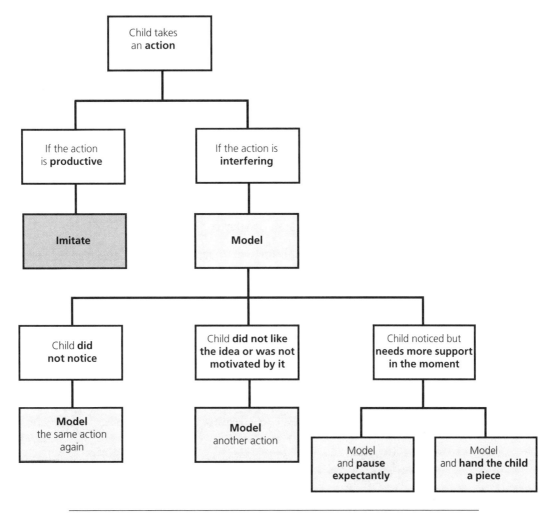

FIGURE 9.6. Notice and respond to the child's action by imitating or modeling.

Will the situation resolve if I wait?

If you are uncertain about the appropriateness of the child's actions, wait a moment or two before you model to see what happens next; however, if you suspect the child is about to lose engagement, you should model quickly to maintain the routine.

Does the action interfere with engagement?

Some actions are not intrusive. If the child's action does not interfere with engagement or disrupt the routine, then you may choose to continue monitoring instead of modeling right away. For example, if the child demonstrates a sensory action, such as tapping the toys on the table before she takes her turn, you might choose to wait to model, because the child is still playing and is engaged. If the child's action increases to the point that it interferes with engagement or disrupts the routine, you should model to redirect the child back to the routine with a more productive action.

Can the child do it on her own?

Some children need more time to take difficult play actions or to complete challenging motor skills. Do not rush to model or provide support if the child can do the action on her own. The time to intervene is after the child has had an opportunity to try but before the child loses engagement. Remember, you may be able to help the child take her turn by adjusting the angle of the toy so it is easier for the child to access (see Chapter 7, Section 7.5.2). Practice choosing the correct strategy, imitating or modeling, based on the child's actions in Exercises 9.3 and 9.4.

EXERCISE 9.3. **Imitate or Model?**

Identify whether the adult should imitate or model based on the child's action, assuming the child's mastered play level is presymbolic.

Child's action	Adult's response	
1. The child pretends to walk the figures onto the bus and drives them to school.	Imitate	Model
2. The child repeatedly rolls the bus back and forth.	Imitate	Model
3. The child tosses the figures into the school.	Imitate	Model
4. The child pretends his figure is the teacher at the school.	Imitate	Model

---

EXERCISE 9.4. **What Comes Next?**

Match each scenario to the most appropriate action for the adult to take next.

Description	Adult's response
1. You and the child are pretending to have a picnic with some dolls. The child takes the doll, places it in the picnic basket (pretending it is a bed), and says, "Good night!"	A. You put a blanket on the doll and say, "Good night, baby." B. You put another doll in the basket and say, "Good night, baby." C. You say, "That's not a bed" and model feeding the doll.
2. You and the child put a cake into an oven. The child repeatedly pushes the buttons on the oven.	A. You take the oven away and say, "All done with oven." B. You imitate pushing the buttons on the oven and say, "Push more." C. You model taking the cake out of the oven and say, "Cake is done!"

9.7 Common Challenges with Imitating and Modeling

Next, we address some common questions and provide case examples specific to a child. If you are having consistent trouble finding a balance between imitating and modeling, you can also use the ACT framework from Chapter 8 to troubleshoot.

9.7.1 Common Questions

In this section, we address common questions regarding imitation and modeling.

What if the child does not notice my turn?

It is okay if the child does not always notice your turn. If this becomes a consistent problem, make sure you are within the child's line of sight. Notice where the child is looking and then take your actions within the child's view. Check the environment. Ensure that you are face to face with the child and the shared object is still directly in between you and the child. You can also highlight your turn by pairing your actions with language and gestures. For example, you could comment, "Stack" and point to the structure as you take your turn (see Chapter 12). As you take these steps, avoid prompting for the child's attention.

What if the child keeps taking the same action?

You might wonder what to do if the child keeps taking the same action repeatedly in the routine. Should you keep imitating? It depends on the routine. It is appropriate to stack blocks for about 8–12 turns before you restart but less appropriate to pretend to add soap to the doll's hair 8–12 times before you do something new. If it feels as if the child keeps taking the same action over and over again to the detriment of the routine or the child's engagement, this may be a sign that the action has become rigid and repetitive or that the child is bored. In this case, you can introduce new related choices or expand the routine and show the child something else to do (see Chapter 11).

Should I keep modeling if the child is not initiating or imitating?

We typically do not want to model something repetitively without response because we risk losing the child's engagement and becoming overly directive in our role. If the child has not imitated or initiated after a few models, start by evaluating the child's engagement (e.g., Is the child ready to move on to something new?). Then evaluate your environment and toy choice (e.g., Is the environment so cluttered that the child cannot notice you modeling? Is this toy at the right play level? Do you need to introduce new toys into the environment? Does the child understand how the toy works?). Next, consider the clarity of your model (e.g., Are you modeling something that is too high in play level? Are you modeling in the child's attentional focus?). As you evaluate each of these aspects and make adjustments, the child will be much more likely to successfully imitate your model or initiate something new.

9.7.2 Case Examples

The following fictional case examples address challenges with imitation and modeling specific to a child.

To Imitate or Not to Imitate

Dear JASPER,

The student I work with loves toys and has lots of fun ideas about how to play with them. During the SPACE, she showed many different actions at the general combination level, and she even had some presymbolic play too. I also noticed that she spent a lot of time on very early play actions like rolling the truck back and forth and tapping several toys. We are now on our third session but still struggle to make progress in our routines. I have general combination toys such as Lego blocks that she likes to stack into a tower. This could be a base routine, but after stacking a few blocks she will take two blocks off and start tapping them together. I want to imitate her ideas, so I take one block off the tower too, but then we get stuck tapping the blocks. This same cycle seems to repeat with each of the building toys that I try. Should I keep imitating?

Thanks,

To Imitate or Not to Imitate

Dear *To Imitate or Not to Imitate,*

It sounds as if your assessment is accurate that it's difficult to get a solid routine established and you may need more help knowing when to imitate. The Lego stacking base sounds appropriate and productive so you are correct to imitate. However, the child's "expansion" of tapping the toys is not productive, and therefore we would not imitate this action. Try imitating quickly by immediately putting your block on the tower. Sometimes taking your turn faster can be enough to "skip over" that repetitive step in the routine. Make sure you have enough Lego blocks available in the environment to keep the routine moving forward. It's also possible that the child may be ready for an expansion to this routine. Perhaps you could add some Lego figures to put on top of the stack. If you find these strategies are not working, do not be afraid to model a new step!

Good luck!

JASPER

Weaning the Bottle

Dear JASPER,

I'm working with a child who really loves to play with baby dolls. When we start our sessions, he goes straight for them. We have a routine where we dress them, cradle them, and feed them a bottle. However, he really loves to just feed them the bottle over and over. It becomes really difficult to try to restart or add more steps our routine. I want to imitate, because it's such a great play act at his target play level, but it becomes all that he wants to do! I keep trying to model a bunch of different things, but he always goes back to the bottle.

Sincerely,

Weaning the Bottle

Dear *Weaning the Bottle,*

We love that you are trying to make this routine more complex and reach the child's target play level. You have done some work to troubleshoot this challenge using primarily modeling, so we will offer some tips focused on the environment. First, let's assess. Sometimes when the environment does not provide a clear visual cue for what the child can do with the toys or there aren't enough options available in the child's reach and sight, children will keep doing what they're used to. It may help to create a plan that gives the routine a clearer direction. For example, you could bring in a bathtub or some beds to help the child think of something else to do with the dolls. If the child does not generate an idea with these materials, you can then try to model. If these strategies are not enough, it may be necessary to set the bottles aside for a while until you establish more diverse steps in the routine.

You can do it!

JASPER

9.8 Conclusion

Imitating and modeling are essential strategies for establishing and maintaining the routine. Take a moment to review these strategies in Figure 9.7. When the child is first learning routines, he may require more models to understand the play actions and to maintain engagement. Over time, the goal is to see improvement in the child's ability to initiate productive play actions and a decrease in interfering behaviors, allowing you to imitate more and model less. You should also see an increase in the child's skills, as your imitation provides reinforcement and your models show the child new actions. Now that you have the guidelines of how and when to imitate and model, you can use these strategies in the next chapter to establish the base.

Chapter 9 Summary

PRIORITIZE **IMITATION**	**MODEL** TO PROVIDE SUPPORT	**BALANCE** IMITATION AND MODELING
○ Imitate the child's productive play acts ○ Imitate immediately and consistently ○ Play out your role ○ Do not imitate interfering actions	○ Model when the child needs support ○ Model an action the child is likely to imitate ○ Pause for the child to react	○ Try to imitate more than you model ○ Return to imitating after you model ○ Match the child's pace

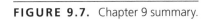

FIGURE 9.7. Chapter 9 summary.

Establishing the Base

10.1 Introduction

Once you and the child are playing together, the goal is to establish the base of the routine. As you may recall from Chapter 5, the *base* includes a familiar step (or steps) at the child's level. It should be easy and predictable enough for the child to initiate and maintain. In this chapter, we will discuss the strategies to establish the base of the routine. We will start with the features of the base. Then we will explain your role in the routine as well as signs of an established base. And finally, we will explain how to restart the routine if the child needs more practice to establish these steps. At the end of the chapter, we will address challenges that may arise along the way. Many of the strategies should look familiar by now—managing the environment, learning to play an equal and active role, and imitating and modeling. These strategies all come together to establish and sustain engagement in the routine.

10.2 Fundamentals of the Base

The base includes the first few play steps that serve as a foundation for the rest of the routine. Before going into the mechanics of how to establish the base, we will describe the features of the base in more detail.

10.2.1 Features of the Base

The base should include steps at the child's *mastered* play level to ensure the child is comfortable and confident in starting the routine.

The Base Launches the Routine

The base begins by following the child's interests within the choices you have prepared in the environment. This ensures the child will be motivated by the routine and facilitates entry into joint engagement. Some children may have a base of just one step, while others may have a base routine with several steps. Either way, the actions should be repeatable to establish back-and-forth turn taking that sets the tone for the routine. For example, if the child chooses a set of nesting boxes and puts one inside another, you could establish a base of nesting boxes inside of each other (presentation combination) and then stacking them on top of each other (general combination). By taking turns completing each of these actions together, you establish a starting point for your routine.

The Base Is a Comfortable Place to Return To

Like a "home base," this is a step (or set of steps) that the child can feel confident returning to throughout the routine. To continue the nesting box example above, you might *expand* your base by adding figures into the openings of each nesting box in your tower (child as agent). If you notice the child becomes less engaged or less motivated during this more difficult step, you could return to the base and *restart* the routine by repeating the familiar steps of nesting or stacking the boxes to increase the child's engagement and confidence.

10.3 Your Role in Establishing a Play Routine

To establish the base, you must take an equal and active role in the play steps and support the child's play. Your role as an equal and active play partner includes the following steps: leaving room on the child's turn, imitating and modeling play acts on your own turn, and managing the environment throughout the routine. In this section, we will explain the guidelines for these strategies as you establish the base, and they also apply as you maintain and grow the routine.

10.3.1 Leave Room on the Child's Turn

There should be quiet time and space for the child to initiate play actions and language on his turn. This means *you should not talk or take play actions during this time*. Children may need time to formulate ideas of their own before they are able to share with you. If you fill the space with your own words or actions, it will be more difficult for the child to initiate. Instead, your role during this time is to *notice the child's actions and communication* and *prepare to respond*. You can smile and look at the child expectantly to show him you are ready to receive what he has to share, but do not recruit attention or prompt in any way. In Figure 10.1, the adult closely monitors the child and is ready to act immediately when his turn comes.

Notice All Signs of Intent

The child's actions may not always look as we expect. She might look at a toy, pick it up, or try something unconventional. She might look at you, gesture, or use a word approximation. The child may not always use words to express herself, but that does not mean she is not communicating something. Take note of other signs and behaviors as well. You might notice the child is motivated and excited or bored and losing engagement. You might even see early signs of dysregulation or challenging behaviors. It is your job to actively monitor these subtle signs and adjust accordingly so you can keep the routine moving forward.

Be Patient as the Child Tries New Skills

Do not rush through the child's turn. If the child is trying to say or do something, give the child enough time to try it on her own. For example, if the child is fumbling to put a figure in a chair,

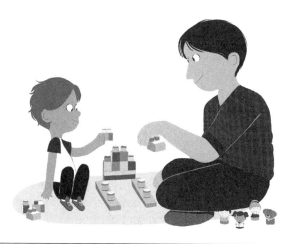

FIGURE 10.1. The adult does not talk or take actions on the child's turn.

allow her a moment to try before assisting or asking if she wants help. If the child begins to speak and trails off, give her an opportunity to complete her communication. By being patient, we allow the child to practice new skills she might not otherwise attempt. While it is okay to occasionally provide assistance, this should be provided only in cases where the child needs support to maintain engagement and regulation.

10.3.2 Use Your Turn to Imitate and Model

Once the child takes an action, you will respond with one developmentally appropriate action of your own that contributes to the routine. As introduced in Chapter 9, you will imitate if the child takes a productive play action or model if the child needs support. This is your opportunity to play the role of a fun, engaged, social partner. (You will also communicate on your turn by responding to the child or modeling language and a gesture; see Chapter 12).

10.3.3 Continue to Manage the Environment

As you play, the environment will change; the toys will get mixed up, the child will move around, and the well-prepared environment you created might no longer offer the support you intended. Check the play area regularly to make sure the arrangement is optimal for the child. For example, in Figure 10.2, the adult notices that the child is running out of blocks and discreetly pushes more over while she takes her turn. This is where the environmental arrangement strategies from Chapter 7 come into play. Manage the clutter and group similar toy pieces together, so the child can access pieces more easily. Replenish toys as you go so that the child has the materials needed to continue the base steps. This should be subtle and should not distract from the routine—nor should it take the place of your play turn.

10.4 Monitor for Signs of an Established Base

After you start the routine, the goal is to *establish the base*. By this, we mean that the child is comfortable with the base steps and is able to maintain them with relative ease. As you are playing,

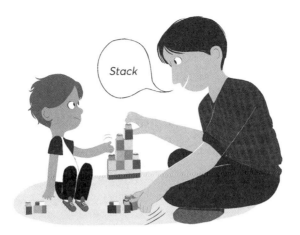

FIGURE 10.2. The adult takes his turn and discretely manages the environment to help establish the base.

you should monitor the child's engagement and familiarity with the base steps. Does it appear as though the child is comfortable with the base steps? Or does he need more time to practice? Figure 10.3 shows signs that indicate the stability of the base.

10.4.1 Determine Whether to Restart or Expand

If the base is established, you can expand the routine to add new steps. However, if the base is still unstable, you will restart the routine to continue practicing. Recall from Chapter 5 that *expanding* is the process of adding one new step to the routine, and *restarting* is the process of returning to an earlier step in the routine. In most cases, children with ASD need some time to build a strong base before they are ready to expand. Therefore, you may need to restart the base several times before you add something new. We will talk more about the mechanics of restarting a routine in the following section (and expanding will be addressed in Chapter 11).

SIGNS OF AN ESTABLISHED BASE	SIGNS OF AN UNSTABLE BASE
o Repeatable steps that build a coherent sequence o Multiple repetitions of each step o Some child-initiated play turns o Equal participation from both players o Facilitates joint engagement	o Child is shifting among toys o Disjointed sequence o Few repetitions of each step o Lack of child-initiated play turns o Unequal roles (e.g., adult models frequently) o Limited or fragile joint engagement

FIGURE 10.3. Signs of an established versus unstable base.

Before moving on, take a minute to work through Exercise 10.1 to identify whether a base routine has been established.

EXERCISE 10.1. Identifying an Established Base

Identify whether the base is unstable or established.

1. You and the child are stacking boxes into a tower. You crash the tower and the child looks up at you and laughs, and then begins rebuilding it. Unstable   Established

2. You and the child are sticking pegs into a pegboard. After you model and hand the child a piece, he slowly takes his turn. You take another turn and he visually inspects the holes in the pegboard. You hand him another piece, and he takes his turn. Unstable   Established

3. You and the child put pizza slices on a plate and put two shapes into a sorter. Next, you model stacking up foam blocks. Unstable   Established

---

10.5 Restart the Routine

Restart as needed to establish the base. As you may recall from Chapter 5, you can restart after the base steps (to establish the base) or after an expansion. You can also restart to maintain engagement or when natural opportunities arise. In each of these circumstances, you can follow the steps in Figure 10.4 and explained below to restart the routine. See Figure 11.11 for signs that it may be time to restart.

10.5.1 Return to an Earlier Step

To restart the routine, look for a clear way back to an earlier step in the routine. This should feel like a natural part of the interaction, and it should make sense within the broader context of the routine. One of the most common ways to restart is to disassemble something you previously put together—crash the structure, dump out the puzzle pieces, or break apart the Velcro food (see Figure 10.5). Try to reset the pieces all at once, rather than taking them apart one at a time. For example, if you have placed all the cupcakes into a baking tin, quickly pour them out and organize the materials. If you remove each cupcake one at a time, the child may feel you are undoing his actions and the time spent may break the child's engagement.

At higher play levels, you can often make the restart part of the "story" of the routine. For example, if the routine involves putting figures in a car, driving them to school, and then seating them at their desks, you can restart by putting the figures back into the car (restart) and driving them home. This restart is particularly flexible and creative because it repeats a familiar step (driving) in a new creative way (traveling to new locations). This allows the child to take many familiar steps and maintains the goal of the base and restart, while keeping the steps creative. There are

---

GUIDELINES FOR RESTARTING ☑

☐ Return to a previous step (e.g., crash down pieces, figures return to the market to buy items for another meal)

☐ Quickly reset materials (e.g., prebuild toys, put pieces next to the child)

☐ Clean up the environment (e.g., move extra pieces to the side)

☐ Support the next steps (e.g., imitate, hand the child a piece, or model)

FIGURE 10.4. Guidelines for restarting.

many ways to restart based on fun ideas or natural opportunities that arise in the routine. For example, if you have a routine that involves putting cookies on the cookie tray, you could have the Cookie Monster come and "eat" all the cookies while pulling them off the tray.

10.5.2 Reset the Environment

Once you restart the routine, quickly reset the environment. Partially assemble some toys (e.g., restacking a few blocks to restart a tower), and make sure there are materials available for the child. Reorganize the toys, disassemble pieces, group toys back together so they are easy to notice, and set any extra expansion materials off to the side. If the materials are a mess when you restart, the child will not be able to initiate the next step, or she may find it difficult to stay engaged in the routine. This must happen quickly, so you can get the base started once again.

10.5.3 Support the Next Step after the Restart

Some children lose engagement at this step or may not understand that they can continue to play with the toys after you restart. Therefore, it may be necessary to support the child through this next step. If the child initiates the first step herself, you can imitate. If she does not, you should be

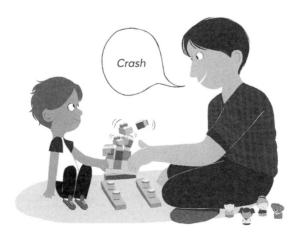

FIGURE 10.5. The child and adult crash to restart and return to the base routine of building a tower.

prepared to quickly model. Once the child is more comfortable with the routine, she may not need as much support to restart the base.

10.5.4 Common Questions

Here are some common questions related to restarting the routine.

At what step in the routine should I restart?

You do not have to restart at a particular step in the routine. The most common time to restart is after you run out of materials, complete the steps in the base, or after expanding; however, you might also choose to restart any time in between depending on various factors, such as engagement or regulation. Similarly, you do not have to return to the very first step in the routine.

Should the child participate in restarting the routine?

It depends on the child and the routine. The child can participate in restarting if it is an essential step in the routine, such as putting figures back in cars to go home. However, in cases where restarting involves merely resetting the materials (e.g., dumping shapes out of a shape sorter), the child may or may not be involved depending on if he finds it motivating. As you repeat the routine, the child may initiate the restart on his own. For example, the child might say, "Crash!" to signal that he is ready to knock down the tower.

Does the routine always have to restart?

There is usually some aspect of the restart in every routine; however, it can be flexible, especially for children at higher levels. Restarting is simply a way of maintaining engagement. If the child is initiating many of the expansions and leading the interaction, then you may not need to restart as frequently.

How often should I restart?

Finding the right balance of restarting or expanding allows you to maintain the child's motivation and engagement in the routine. In addition to monitoring for signs of an established base, there are several factors to consider when determining if you should restart or expand. For newer routines, it may take more repetition to establish the base, but for familiar routines, you will likely be able to establish the base much more quickly. When determining if you should restart or expand the routine, consider the following:

- Length of the base
- Level of the base (e.g., are these steps and ideas well mastered?)
- Number of times you have already restarted
- Number of times you have used this routine in this session and across sessions
- Similarity of this base routine to other routines

Each of these factors will affect how much practice it takes to build an established base. See Figure 11.11 for additional indicators.

10.6   Support the Child's Pace

As you establish the base and throughout the rest of the routine, you must support the pace of the routine. By *pace* we mean the timing, speed, and fluidity of the interaction, often measured by the rate of play actions and communication. All children have a natural pace at which they play. Some children have a very quick style of play, whereas others are slower and more methodical by nature. If a child moves at a fast play pace, she may have a lot of ideas for what should happen next. You should keep the toys replenished, be ready to take your turn, and try to keep up. Alternatively, if the child has a slower play pace, she might need more time to think about each step. She might have motor delays, have repetitive behaviors, or spend more time observing the objects and making decisions about what to do. In this case, you must be patient and leave time in the routine for the child to absorb everything that is happening. While we introduce this strategy here, as part of establishing the base, it is also a vital part of your role throughout the routine, particularly as you support engagement.

10.6.1   Monitor the Pace

The child's pace might become too fast or too slow, or there might be a significant change in pace; these are typically indicators of a change in engagement and signs that the child needs support. Figure 10.6 provides indicators that the pace is too fast or too slow. In the following section, we will provide tips for adjusting the pace for slower and faster players.

10.6.2   Modulate the Pace

When the child is playing too fast or too slow, you must *modulate the pace*. This is the process of adjusting your turn to help the child return to a more sustainable rate of play.

SIGNS THAT THE PACE IS TOO FAST	SIGNS THAT THE PACE IS TOO SLOW
• The turns feel frantic and out of control • The child appears to be object engaged • The actions feel repetitive • The child takes rapid steps with little room for your turn • You cannot take an action without overlapping with the child • The overall quality of the interaction declines	• The child appears distracted, bored, or weary • The child fidgets with the toys instead of playing productively with them • There is considerable time in between the child's turns • You struggle to move the routine forward • It feels as if you are losing momentum

FIGURE 10.6. Signs that the pace is too fast or too slow.

Adjust When the Pace Is Too Fast

When the pace becomes too fast, this is often a sign that the child is highly motivated by the toys or to complete the routine but is less interested in sharing that experience with you. It may be difficult for you to fit your turn in or prepare materials quickly enough to keep the routine going. If the child is moving too quickly, *the goal is to slow down the pace of the play enough to help the child connect with you.* Strategies when the pace is too fast include the following:

- Slow down your play turn. (You will need to be quick initially to get your turn in, but you can then slow down the action you are taking to complete your turn).
- Use a calm affect.
- Slow down the speed of your language.
- Partially limit access to materials so the child moves through the toys more slowly (e.g., only provide three pieces at a time).
- Use toys that require more motor control (e.g., building blocks that have to fit together a specific way).

Adjust When the Pace Is Too Slow

When the pace becomes too slow, this is often a sign that the child's motivation and engagement are declining and you are losing momentum in the routine. For slow players, you should make materials clearly available and increase your affect to keep enough momentum so you do not lose the child's interest. In this case, the *goal is to increase the child's motivation and engagement in the routine.* Strategies when the pace is too slow include the following:

- Imitate the child's turn immediately, clearly, and in his line of sight.
- Give the child a piece, so it is easier for him to take the next turn (i.e., using a suggestive environmental prompt).
- Provide support in the environment (e.g., orient toys to face the child and ensure materials are close at hand).
- Increase your affect to encourage motivation in the routine.
- Share in what the child is exploring by modeling joint attention language and gestures (e.g., point to and comment on the toys the child is looking at).
- Provide expansion choices if the child is bored.
- Provide new routine choices.

10.7 Common Challenges Establishing the Base

It may not always be easy to establish the base. In this section, we will address some common challenges you may encounter in establishing the routine and provide a few additional strategies you can use to push through difficult moments. If you struggle to establish the base, return to the ACT framework from Chapter 8 to assess the possible cause and create a plan.

10.7.1 Common Questions

In the section below, we address common questions related to establishing the base.

What if the child is distracted by extra choices?

Once the child makes an initial toy choice at the start of the session, you can move additional choices out of reach. If the child is still distracted by the peripheral choices and it is difficult to establish a base routine, you can move extra choices completely out of sight. When you restart or expand, adjust how and when you add new toys to the environment. If the child is easily distracted by extra pieces, it is often best to wait until after the child has started the base to put out the extra steps.

What if the child becomes unengaged during the restart?

You may need to increase your pacing and use your environment to further support the child staying engaged with you through this moment. For instance, quickly reset the materials for your base routine and remove any distractions. Make sure to have more pieces readily available so you can quickly present more materials in the environment or hand the child another piece to encourage him to take his turn again. If this does not work, then quickly model and try handing the child another piece. You may also need to restart in more subtle ways, so it feels as if the routine is continuing, rather than signaling a break. For example, instead of dumping all the coins out of a piggy bank in front of the child, you could quickly dump them out of his sight and then present the materials back on the table to repeat the base step. Alternatively, you could take turns taking the coins out of the pig so that this becomes more like a step in your routine than a clear restart and presumed stopping point.

What if the child deconstructs the base before you can get it established?

If the child keeps deconstructing the base (e.g., taking the pizza pieces off the plate over and over), you can use a mix of your environmental and pacing strategies to increase the amount of support and help to get the routine off the ground. Try using materials that cannot easily be crashed or taken apart (e.g., blocks that stick together or toy food with magnets or Velcro). You can also increase your pace so that you quickly imitate any of the child's appropriate actions, and then try moving a toy forward or handing her a piece as a suggestive prompt to continue the routine. If the challenge is related to rigidity or other repetitive behaviors, consult Chapter 17.

10.7.2 Case Examples

The following fictional cases examples address challenges establishing the base.

Frenzied Fran

Dear JASPER,

I think I am paired with Lightning McQueen—this child is *so* fast! I am excited that she's such a great presentation combination player. Our base starts out okay, but after a few minutes there are pieces flying everywhere and I feel I can't keep up. She moves so fast that I think even she gets upset with the rate of the play! I have a very difficult time connecting with her when the pace gets so out of control. She doesn't seem to hear my language or notice my actions, and sometimes I question if she even notices that I'm there with her. How do I help her stay engaged and regulated as we establish our base?

Best,

Frenzied Fran

Dear *Frenzied Fran,*

We hear you describing that the child becomes object engaged at this high pace. Let's create a plan to help slow down the child's pace. First, try monitoring the number of pieces in the environment. By having only a couple of pieces in the child's reach at any given time, it will be tougher for her to speed through many pieces. Second, you could also try physically slowing your turns. Rather than trying to match her pace, you can model a slower pace. You will need to move quickly to get your toy into the child's line of sight, for example, quickly putting the ring above the stacking post; once you are there, slowly place your ring on the post. Modeling this calm, positive, slower pace can help the child to slow her own pace. Third, when things get frantic, don't forget to modulate your affect and language. It can be helpful to use a calmer affect as you slow down the pace of your turn. Last, since it appears the presentation combination base is well mastered, you can also try a base step at the next level, general combination. This novel, challenging play act will likely require more concentration and effort for the child to complete. Using a novel play act may help her to notice you and to move back to a state of joint engagement.

Keep it up!

JASPER

Silly Zilla

Dear JASPER,

I work with a child whose target play level is physical combination play. He's made so much progress that now we are able to stay within a routine for 15 minutes! He loves building with big blocks, and we both get so excited when he makes a tall tower that he can push over. We both crack up when the tower falls! It feels like a really great moment of engagement, but then I tend to lose him almost immediately after that. He starts to push over other toys and dump toys out of containers. It's hard for me to help him calm back down to play again. The block tower routine is so fun and it feels so engaging, but it is difficult to maintain and grow. How do I keep this routine going and try to make it more productive?

Sincerely,

Silly Zilla

Dear *Silly Zilla,*

It sounds as if sessions are a lot of fun, but the child is becoming dysregulated when there is too much excitement. It is important to build a block tower that you can control, especially when knocking it down. You want the child to take part in knocking the tower over, but you should control it so that it doesn't become too dysregulating and cause him to disconnect from you. It also sounds as if the child has quite high affect. Even though the moment of the tower falling is fun and exciting, you can model a calmer positive response to help balance out his very high affect. You may notice that when you diminish your response, the child tries to seek a bigger response from you. Instead of using your response to reinforce the crashing that is becoming dysregulating, use your affect to reinforce when the child initiates to reinforce a new step in the routine or when the child imitates something you have modeled.

Keep it up!

JASPER

10.8 Conclusion

The base provides a crucial foundation for the goals of the intervention. Most notably, it allows you to establish and reestablish engagement in the routine. It also provides a comfortable and familiar starting point for the child to practice initiations. You will continue imitating, modeling, managing the environment, and restarting until you establish the base. For some children, this will happen quickly. For others, it may take time. Once the base is established, you can expand the routine. As the child becomes more familiar with the routine over time, it should get easier to establish the base. Before moving on, take a minute to review strategies for establishing the base in Figure 10.7.

Chapter 10 Summary

ESTABLISH THE BASE

- Use repeatable steps to make a coherent sequence
- Add multiple repetitions of each step
- Promote child-initiated turns
- Foster equal participation from both the child and the adult

IMITATE OR MODEL ON YOUR TURN

- Take your actions within the child's attentional focus
- Imitate or model to establish momentum
- Pair actions with language and gestures

LEAVE ROOM FOR CHILD INITIATIONS

- Do not talk or play on the child's turn
- Watch for the child's actions and communication so that you can respond

SUPPORT THE BASE

- Manage the environment
  - Control clutter
  - Replenish toys as you go
- Restart the routine
  - Return to an earlier step
- Reset the environment
- Modulate your pace to support the child

FIGURE 10.7. Chapter 10 summary.

Expanding Routines

11.1 Introduction

Once you establish the base, the goal is to *expand* the routine by adding one new play step at a time. As we introduced in Chapter 5, expansions add new steps to the routine. Like restarting, expanding supports our goals in that it extends the amount of time the child spends playing and engaged in the routine. Expanding also keeps the routine motivating. If you never added new steps, the routine would become repetitive, and the child would likely get bored and move on to something else. Instead of ending the routine, we can use the expansion to help the child practice new play steps within the comfortable setting of the established routine. This also encourages flexible initiations and increases the child's diversity and complexity of play acts over time. Expanding a routine can sometimes be difficult. These are often new steps the child has not tried before, and it requires flexibility to use the toys in novel ways. Therefore, it is best to provide support to help the child with these next steps. In this chapter, we will explain how to prepare the expansion toys, set up the environment for expansions, and leave plenty of room in the routine for the child to expand. If the child expands the routine, you will imitate the expansion to incorporate the new step into the routine. If the child does not expand, we will explain how to add support.

11.2 Fundamentals of Expansions

Expanding is one of the primary ways that children learn new play skills, share ideas, and practice more diverse and complex skills. Here is an example of expanding:

> *You and the child build a base routine playing "house" where you are the mom and the child is the daughter. After pretending to eat breakfast together, the child says, "Mom, it's time for school!" and brings over blocks to substitute as a car to drive to school.*

When the child initiates these steps, it builds on the child's motivation and extends engagement in the routine. Over time, you can connect several steps (and even routines) together. Before we discuss the guidelines for how to expand, we will first explain more about the types, features, and timing of expansions.

11.2.1 The Types of Expansions

There are two types of play expansions: horizontal expansions and vertical expansions. A *horizontal expansion* is a new play step at the same play level as the current step. For example, in Figure 11.1, the adult and child start out stacking nesting boxes, which is a step at the general combination level; then they add a different type of stacking block, which is another general combination act.

A *vertical expansion* is a play step at a level higher than the current step. For example, if the child is playing at a general combination play level, a vertical expansion would be an act at the presymbolic level, such as conventional combination or child as agent. In Figure 11.2, the child starts by stacking blocks at a general combination level and expands with a child as agent (presymbolic) action of adding figures onto the structure.

Horizontal expansions improve the *diversity* of a child's play by increasing the number of play acts within a current play level. Vertical expansions improve the *complexity* of a child's play by

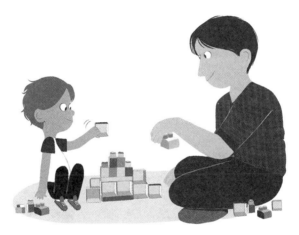

FIGURE 11.1. Blocks are added to the nesting boxes to expand horizontally at the general combination level.

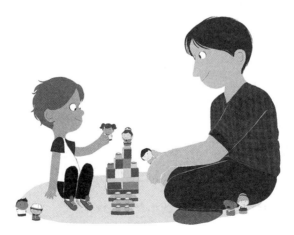

FIGURE 11.2. Figures are added to the structure to expand vertically at the child as agent level.

increasing the number of play acts at higher play levels. Horizontal expansions are often easier for the child than vertical expansions because they are more familiar and closely related to actions the child is already able to take, while vertical play acts are often more challenging because they are at higher play levels. Your routines should incorporate both types of expansions so that you build variety in play at both the mastered and target play levels.

11.2.2 The Features of Expansions

In order for expansions to be successful, they should be natural additions that support the qualities of a play routine (see Chapter 5, Section 5.4). Consider the following features.

Expansions Support a Purposeful Direction to the Routine

Expansions should always be clearly connected to the base, and they should make sense within the "story" of the routine. At higher play levels, this can feel more like a narrative. For example, baby dolls might take a bath, brush their teeth, read a book for bedtime, and go to sleep. At earlier play levels, you are weaving together a set of steps that are logically connected for the child. For example, you could put coins into a piggy bank, stack the coins on top of boxes, and then continue stacking boxes into a tower. It is important to maintain links among the steps, so you build a cohesive sequence that the child can sustain throughout the session, rather than haphazardly jumping around from one play act to another. One of the most common errors is to introduce a play act that is not logically connected to the prior steps. For example, you should not put coins into a piggy bank, then stack ice cream, and then put shapes into a shape sorter. While these are all steps at a presentation combination play level, they do not form a cohesive sequence. If the child does not see a very clear and obvious connection to what you are currently doing, he will likely not be able to take the next step.

Expansions Are Tailored to the Child's Interests and Experiences

Expansions should always be clear and logical to the mind of a child. For example, you start a routine adding figures to a boat. You mistakenly assume the child understands the concept of "fishing," so you choose to expand by adding in fishing poles and cooking materials to grill the fish. These are logical expansions to a symbolic fishing routine, but because the child is not familiar with fishing, he becomes less engaged and is unable to initiate other steps to keep the routine moving forward.

Expansions Can Include Small Changes

Expansions do not have to be major additions to the routine; they can be slight alterations to previous steps to increase the flexibility and diversity of the child's play. For example, you can build a structure into a different shape (e.g., a tall and narrow structure versus a short and wide structure), add a new building material (e.g., blocks mixed with nesting boxes), or take the same action with different figures (e.g., brush to self and then brush to a doll).

Expansions Encourage Child Initiations

Every time there is an opportunity to expand in the routine, the child has a chance to share a new idea. While both you and the child can add expansions to the routine, it is ideal for the child to expand the routine because this encourages child initiations and ensures the routine is motivating to the child.

11.2.3 The Timing of Expansions

Expansions should take place after the base is established and before the child's engagement decreases. Most of the time, the child will indicate that he is ready for something new by looking around the room, looking for other toys, or appearing less interested than he was before. The goal is to have the materials in place and expand *before* this point. As we discussed in Chapter 10, sometimes children are ready to expand soon after starting the routine; other times children need more time to establish the base before they are ready for new steps. In Figure 11.3, we provide some indicators that it is too soon or too late to expand.

11.3 Prepare the Environment to Expand

Prepare the toys and the environment ahead of time to support expansions. This ensures you have what you need when it is time to take the next step. Ideally, the child will spot a new toy or think of a new idea, and she will expand the routine on her own.

11.3.1 Choose Toys for Expansions

As we discussed in Chapter 6, you should prepare toys and actions for expansions. Figure 11.4 presents some guidelines, and Table 11.1 provides examples of horizontal and vertical expansions for each play level given a particular base step.

11.3.2 Set Up the Toys for Expansions

Place a few expansion options in the environment. These toys should be within the child's sight and reach, without distracting from the ongoing base steps. In the pizza routine in Figure 11.5, the adult has two different expansion options available, an oven and a bunny.

Too soon	Time to expand	Too late
o The base is not yet established o The routine feels fragile o The child has low engagement o The child needs more time to practice the steps	o The base is established o You have completed several repetitions of the current step o The child is ready to add a new step	o The child has lost engagement o The child is becoming dysregulated o The child is looking for something new to do o The child has shifted away from the toys

FIGURE 11.3. Timing of expansions.

GUIDELINES FOR PLANNING EXPANSIONS ☑

☐ Choose toys and actions that are developmentally appropriate

☐ Include horizontal and vertical expansions

☐ Choose toys and actions that encourage flexible and diverse actions

☐ Clearly link new toys and actions to the steps in the routine

☐ Support a purposeful direction

☐ Support the child's interests and experiences

FIGURE 11.4. Guidelines for planning expansions.

TABLE 11.1. Expanding Routines

Toy and play level	Base step	Horizontal expansion	Vertical expansion
Snap beads (simple play)	Drop beads down ramp (discriminate)	Drop beads into boxes (discriminate)	Put beads together (presentation)
Ring stacker (presentation)	Put wood rings on stacker (presentation)	Add plush rings to stacker (presentation)	Stack boxes on stacker (general combination)
Blocks (general)	Build boxes out of blocks (general combination)	Put cars into boxes (general combination)	Build garage with blocks (physical combination)
Utensils/dolls (presymbolic)	Bring cup to self (pretend self)	Spoon to self (pretend self)	Bring spoon to a doll (child as agent)
Tea set (symbolic)	Pretend to pour "tea" into cups (substitution without object)	Pretend to add sugar into tea (substitution without object)	Dolls mix "sugar" into "tea" and drink it (multi-scheme)

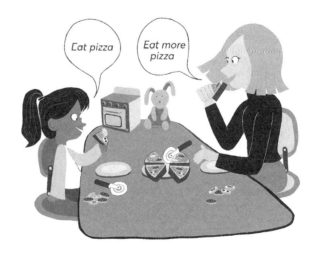

FIGURE 11.5. The adult prepares the environment for a child-initiated expansion by setting out an oven and a bunny.

Put Out the Toys before the Child Is Ready to Expand

You should place these toys in the environment *before* the child is ready to expand. This could be before the routine begins or after you establish the base steps. Do not make the child wait for materials or allow the child to lose engagement. These are signs that you should have put the toys out sooner.

Provide Choices to Expand

The number of expansion options you provide depends on the child. We typically recommend two options, because we prefer to give the child choices for how the routine could expand. This allows him to choose a step that is motivating and makes the most sense to him.

11.4 Leave Time for the Child to Expand

Once you set up the environment, leave time for the child to expand the routine on his own. There should be quiet time and space after the base is established for the child to notice the toys and think of a new step. This quiet time means we are waiting expectantly for the child to show us his idea. No tapping, banging of objects, gasping, or other verbal prompting should occur during this time.

11.4.1 Watch for New Actions and Interest

Watch closely for signs that the child is ready to expand. Ideally, the child will see one of the toys nearby and come up with an idea for the next step. In Figure 11.6, the child notices the oven nearby and expands the routine by pretending to cook one of the slices. Sometimes the child's expansion step may be quick or unclear, or the child might look at a toy or pick it up but then not know what to do with it. Pay close attention to all signs of interest so you are ready to respond!

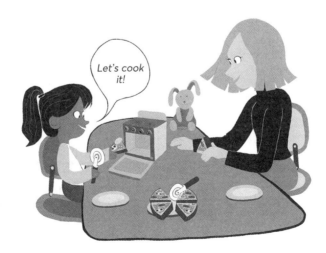

FIGURE 11.6. The child expands the routine by putting the pizza in the oven.

11.4.2 Imitate the Child's Expansions

If the child initiates a productive expansion that can be connected to your existing routine, you should imitate to reinforce the child's idea! For example, in Figure 11.6, the adult should immediately imitate the child by also placing a piece of pizza in the oven. (If the action is not clearly connected to the routine or is possibly interfering, you can respond in a way that builds on the child's idea and connects it to the routine.)

11.5 Provide Additional Support to Expand

If the child does not expand on her own, you can provide additional support to help expand the routine. This is illustrated in Figure 11.7 and explained in the sections below.

11.5.1 Rearrange the Environment

Rearrange the expansion toys so the child notices the options available. You can make the choices clearer by cleaning up the base toys and moving the expansion choices closer to the child. As is

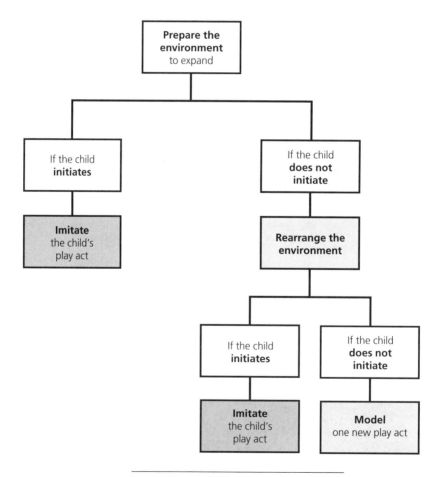

FIGURE 11.7. Expanding decision tree.

always the case with environmental prompts, this should be done quickly and discreetly. If the child does not take the first step on her own, you can increase the level of support further by bringing one expansion toy forward. For example, in Figure 11.8, the adult moves the bunny to the middle of the table and waits to see what the child does. This helps the child choose how to expand the routine without you modeling what to do.

    If that is still not enough support, you could hand the child a piece (e.g., a piece of food to feed the bunny).

11.5.2 Model an Expansion

If the child does not initiate an expansion after the environmental strategies you have provided, model one new play act. In Figure 11.9, the adult models feeding the bunny a slice of pizza. The

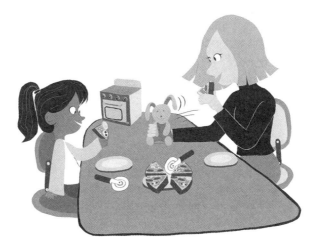

FIGURE 11.8. The adult pushes the bunny forward to support the child to expand.

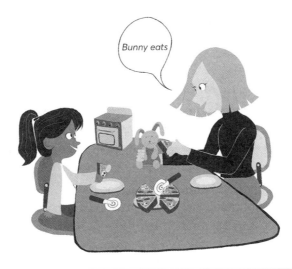

FIGURE 11.9. The adult models feeding the bunny to expand the routine.

goal is for the child to imitate your expansion and for the step to become incorporated into the routine.

Make Sure the Expansion Was Clear

Make sure that the expansion you modeled is something the child could easily notice and repeat. Signs that the expansion is clear include the following:

- Developmentally appropriate
- Within the child's line of sight
- Timed appropriately (on your own turn, immediately after the child's turn)
- Tailored to the child's interests, experiences, and motivations
- Clearly and coherently linked to the previous steps

You may realize that the expansion you modeled was not clear or easily reproducible. The play level was too high, you expanded too many times, or you realized it was not motivating to this child. In any case, it is okay if the child does not follow your model. Simply let the moment go and try again another time. If your expansion model *was* clear and the child still did not respond, move on to the next step.

11.5.3 Model Again

The child does not *have* to imitate your expansion step. She might not be interested in that particular step or be ready to try it out yet. At this point, you have a choice. On your next turn, you can repeat the same model, model and hand the child a piece, or try a different expansion idea.

11.5.4 Try Again Later

If the child still does not expand, there is no need to prompt or continue adding support (see Box 11.1); simply try again at another point in the routine. Keep giving the child opportunities to expand following the levels of support outlined in Figure 11.7 until the child imitates your expansion or tries an idea of his own. Here is an example of how all these steps work together in a routine.

- *Establish the base of the routine.* You and the child build a school.

- *Prepare the environment.* You place a couple of desks and some figures within the child's reach as you continue taking base steps.

- *Return to the base.* After adding more rooms to the school, the child appears confident in the steps and shows signs that he is ready to expand.

- *Rearrange the environment.* You bring desks and chairs forward as possible expansion materials. The child notices the new toys and picks up the desk. You wait to see what the child will do, but he just continues to look at it.

- *Model.* After waiting a couple seconds, you model placing a desk into the classroom. The child notices but does not take an action.

BOX 11.1. **Can I Use Directive Prompts to Expand?**

In general, we avoid using directive prompts to expand. In our experience, these prompts are too intrusive, and other strategies are better suited to teaching these skills. Why? Directive prompts do not typically produce spontaneous play acts. They end up feeling more like "drills" than play, which takes away from the playful feel of the interaction. Finally, they make the child look for the "right answer" instead of flexible, spontaneous ideas of her own. Instead of verbal, gestural, and physical prompts, we rely on suggestive prompts, such as environmental arrangement and modeling, to provide subtler prompting of expansions. This is typically enough support for the child to initiate a new play act. If the child is not expanding, typically this means something else is going wrong, *not* that the child needs an intrusive prompt. (See Section 11.8 for more reasons the child may not expand.)

- *Increase support.* You give the child a desk and wait. The child puts the desk down.
- *Try again another time.* Since the child did not follow the expansion, the adult restarts the routine by rebuilding the school, reestablishes engagement, and commits to expanding again in a few turns (either in the same manner or by trying a different expansion idea).

In this example, the adult gives the child ample opportunity to expand, yet the child does not expand. The child may not be motivated by the expansion step or may not understand what you are expecting. Continue trying, by either repeating the same step later in the routine or by modeling a different expansion (e.g., putting a pillow or blanket on the bed first). If you are consistently unable to expand, you should troubleshoot by using the ACT Framework and completing Form 8.1 until you make progress in growing your routines.

Practice identifying how to expand the routine using Exercise 11.1.

EXERCISE 11.1. **Expanding Routines**

Identify the best action for the adult to take in the following scenarios given JASPER guidelines.

1. You and the child establish a base of connecting train tracks into a circle, driving a train on the tracks, and crashing the train tracks. You have moved through this sequence three times and notice that the child is starting to take her turns more slowly and shift her body away from you. Which of the following steps should you take first?

    A. Put the train tracks away and get a new toy out.

    B. Withhold pieces on each turn so the child must communicate for them.

    C. Move figures and nesting boxes close to the child as potential expansions.

    D. Model stacking boxes on top of the train tracks.

2. You and the child establish a base of putting pizza pieces together and cutting them apart. The child then expands by stacking pizza pieces on top of each other like a tower. What is the best next action (assuming the child has a mastered play level of presentation combination)?

    A. Return to the base of the routine by reassembling the pizza pieces.

    B. Hand the child more pieces so he can finish his idea on his own.

    C. Take your own turn stacking pizza onto the tower.

    D. Model a different step of putting the pizza pieces on plates.

3. You and the child begin a routine of walking animals into a barn. The child then starts repeatedly opening and closing the doors to the barn. What can you do to keep the routine going (assuming the child's mastered play level is single-scheme sequence)?

    A. Imitate the child's expansion of opening and closing the doors.

    B. Model a productive step with the doors (e.g., have the animal knock on the door).

    C. Bring in new materials for the child to expand with (e.g., food for the animals).

    D. Either B or C.

11.6 Continue the Routine after an Expansion

Once you have successfully added an expansion step, continue the routine with this new step until you run out of materials, you both take a reasonable number of turns, or the child is ready to do something else. At this point you can decide to restart or expand again. This is the process of growing the routine.

11.6.1 Monitor Engagement

Notice whether the child's engagement increases or decreases when you expand the routine. This will help you determine what steps to take next. If the child is less engaged, it may be time to restart again, such as in Figure 11.10. If the child is more engaged, this is a sign that the child may be able to maintain the routine at this level or even expand again. Eventually, the routine may come to a natural end or the child may signal that she is no longer interested. At this point, you can use environmental arrangement to support the transition to a new routine. See signs to restart, continue expanding, or transition to a new routine in Figure 11.11.

11.7 Continue Adding Depth to a Routine

As you expand your routines, consider adding flexibility and variety to your steps. This is how you build the diversity and complexity of the child's skills and keep routines from becoming boring, rigid, or repetitive.

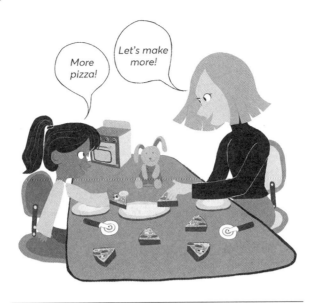

FIGURE 11.10. The adult and child restart the routine.

SIGNS TO RESTART	SIGNS TO EXPAND AGAIN	SIGNS TO TRANSITION TO A NEW ROUTINE
• The child does not seem comfortable with the current steps • The child shows signs of lowered engagement (e.g., less eye contact, slower turn taking) • The child shows fewer initiations • The child is not using as many joint attention or requesting skills as before • The adult is modeling more often • The routine is losing direction • The story of the routine naturally leads to being repeated	• The child is engaged and excited about the routine • The child is comfortable with the current step • You have played with this routine in past sessions • The child starts to indicate boredom or slows pace • The child tends to engage with toys for a short period before moving on • The child often loses engagement when you restart	• The routine has come to a natural stopping point • You have already explored creative and flexible ways of expanding the routine • The "story" of the routine has been played out or is becoming too repetitive • The routine is becoming too complex for the child's developmental level (e.g., multiple vertical expansions) • The child's pace, engagement, and communication decrease, indicating loss of interest • The child engages in more repetitive behaviors

FIGURE 11.11. Adjust the course of the routine based on the child's engagement.

11.7.1 Increasing Flexibility by Play Level

The way you add variety to your routines can look different, depending on the child's play level. You can increase flexibility with even small changes or additions to the previous steps. In Figure 11.12, the adult and child start the routine by putting coins in a piggy bank and expand with a similar step of adding cookies to the piggy bank. By adding and mixing these different materials, the child builds flexibility in the routine. Here are some additional examples of how to expand for each play level.

Simple Play Routines

Most toys that lend themselves to simple play acts are cause-and-effect toys with one obvious action that can be taken. These toys are not typically designed to be played with in multiple ways or combined with other toys, so it may require some creativity to expand. In most cases, expanding simple play routines involves taking similar actions in a sequence across different toys. Here are some ideas:

- Introduce multiple ways to use cause-and-effect toys (e.g., roll different kinds of vehicles on the floor, on a track, and then down a garage structure).
- Include variety in the items you choose (e.g., roll various kinds of balls back and forth between the two of you and then roll them down a ramp).
- Take similar actions across different toys (e.g., bang on a drum and then a xylophone).

Combination Play Routines

Combination routines typically involve stacking or putting materials together. At this play level, it is okay to mix materials together. Because the child is mostly thinking in terms of combinations rather than the symbolic function of the toy, it is developmentally appropriate to mix materials with less regard for what the materials represent. In Figure 11.12, the adult and child put cookies and coins into a piggy bank. Similarly, you could put the animal pieces from the puzzle into a dump truck or stack them on top of nesting boxes. Rather than thinking of what makes sense at an adult

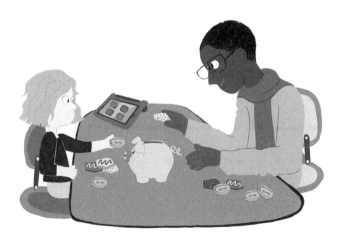

FIGURE 11.12. The adult and child put coins and then cookies into a piggy bank.

level, you are thinking about what makes sense to the child. You can also add slight variations to the toys, layout, or sequence. Here are a few ideas:

- Mix different presentation combination toys to make general combinations (e.g., put shape sorter pieces into nesting cups).
- Add another type of material to a structure (e.g., stack blocks on top of nesting boxes, wooden blocks, foam blocks, or shoeboxes).
- Add new shapes to a structure (e.g., add triangles or rectangles to a structure made of squares).
- Build different-shaped structures (e.g., build a tall, narrow tower and then build a short, wide tower).
- Mix food toys together (e.g., stack ice cream on top of a cake).

While it is okay to mix materials at this level, there should still be a sequence and a sense of order to the steps. Do not haphazardly dump materials together without reason. If all the materials get mixed together and then you add them to a truck, this is not an expansion. There must be a purpose behind the action and progress in the direction of the routine.

Presymbolic Play Routines

Presymbolic routines are often made up of many individual acts within a common theme, for example, taking dolls out of a bed, putting clothes on them, and feeding them breakfast. Expanding these routines often involves some addition to the theme of the routine (e.g., brushing the doll's teeth, sitting the dolls in chairs for breakfast, or making pancakes). It could also include variation in the routine (e.g., putting the dolls in a bed and adding blankets or sitting them in a school bus). Here are some additional ideas:

- Build each element of a setting before adding figures (e.g., build a house, set up fences around the house, add trees and flowers to the garden, and then put people in the house).
- Feed different items to the figures (e.g., bring a spoon to the baby doll's mouth and then a bottle of milk).
- Add many small steps from daily routines (e.g., cut vegetables, put them in the microwave, put them into a bowl, mix them with a spoon, and then pretend to eat them).
- Build creative locations and contexts (e.g., swimming pool, school, space station, grocery store, castle).

Symbolic Play Routines

Similar to presymbolic routines, the expansion steps in symbolic routines typically continue the theme or traditional procedure of an interaction (e.g., tea party, treasure hunt, bath time, amusement park). However, now you can build in even more creativity as the child is able to give life to the dolls, take certain roles herself, and substitute objects. For some children, you will not have a clear restart or return to the base of the routine, but you may come back to familiar steps or ideas in between expansions as your routines grow to include multiple themes. For example, you might have a recurring step of figures walking down a path in between the home, school, and playground. Over time, each play theme should grow to include more varied actions. This allows the child to layer in more diverse and complex play ideas and ultimately helps the child stay engaged for longer periods of time rather than jumping between ideas. Here are some more ideas:

- Use exciting events from your child's experience to create multiple steps within a story (e.g., you and the child build a house, and then have people figures come to the house for a party, bake a cake, tie up balloons, and play freeze dance before opening presents).
- Use children's books to inspire themes for your routine (e.g., pirates discover pieces of treasure, gather their treasure in a chest, load the chest onto a boat, build an ocean out of tiles, sail the boat to an island, climb the trees to harvest fruit, use their treasure to pay for tea, and then have a tea party).
- Introduce different types of figures to act out the story (e.g., animals make waffles, sit down at the table, eat breakfast, line up for the school bus, ride on the bus to school, and go to class).

11.7.2 Bridge Routines Together

Once you have several well-established routines with a number of expansions, flexibility, and variation to the steps, another way to continue to expand play is to "bridge" separate routines together. *Bridging* is the process of connecting two or more routines into one larger, more complex routine. Bridging is not an immediate goal for all children. The child must already be very comfortable with the routines you are trying to bridge, and you should already have a variety of expansions in each routine. When you are considering bridging, choose routines that have similar actions and a common theme that is logical to the child. In Figure 11.13, the child has two separate routines: The routine on the right involves dolls playing on the playground, and the routine on the left involves dolls going to bed in the dollhouse. Since these two routines are well established and have similar steps, you can connect them to create a longer story. For example, you could begin by playing in the first routine with the figures on the playground. Then you could put the figures into the cars and drive them to the house where they could go to bed.

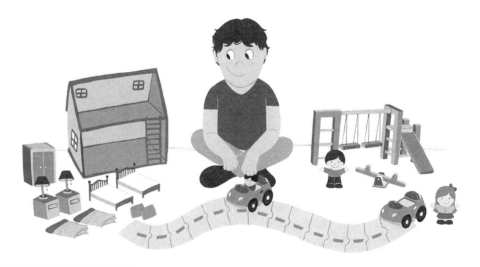

FIGURE 11.13. The road creates a clear visual cue to help the child bridge the house routine and the park routine together.

It is only appropriate to work toward bridging routines together after the child has several established routines with multiple expansions and is able to make bigger connections between play ideas. If your child is not ready to start bridging yet, it is perfectly fine to continue working on expansions within your routines.

If the child is ready to bridge routines, follow the instructions below:

1. Choose two (or more) established routines to connect together.
2. Before the session, set up each routine separately but near one another.
3. Come up with a few different ideas for how you might bridge the routines together and gather any necessary materials to create the bridge.
4. As you begin session, start with the routine of the child's choice. Make sure that the first routine is firmly established before you attempt to make the bridge to the second routine.
5. After the first routine is established, expand to bridge the routines together. If the child comes up with an idea to bridge the routine, follow his idea. If the child does not initiate the bridge, either model the first step or provide more support to help the child initiate the next step.

When you are first bridging routines, it is often helpful to create a clear visual connection or physical "bridge" that links the two routines together when you set up the toys. For example, in Figure 11.13, the adult set up two distinct routines with a road in between. This helps the child make the connection from the playground to the dollhouse. Certain toys help to create a visual connection between different routines. Some optional bridging toys include the following:

- Objects that can take on life (e.g., agents such as dolls, animals, or figures)
- A path for agents (e.g., slide, stairs, ladder, walkway)
- Large vehicle for agents (e.g., boat, car, airplane, train)
- A path for vehicles (e.g., roads, tracks, tunnels)

At first, you may need to help the child bridge the routine. As the child becomes more comfortable connecting bigger themes together, the child may initiate steps to bridge routines together on her own.

11.7.3 Increase Child-Initiated Expansions over Time

As you continue expanding and changing your routines over time, it is important to consider the balance of adult- and child-initiated expansions. When you are first building routines, there may be a mismatch, with either the child initiating most of the expansions (often a sign of rigidity) or the adult primarily expanding (often a sign that the child needs to work on initiations). Ideally, there will be a balance between the two roles. This reciprocal interaction should improve over time in order continue building flexible routines.

11.8 Common Challenges Expanding

Expanding can be a difficult step for children. The child may not be ready to expand, or he might enjoy the way that he is playing with the toys and not want to change. As you work toward expanding with increased flexibility, you can expect some resistance. When you are first learning

JASPER, it may be tempting to give in every time the child gets upset. But you should work through the child's resistance since this is where we see change. As the child gets more familiar with the routines and the structure of the session, you should expect the child to show more diversity, creativity, and flexibility in his play skills. It may require a few different attempts before the expansion feels comfortable and fluid. The following sections contain some common questions and scenarios on challenges expanding a routine. In these moments, you can use the ACT framework from Chapter 8 to troubleshoot. Keep trying and adjusting your plan as necessary.

11.8.1 Common Questions

In the following section, we address some common questions and challenges that may arise as you try to expand your routines.

How do I maintain a clear direction in the routine?

The direction of the routine can change based on the child's expansion. The child might come up with an idea you did not expect or prepare for, or he might take a step that does not quite fit with the plan you had envisioned. Support the child's productive ideas and follow the direction the child has in mind, even if that means abandoning your vision for the routine. You may need to provide new materials to connect the child's idea to the routine or to take the routine in a new direction. Here are some things to consider:

• Think one step ahead. Identify what materials you may need for the steps ahead and prepare steps you could use to support the story of the routine. As the child adds new ideas to the play, you should be flexible and follow his lead, while also having "backup" ideas to keep the routine going.

• Use your turn to shape or scaffold the child's idea to fit with the routine. For example, if you are putting together Velcro food, and the child picks up a baby and rocks it, you could rock the baby and then model feeding the baby the food. This allows you to reinforce the child's initiation while continuing your current routine.

• Adjust the toy choices in the environment so the child's ideas are likely to be connected. Some children seem to initiate a lot of ideas but then are only able to sustain one step at each idea before moving on to a new toy. In these cases, you may need to limit the environmental choices to just a few immediate options. This lets the child choose between expansions while also allowing you to stay in control of the environment and, therefore, the direction of the routine.

• Consider restarting the routine. If the direction of the routine gets lost or confusing, return to the base or an earlier step in the routine and rebuild in a clearer direction.

What if I run out of ideas?

Although you may feel you have a good grasp on the concepts of play routines and expansions, coming up with specific steps and expansions in the midst of a JASPER session can be difficult. It is common for interventionists-in-training to "blank" on new expansion ideas while playing with a child. A great exercise is to write down 5 to 10 different expansions you could take across various play levels with a commonly used toy. For example, using a pizza toy, we have described a few potential expansions by play level:

Combination

- Putting toppings on the pizza
- Putting the pizza slices together
- Stacking the pizza pieces up

Presymbolic

- Cutting the pizza
- Placing the pizza in a toy oven
- Feeding the pizza to a figure
- Putting toppings in a bowl and mixing with utensils
- Pretending to eat the pizza
- Building an oven from blocks
- Placing the pizza onto plates

Symbolic

- Adding blocks on top of the pizza as a substitution for other pizza toppings
- Pretending the pizza is hot and blowing on it
- Buying the pizza at a restaurant with a cash register

Remember to take inspiration from the children you work with! Ideally, we want children to be initiating play acts for us to imitate, so if they come up with a fun and productive new idea, add it to your expansion repertoire.

What if the child does not like my expansion idea?

At times, you may feel your expansion ideas fall short. Do not feel discouraged! This will happen, and it is okay. Save that expansion idea for another time or a different routine and brainstorm other fun ways to keep the child engaged. When you feel stuck, look around your environment and see if you can use other toys to expand with. Sometimes briefly pausing and collecting your thoughts will help spark a new expansion.

What if the child moves quickly through the routine?

If pacing is not an issue (refer to Chapter 10, Section 10.6), consider the length of time you spend at each step. It is a common challenge, especially with the presymbolic and symbolic routines, to quickly fly through your expansion ideas (e.g., brushing a dog, putting out food bowls, filling the bowls with food, and then having the dog eat). Even though you may have taken several steps, you find yourself with nothing left to do within a matter of minutes. In addition to brainstorming additional expansions, you can also find ways to lengthen the individual steps within a routine. Consider the following tips:

- Increase the number of figures so that both you and the child can take numerous turns extending the action to various figures.
- Break big ideas into small steps. For example, in a bath routine, you might plan to put the doll in the tub and then take the doll out, but there are many other steps you could add in between, such as scrubbing the doll with soap, washing the doll's face, adding shampoo, and

drying off. The more steps you add in between, the longer you extend the routine before you transition to the next big idea, such as putting the doll to bed.

• Mix advanced combination actions (which generally require more time spent turn taking) with actions with the dolls. For example, build a schoolhouse for the dolls and then take actions with the dolls at the school to play out a school-themed routine.

11.8.2 Case Examples

The following fictional cases examples address challenges expanding.

Camp Counselor

Dear JASPER,

I've built the most amazing camping routine with this little girl, but I can't seem to expand past a certain point! We start by building a campfire out of brown blocks and place red blocks on top to make the fire. Then we pretend we're roasting marshmallows over the fire for s'mores. We also pretend to eat them and have figures eat them. We're very successful making it to this point in the routine. There are so many choices for where we could go next, but the child simply takes everything apart and starts the same routine again. It seems she just really likes these first steps. I want to follow her lead, but I also want to add new steps since she is so comfortable with the routine as it is. I have tried modeling some new ideas, and I have expansion materials in her reach, but she either doesn't notice or maybe is just not interested. How can I help her to expand our routine?

Sincerely,

Camp Counselor

Dear Camp Counselor,

What an exciting routine you have! We agree it is time to expand since she appears to be fluent in the current steps. Here are a few ideas to help you expand. First, note the timing of your environmental arrangement. Plan to have the expansion options within reach before she finishes making the s'mores. This way, she will have visual cues for next steps before she has the chance to begin to take the toys apart. Second, choose expansion toys that provide clear next steps. For example, you could try putting hot dogs or fish that you could roast nearby. If timely environmental arrangement does not spark an initiation, then model the play act before the child restarts the s'mores step.

Additionally, it sounds as if you have a lot of vertical expansions and could benefit from more horizontal expansions at a presymbolic level. For example, you could use triangle-shaped blocks to build tents for the dolls (physical combination) and add sleeping bags and pillows (conventional combination). Adding horizontal expansions, such as putting candy on top of the s'mores or feeding different kinds of figures (e.g., stuffed animals instead of dolls), can also serve as a way to move beyond the established steps. If these strategies are not enough, the child may be particularly attached to this pattern in ways that are rigid, in which case you may need to build in flexibility (e.g., mixing up the order of the base steps, starting with a different base step).

Good luck!

JASPER

Combination Conundrum

Dear JASPER,

I'm stuck in the land of general combinations, and I can't get out! I am supporting a student who otherwise has well-mastered combination play skills and also has some great presymbolic skills. For example, he will extend the toy fruit to himself, to me, and to animals. He also puts people in chairs, vehicles, and different structures. But I can't seem to make movement on the physical combinations. I have tried building long roads, houses, vehicles, buildings, and tons of other things out of blocks, but these don't seem to be anything more than general combination to my student. Should I just keep trying?

Sincerely,

Combination Conundrum

Dear *Combination Conundrum,*

You've done a great job of assessing the child's next step (moving into physical combinations) and working to get there. This can be a difficult step up in play level as the child transitions to understanding more abstract ways of building toys. When we are trying to help a child into physical combination, one strategy is to use toys that can create clear and concrete representations of specific objects. For example, use blocks that allow you to make something that physically resembles your intended end product (e.g., use circular blocks for the wheels of a car). The more concrete the structure is, the easier it will be for the child to understand. Another strategy is to try to find something that is motivating and that the child has experienced in his life that you can represent as a physical combination. For example, if the child enjoys trips to the post office, you could build a structure, add the post office logo, and then build mailboxes and packages that go inside. You can also pair a concrete version of the object with the physical combination. For example, you could start with toy chairs, and then build additional chairs to seat each of the figures in your routine. If you've been trying for a while and it doesn't seem as if the child is understanding physical combinations, your student may just not be developmentally ready yet. Advance the complexity of your routines through other presymbolic play acts first and then come back to this a little later.

Good luck!

JASPER

Short Start

Dear JASPER,

I'm supporting a tiny tot who is 18 months old and who is just learning to play. We are working on simple play and have just emerged into presentation combination, which is so exciting! However, I'm worried that our routines are too short. I usually have about five choices in the environment, and he can move around and make his own selections. We have some good moments where he puts rings on a stacker, and he loves musical instruments like drums and xylophones, but these routines only last for one or two steps. Is this okay?

Regards,

Short Start

Dear *Short Start,*

We agree that these actions are exciting, and we encourage you to continue building upon them! It sounds as if the child is interested and engaged, and we encourage you to keep building on these great moments! Remember that routines can be shorter for very young children than they would be with older or higher level players. It is developmentally appropriate for your child to be working on increasing attention and engagement, so it may be time to create a plan to lengthen your routines by changing your environment and your own actions.

- If the child is jumping from toy to toy, try reducing the number of choices in the environment down to two to three clear choices.

- Add choices at the emerging presentation combination level. This may provide a range of new options for novel expansions. You can also set up many presentation toys with a take-apart base step to begin at the mastered level and expand to the target level.

- Prepare expansions. Pick materials that you can combine. Try to make a natural connection, rather than an abrupt change. For example, in a piggy bank routine, keep other materials nearby that could also be placed into the bank (e.g., coins, cookies, pizza toppings).

- Lengthen your routines with musical instruments by incorporating a familiar or favorite song (e.g., tap the drums while singing "If you're happy and you know it").

- When you restart, increase the pace and model with high affect to lengthen the duration of one routine rather than switching to an entirely new one.

Keep it up!
JASPER

Needs Some Glue

JASPER,

I have a little gal who has tons of symbolic play ideas! I want to encourage and support her ideas, but I feel a bit funny following her sometimes, because we don't seem to be going anywhere. She's playing, but nothing feels connected. For example, I'll bring out her favorite cats. We have several stations where the cats can climb trees and chase birds, a house where they eat and sleep, a rescue station where they can bring other cats to the doctor, and more! She can do all these things, but it feels as if we're jumping from action to action and station to station. These are all great ideas, but there doesn't seem to be any glue holding them together. Should I just keep following?

Yours truly,
Needs Some Glue

Dear *Needs Some Glue,*

It sounds as if your creative cat routine needs some structure to pull all the play actions together into a more cohesive routine. Create a plan to lengthen the number of actions you take at each station before you move on to the next one. Each station could be its own discrete and complex routine. You can think of these as "chapters" that come together to build a larger "story." By lengthening the chapters, we increase the duration and complexity of the story. For example, if the tree station currently has two steps, climb trees and catch birds, try preparing materials for at least 10 more steps. You can then add in a step or toy to "bridge" the chapters together. For example, you could build a path that the cats walk on between each station. Finally, consider the following strategies:

- Check the materials within each station: Are there enough materials to facilitate several steps within that station? Are there materials available for new and novel steps?

- Check the number of stations and proximity of each in the environment: Is there enough distance between the stations, so the child focuses on the materials in front of her? Are there materials to naturally bridge one station to the next?

- Check pacing of imitation and modeling: Does she pause or appear unsure what to do next before she moves to another station? Does she need you to model to extend the current part of the routine?

Keep up the good work!

JASPER

11.9 Conclusion

This concludes the play chapters in Part IV. In a sense, the strategies we have discussed so far reach a pinnacle moment when it comes to expansions. The way you set targets, set up the environment, and establish the base all lead to these moments when you can increase the child's initiations, play skills, flexibility, and engagement through expansions. In addition to helping the child learn new skills, expansions also keep the play fun while leading to more complex, diverse, and longer-lasting routines. For a summary of strategies to expand the routine, see Figure 11.14.

In Part V, we will introduce the next element of the routine—communication. Communication strategies layer on top of the play strategies and should be incorporated alongside the strategies in Part III.

Chapter 11 Summary

PREPARE EXPANSIONS

- Plan *horizontal expansions* to add diversity at the same play level
- Plan *vertical expansions* to add complexity at a higher play level
- Make appropriate expansion toys available as the base is established

SUPPORT EXPANSIONS

- Rearrange the environment as a suggestive prompt
- Model if the child does not initiate
- Ensure the model is developmentally appropriate, clear, and in the child's sight

IMITATE THE CHILD'S EXPANSIONS

- Leave room for the child to expand
- Imitate the child's productive expansions
- Scaffold emerging play ideas

INTRODUCE CHANGES OVER TIME

- Increase flexibility through including small changes to the routine
- Work to balance the child's and the adult's expansion ideas
- Bridge different established routines into one complex routine

FIGURE 11.14. Chapter 11 summary.

PART V

COMMUNICATION

In this section, you will learn how to respond to and expand the child's communication, use programming, and include a speech-generating device to support early language learners.

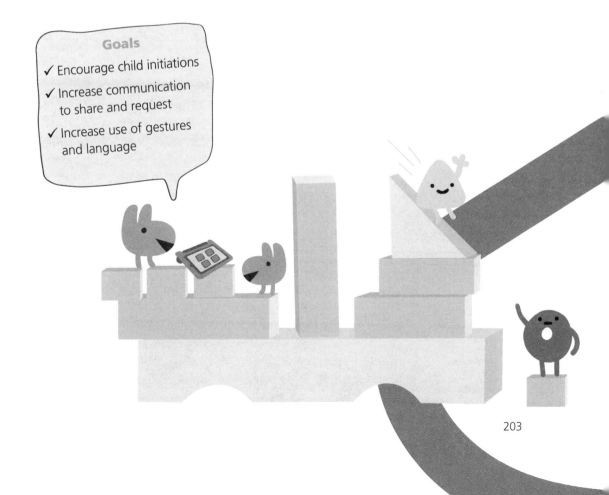

Goals

✓ Encourage child initiations

✓ Increase communication to share and request

✓ Increase use of gestures and language

CHAPTER 12

Core Communication Strategies

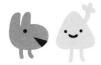

12.1 Introduction

In this chapter, we will explain how communication is layered into the routine. Here is an example:

The adult and child have a routine with animal figures, a tractor, and a barn. The child adds an animal to the tractor and looks up at the adult. The adult shows his animal to the child before putting it in the tractor, saying "Horse!"

Similar to the strategies for play, you will take the role of an equal and active communication partner. You will leave room for the child to communicate, monitor the child, and use modeling and imitation (along with language expansions). You will use these communication strategies along with your play strategies to encourage more social communication in the routine. In the first half of the chapter, we will explain how to reinforce the child's productive communication through *imitating and expanding*. We will then discuss *modeling* communication. Last, we will provide some tips on how to respond to communication challenges, such as unconventional communication, requests outside of the session, challenging behaviors, and expressions of dysregulation. Before we discuss the details of imitating, expanding, and modeling communication, take a moment to review the communication guidelines we have introduced so far in Figure 12.1.

STRATEGY REVIEW

Be an equal and active communicator

✓ Do not be too passive or too directive

✓ Leave room for the child to communicate

✓ Do not talk or gesture on the child's turn

✓ Pair your play acts with language and joint attention gestures

✓ Limit verbal praise

Choose language that the child can use

✓ Match the child's language level

✓ Use commenting language

✓ Avoid directives

✓ Be flexible and natural in intonation and tone

✓ Balance the consistency and diversity of your words
(See Chapters 5, 6, and 8.)

FIGURE 12.1. Strategy review.

12.2 Monitor for Signs of Communicative Intent

Just as you leave room for the child to play, you should also leave room for the child to communicate in the routine. This means you should not talk during the child's turn, nor should you recruit the child's attention or prompt. Instead, you should watch and wait for communication and monitor the child for signs of communicative intent. This is especially crucial on the child's turn when he is most likely to communicate. Pay close attention so you can notice and respond to all of the child's communicative bids, including those subtler ones. Figure 12.2 includes some signs of communication you may notice in the session.

12.3 Imitate and Expand Productive Communication

Throughout the routine, you should respond to the child's communication by *imitating and expanding*. Imitating communication is the process of flexibly repeating the child's communication, and expanding is the process of adding one or more new words. For example, in Figure 12.3, the child says, "Pig in," and the adult imitates and expands by saying, "Horse goes in!" adding one new word.

Imitating and expanding reinforces the child's communication and also shows the child skills he can try out on his own. As illustrated in Figure 12.4, whether the child looks at you, gestures, or uses language (in this case, an approximation), you can show the child a variety of skills she could use to communicate the same message. By building on the child's initiation, you are taking advantage of a moment when the child is likely to notice and understand. In the following sections, we will introduce some guidelines to imitate and expand effectively during the routine.

TARGET SKILLS	EMERGING SKILLS	UNCONVENTIONAL COMMUNICATION
○ Eye contact, gestures, and language ○ Communication to share and request ○ Ability to initiate and respond ○ Combinations of nonverbal and verbal communication	○ Fleeting glances ○ Partially formed gestures ○ Word approximations or sounds with clear intent to communicate ○ Words that are spoken too quietly or quickly to understand ○ Communication that is not clearly directed at you but is related to the routine	○ Scripted language ○ Echolalia ○ Leading an adult by the hand to access an item ○ Communication that is ambiguous, not directed at others, repetitive, or poorly articulated ○ Screaming or crying persistently

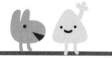

FIGURE 12.2. Monitor the child for all types of communication throughout the session.

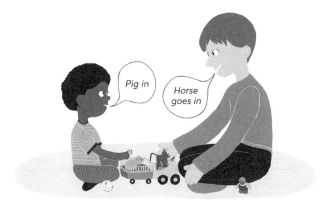

FIGURE 12.3. The adult imitates and expands upon the child's language on his turn.

12.3.1 Imitate and Expand at the Child's Developmental Level

When you imitate and expand, adapt to the child's developmental level. If the child speaks in one-word utterances, your responses will be two words, including imitation and an expansion (language expansions are underlined below).

- If the child says, "Car," you can say, "Yellow car!" or "Fast car!"
- If the child *points* to a puppet, you can *point* and say, "Puppet!"

If the child has longer utterances, you can imitate and expand in full sentences.

- If the child says, "We're going fishing," you can say, "We're going fishing on the boat!"
- If the child says, "I'll be the captain," you can say, "I'll be the fisherman!"

Consider the language expansions in Table 12.1.

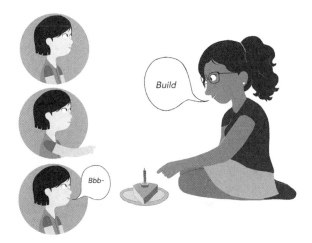

FIGURE 12.4. The adult provides a communication-rich response to the child's various communication attempts.

TABLE 12.1. Imitating and Expanding Communication

Child's communication		Adult's expansion
Child uses a sound and/or eye contact	➜	Expand to one word and add a gesture
Child uses a gesture	➜	Imitate the gesture and add one word
Child uses a gesture and one word	➜	Imitate the gesture and expand to two words
Child uses one to three words	➜	Expand to two to four words and add gesture
Child uses a short phrase	➜	Expand to a longer phrase and add gesture
Child uses a long phrase and gesture	➜	Imitate the gesture and expand to a sentence
Child uses sentences	➜	Play out your role in the conversation
Child uses the same words repeatedly	➜	Rephrase the message

Respond Immediately

Respond immediately so the child understands that you noticed and received his attempt to connect. If the child has to repeat himself in order to get a response, he may think that his communication is not good enough, that it is not understood, or that it is simply not worth the effort. For a faster-paced player, your response can occur as you take your next play turn. For a slower-paced player, or a child with very infrequent communication, you may need to make an exception to the general rule and respond during the child's turn to effectively reinforce the child's communication. (In this case, you can be quiet on your next play turn to maintain an equal and active role.)

Respond Even When Language Is Unclear

Try to build on what you think the child is saying. As the child is learning to communicate, there will be times when the child uses a sound or an approximation, her language is unclear, or you are not sure what she said. In these cases, you should respond with one clear word as described in Chapter 6, Section 6.3.1. Do not tell the child to repeat herself or ask her to say it better. Instead, take your best guess and respond with the word you believe the child is trying to use. This helps the child learn the correct words and shows that her communication is effective. For example, in Figure 12.5 the child approximates "Ah-" and the adult builds on the child's communication by modeling the full word: "On!"

Similarly, you can build on sound effects if they seem productive to the routine. If the child uses a sound effect that is related to his play action, you should imitate the sound effect and add a content word. For example, if the child says, "Vroom" as he pushes a car, you can say, "Vroom! Drive!" If the child rolls a ball toward you and says, "Wee!" you can respond by saying, "Wee! Ball!" However, if the sound effect is unrelated to the routine, scripted, or highly repetitive, you might choose to ignore it or model something more appropriate.

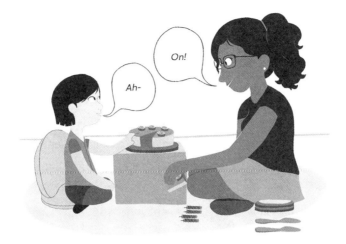

FIGURE 12.5. The adult expands the child's approximation by modeling a full word that is similar to the child's approximation.

Shape Emerging Gestures

The child may begin to initiate a gesture but not be able to form it clearly. In this case, you should choose an appropriate prompt to help the child successfully use the gesture, and then respond. For example, if the child says "Bird!" and attempts a joint attention show but his hand is rotated toward himself rather than you, you can use a partial physical prompt to gently touch the child's hand as a reminder to turn the object outward. Next, respond by pointing and saying, "<u>Red</u> bird." Similarly, if the child uses a partially formed point to request for something out of reach, you could quickly use a full physical prompt to gently shape the child's hand into a point before responding.

Respond with Positive Affect

Use positive affect when you respond. Recall from Chapter 8 that we use commenting language and affect as natural reinforcement (see Section 8.4). Responding to the child's communication with high affect can make it clear that you are excited about her communication and reinforce this skill. It also makes the play feel more fun! However, keep in mind that you must modulate your affect depending on the child.

12.3.2 Play Out Your Role in Conversation

When children communicate at higher levels, you can play out your role in the conversation. For example, if the child says, "The cowboys are racing into the tunnel," you might respond with "Let's go before the sheriff catches us!" or if you are playing the role of the sheriff, you may respond with "You won't escape me!" Direct imitation often sounds redundant, does not serve to advance the dialogue, and may not match your play turn.

Exercise 12.1 provides some examples of a child's communication and an adult's response. Use this exercise to practice identifying an appropriate response.

EXERCISE 12.1. **Imitating and Expanding Communication**

Identify whether the adult responds according to JASPER guidelines. Circle "Yes" if the adult provides an appropriate response and "No" if the adult does not.

Description	Adult's response	
1. The child looks at you while holding a stuffed animal. You point and say, "Bear!"	Yes	No
2. The child puts a car into the garage and says, "Go in." You put a car in the garage and say, "Car goes in."	Yes	No
3. The child says, "I am the policeman. I'm going to get you!" You say, "I am the policeman too! I'm going to get you!"	Yes	No
4. The child puts a tiger in a structure and says, "Tiger in the zoo." You say, "You should put these animals in too!"	Yes	No
5. Child says, "Buh-buh" (for ball). Adult says, "Buh-buh rolls!"	Yes	No

12.4 Model on Your Own Turn

In the same way that we model actions to support the child's productive play steps, we model language to support the child when he is not communicating or is not communicating appropriately. In JASPER, you should model language and gestures on your own turn throughout the routine. This gives the child consistent exposure to words and gestures that he could use on his turn without prompting. In Figure 12.6, the adult models a joint attention show with language, "Pink pig," as he takes his turn. In the following sections, we will introduce guidelines to model effectively during the routine.

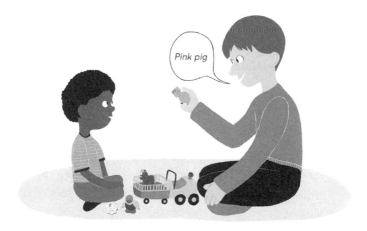

FIGURE 12.6. The adult models a communication-rich response by pairing gestures and language with his play turn.

12.4.1 Model at the Child's Developmental Level

Model commenting language at the child's language level, as described in Chapter 6. The words you choose should be developmentally appropriate and relevant to the routine. Avoid prompts, directives, test questions, and other forms of demands.

12.4.2 Model to Encourage Social Communication

As you are targeting language, try to keep the broader social context in mind. While your models help the child learn new ways to communicate, they are also meant to enhance the social interaction and to highlight motivating moments within the routine. In this way, you are modeling not only communication but also joint engagement, social connection, and the role of a fun play partner. Your models should feel like a seamless part of the routine, rather than an interruption. They should be a moment of connection with the child, rather than an instruction.

In Figure 12.7, the adult and child are building a cake together. The adult hands the child a candle (joint attention give) and says, "Candle!" When presented well, this is a fun moment of sharing together. If timed poorly, this moment will feel like a demand. In cases like these, wait for a moment when it is clear you are sharing, not placing a demand, and use positive affect. If the child does not respond, simply continue the routine.

12.4.3 Model Joint Attention Gestures

Use joint attention gestures during the natural moments in the routine (see Figure 12.8). The goal is to use these gestures frequently and naturally to show the child how they can be used. They should highlight motivating objects and actions and should not distract from the routine. Here are some guidelines to make your gestures natural and noticeable.

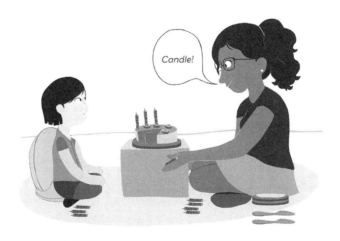

FIGURE 12.7. The adult models language and a joint attention give.

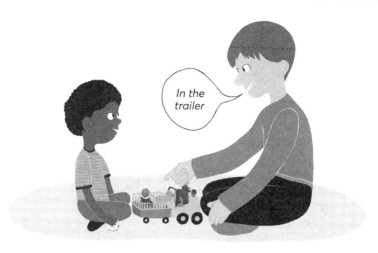

FIGURE 12.8. The adult uses his turn to model a joint attention point and language as he places an animal in the trailer.

Pair Gestures with Language and a Play Act

When you model gestures on your turn, pair them with language and a play act. Here are a few examples of pairing joint attention gestures with language and your turn (gestures <u>underlined</u> below).

- You and the child build a tall tower and take turns placing animals on top. The child looks at an animal. You joint attention <u>point</u> to the animal, and say, "On the blocks!" as you take your turn.
- You and the child take turns feeding a puppet. You joint attention <u>show</u> a piece of food to the child, say "Carrot!" and then feed the puppet.
- You and the child take turns pretending to pour liquid from a pitcher into cups. You joint attention <u>give</u> the child a cup and say, "Here's some juice!" as you take your turn.
- You and the child are pretending to put on a musical concert. The child says, "Where is the drummer?" You say, "I have her!" and joint attention <u>show</u> the drummer figure to the child.

Model Clear Gestures

Make your gestures crisp and clear so they are easy for the child to notice. Model only one gesture at a time, rather than, for example, showing and pointing at the same time.

- When you *show,* hold the object up, with your hand and arm slightly extended toward the child. Do not wave the object in the child's face.
- When you *point,* extend your arm and index finger, and pull back the rest of your fingers to create a fully formed point. Do not tap or touch the toys.
- When you *give,* fully extend your arm and hold the object out to the child with your palm facing up. Do not force the child to receive the object if he does not want to.

Make Gestures Noticeable and Natural

Model gestures in a salient, but natural way. Gesture within the child's line of sight and hold the gesture a bit longer than you normally would (1–2 seconds) to give the child a chance to notice. If the child does not notice or respond, simply move on. The child does not have to look at the toy, imitate the gesture, or take the toy to continue the routine. Avoid taking extra measures to recruit the child's attention. You should not pause too long, shake your hand or the toy, gesture too close to the child's face, or hold the toys unnaturally close to your eyes to evoke eye contact. The goal at this point is simply to provide the child with opportunities to notice these skills. In Chapter 13, we introduce the strategy of *programming* to provide the child with specific opportunities to practice using these gestures.

12.4.4 Pace Your Models

The amount that you model will vary for each child and each routine. We want the child to have numerous opportunities to notice these skills, but this does not mean you should model every turn. There should always be time for the child to communicate. You are modeling too much if you are doing most of the talking during the routine, if you are interrupting the child, or if you are talking over the child on his turn. You do not have to use a gesture every time you communicate either; however, you should use them consistently and naturally throughout the session.

12.5 Common Challenges around Communication

It may be difficult to know how to respond to some communication. When you feel stuck, look closer at the child's communication. It may be subtle, but there are almost always a few opportunities during session that you can respond to. Although it may be difficult, be aware of opportunities to work on language, become an expert at noticing the child's skills, and make the most out of these brief, meaningful moments to respond. In the following section, we provide some common questions and case examples on using core communication strategies.

12.5.1 Common Questions

The following section addresses some common questions related to communication.

How should I respond if the child's communication is unclear?

If the child's communication is unclear or incomplete, do not ask the child to try again or to say it better. Instead, do your best to respond to the child's language as it is. It is most important to continue the emerging conversation by quickly reinforcing the child's attempt. Modeling the correct pronunciation on your turn may encourage the child to say the words or phrase again with more clarity.

How should I respond to scripted language?

Your response depends on the appropriateness of the child's communication. If it seems as if the child is trying to communicate with you or the speech is closely related to the routine, you can try to build on the child's language or model something more appropriate. For example, if the child is playing with trains and starts repeating a scripted phrase, "Here comes Thomas," you can show the child a train and say, "This is Joey! Let's go to school!" as you drive the trains to the school. This response shows the child relevant words he can say that are different from the scripted phrase. If the child's utterance is unrelated to the routine (e.g., scripting, singing an unrelated song), it may be an indicator that the child is less regulated or engaged. Instead of imitating and expanding, you can provide support by modeling a play act or redirecting his communication with an appropriate language model.

Should I always fulfill requests?

As much as possible, we try to fulfill requests to show the child we understand his communication and to create a more motivating play environment. However, our responses are dependent on the function of the request.

Fulfill requests that	Do not fulfill requests that
• Fulfill a reasonable need	• Reduce the child's engagement
• Extend or expand the routine	• Distract from the routine
• Use new or emerging skills	• Enable escape from the activity
• Support the child's engagement	• Increase fixation or rigidity
• Lead to productive play	• Lead to an interfering behavior

It is important to acknowledge the child's attempted request even though you may not always be able to fulfill it. If you can fulfill the request with minimal disruption to the routine, do so quickly. If you cannot, acknowledge the child's language and help redirect him back to play. For example, you might state, "First let's play, then we can read." Children sometimes learn to use requests as a way to escape the activity. This is especially apparent if the child increases the request even after it was fulfilled. For example, if the child continues to request saying, "I want to read! I want to read!" repeatedly throughout a routine, this is likely an attempt to escape the activity, and you should help the child return to the routine. Finally, if a child requests a toy you know will interfere with engagement, you may also need to redirect. For example, you can respond by saying, "We have these toys today," while gesturing to the available choices and then modeling a fun next step. (If any of these steps lead to dysregulation, see Chapter 16 for more support.)

How can I respond to unconventional communication?

If the child communicates in an unconventional way, expand with the skills you want the child to use instead. For example, if the child takes you by the hand and leads you to a toy nearby, you could respond by modeling an appropriate request, such as pointing and saying, "Want toys!" If the child places your hand on top of a jar to request help opening it, you could model a point and say, "Need help." You could also use this opportunity to program for new skills (see Chapter 13).

How can I respond to challenging behaviors and expressions of dysregulation?

Limit your responsiveness in cases when the reply could reinforce an unwanted behavior. For example, if the child seeks attention by screaming and looking at you or if she repetitively sings the alphabet song when you are playing with a barn, these could be episodes of dysregulation or nonproductive scripts that distract from the child's engagement. Instead of imitating in cases like these, we respond based on the function of the child's behavior (see Chapter 16).

12.5.2 Case Examples

Imitate or Initiate

Dear JASPER,

I am confused about how to help a student learn to use novel language. This student is a fabulous imitator. He can imitate anything I say when we play, but I don't often hear him come up with his own phrases. Am I talking too much? Should I talk more? Should I keep imitating when he has just echoed my model?

Regards,

Imitate or Initiate

Dear *Imitate or Initiate,*

You're doing a great job of assessing your student's behavior and noticing that he's relying heavily on imitation. It sounds as if he may need some more space to initiate. Plan to reduce the rate of your communication to provide the child with more time to generate language on his turn. Use your affect and a subtle natural expression (e.g., an expectant pause or encouraging look) when you think he may communicate. Remain natural and do not wait too long. Another helpful tip is to try diversifying your language models to encourage novel words. For example, instead of saying "in" each time you put a person in an airplane, you could model words like *girl, sit, fly,* and *plane.* Even though he is not initiating much, you should still expand on his language. For example, you model, "Eat pizza" and he imitates, "Eat pizza." You can respond by saying, "Eat <u>more</u> pizza" or "<u>We</u> eat pizza." If he continues to imitate, you can continue to respond while making your imitation more flexible (e.g., "Eat the <u>pepperoni</u>").

All the best,

JASPER

Lost for Words

Dear JASPER,

I'm working with a young child who doesn't speak all that much. He is interested in playing and makes some sounds, but I'm not exactly sure what he's trying to communicate. I've tried using simple, single-syllable commenting words, but he doesn't seem to be picking up any of my language models at all. How do I choose the right words? How can I help him talk?

Thanks,

Lost for Words

Dear *Lost for Words,*

It's great that you are providing single-word language models, as he isn't speaking all that much yet. Here are a few more strategies to try out. First, monitor the pace of your interaction and provide lots of space for the child to talk on his turn. When he does make sounds, respond with a clear single word to reinforce each of his attempts. You can use the sounds he is making to guide your word choices. For example, if he makes the *b* sound, then choose simple words that start with those sounds, such as *block* or *build.* If he begins imitating your models, for example, saying "Ba" for *block,* imitate and expand his language by repeating, "Block!" In addition to reinforcing his language, this provides another opportunity for him to hear that word. You may also consider introducing an augmentative and alternative communication (AAC) system to speed up his progress (see Chapter 14).

Keep it up!

JASPER

Stuck in a Loop

Dear JASPER,

I am currently working with a child with emerging symbolic skills. We started incorporating some of her favorite TV characters in our routines. While she has some great higher-level play acts, she seems to get stuck using scripted language. She continually repeats lines that the characters say in her shows, even when I model new phrases that are more related to the routine. I don't want to take the characters away since she is still playing productively and is so motivated by them. How can I help her to use more flexible language?

Thanks,

Stuck in a Loop

Dear *Stuck in a Loop,*

It sounds as if you are making great progress in her play skills, but not as much with her communication. We think it's the right move to stick with what she is motivated by, especially since her play is still progressing. We suggest that you assess your communication goals for her. Does she use only phrases when she scripts? If so, her true mastered length of utterance may actually be much shorter than you think. Create a plan to match your language models to the average length of her spontaneous novel utterances. Another strategy is to shape her scripts. Rather than imitating and expanding upon her scripts exactly, you could respond with flexible language related to the action you are taking. For example, if she repeats the phrase "We're coming to the rescue" as you place characters on a building, you could respond by commenting, "Climb up!" Be sure to use positive affect as you respond, and you can even highlight your comment by combining it with a gesture.

You can do it!

JASPER

12.6 Conclusion

Imitating, expanding, and modeling communication are crucial to the success of the intervention, yet they are only productive when timed appropriately and used in coordination with one another. When you are first learning, you must keep a close eye out for opportunities to imitate and expand and be careful not to model too much. Over time, the child's communication should progress along with your routines. When you repeat words and gestures within familiar routines, it should become easier for the child to notice and then use these skills to communicate back. It may not seem as if the child is paying much attention, but as he becomes familiar with the steps, his engagement should improve. He may start to notice the consistent words and gestures you are using and be more responsive to the opportunities you provide. At first, this might result in more imitation and language responses from the child; over time children begin to express more initiations. See Figure 12.9 for a review of our core communication strategies. In the next chapter, we will introduce the strategies of programming and prompting for communication.

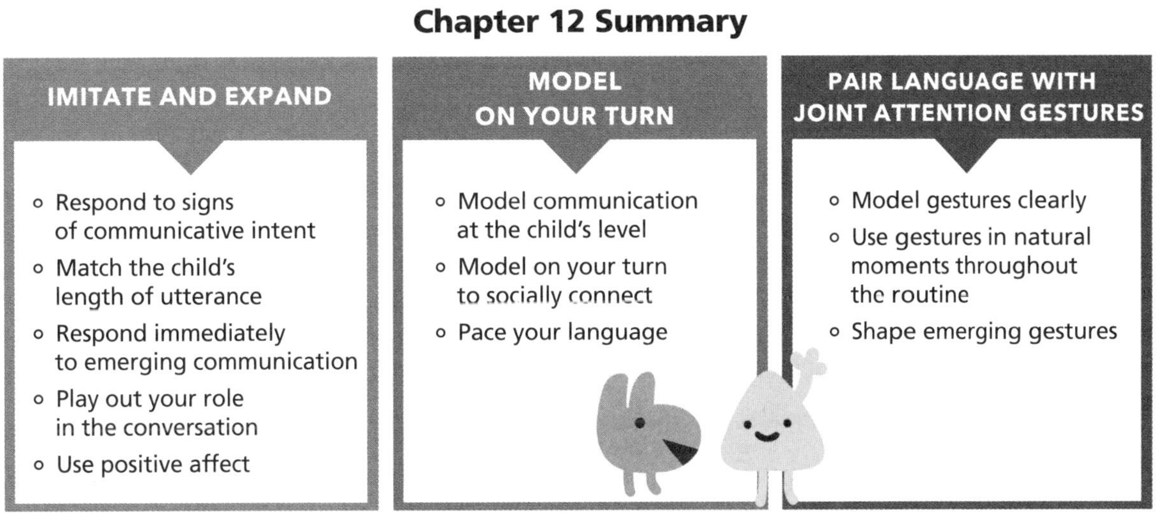

Chapter 12 Summary

IMITATE AND EXPAND	MODEL ON YOUR TURN	PAIR LANGUAGE WITH JOINT ATTENTION GESTURES
o Respond to signs of communicative intent o Match the child's length of utterance o Respond immediately to emerging communication o Play out your role in the conversation o Use positive affect	o Model communication at the child's level o Model on your turn to socially connect o Pace your language	o Model gestures clearly o Use gestures in natural moments throughout the routine o Shape emerging gestures

FIGURE 12.9. Chapter 12 summary.

Programming for Gestures and Language

13.1 Introduction

In this chapter, we discuss the next layer of the communication strategies: programming. *Programming* is the process of providing explicit and systematic opportunities to teach language and gestures within an established routine. The strategies in this chapter go hand in hand with the core communication strategies from Chapter 12. The purpose of programming is to add support to help the child produce the target skill. The process involves the following steps: *modeling* JA gestures and language throughout the routine, *providing a clear opportunity* for the child to use a target skill or *taking advantage of an opportunity* that occurs naturally, *pausing* for the child to communicate, and then *responding* according to what the child does (either providing additional support through prompts or reinforcing the child's communication with your response; see Figure 13.1).

Here is an example of how you could follow this process to program for a joint attention point within a session. To add clarity, the programmed opportunities are underlined in the text throughout the chapter.

> *You and the child are building a castle together and having figures climb the side of the structure to get to the top. Throughout the routine, you choose moments to model a joint attention point as you comment and take your play turn. As you set up to expand the routine, you <u>introduce two dinosaur puppets</u> into the child's sight and reach. You <u>smile, pause, and look expectantly</u> at the child. The child looks at the figure but does not point, so you use the general verbal prompt "What do you see?" and wait. The child demonstrates a joint attention point toward the dinosaurs. You imitate the child's gesture and comment, "Big dinosaurs!" with positive affect to reinforce his communication.*

By introducing the puppets into the environment and pausing expectantly, you give the child an opportunity to share something novel and exciting (preferably by joint attention pointing). While directive strategies like prompting may be necessary in some cases (such as the example above), we always start with programming as a more nature and subtle way of introducing opportunities to share. Throughout the session, you can include programming opportunities like these to help children learn to use targeted communication skills. We will explain the details of programming and prompting below. At the end of the chapter, we will address some common questions and troubleshoot common challenges.

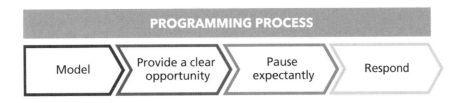

FIGURE 13.1. Programming process.

13.2 Fundamentals of Programming

Before delving into the guidelines for how to program, we will answer some fundamental questions regarding this strategy.

13.2.1 What Skills Should You Program?

Program for the child's target communication skills. In JASPER, we use programming to teach joint attention and requesting gestures and language. See Figure 13.2 to review the communication skills introduced in Chapter 2.

As you may recall from Chapter 2, gestures are an important developmental milestone for all children, even those who are already beginning to use language; thus, we teach both nonverbal and verbal means of communication concurrently. In JASPER, children have target gestures and language for both joint attention and requests. Some children may also have look to share or look to request as targets; however, these targets should always be paired with a gesture target and not prompted for on their own. When programming, try to prioritize the child's target skills from Chapter 4. For example, if the child's target is a joint attention point, you should create several opportunities to program for this skill within your routines. You also can program for other skills

---

TARGET REVIEW ☑☰☑☰

Joint Attention Skills	Requesting Skills
✓ Respond to joint attention*	✓ Look to request*
✓ Look to share*	✓ Reach to request
✓ Show to share	✓ Give to request
✓ Point to share	✓ Point to request
✓ Give to share	✓ Language to request
✓ Language to share	(See Chapters 2–4.)

*If chosen, set an additional gesture target to program. Avoid using directive prompts for these skills.

FIGURE 13.2. Review social communication targets.

beyond the child's targets if opportunities arise. Try to choose a skill that is a natural fit in the context of the routine.

13.2.2 Why Should You Program?

Programming is one of the ways that we teach language and gestures. While some children may learn through observation as you model communication throughout the routine, many children will need programming to provide more systematic opportunities to notice and practice these skills. Programming also helps adults be more aware of the natural learning opportunities available throughout the routine. We are often too quick to communicate and forget to leave room for the child. For example, if something funny happens, we may look to connect with the child right away, or if the child needs help, we might respond immediately to provide assistance. Programming helps us recognize these moments and remember to provide the child with more time and assistance to respond.

13.2.3 When Should You Program?

You should always program within an *established* routine (as defined in Chapter 10). Try to capitalize on opportune moments when the child is motivated and showing signs of joint engagement. For example, if the child looks excited and is initiating many turns, this may be a good moment to program as the child may be more likely to communicate. See Section 13.3.3 for indicators of opportune moments. You can either program during naturally occurring opportunities in the routine or create a clear moment to program, as described below.

Look for Natural Opportunities

Sometimes programming opportunities arise naturally within the routine. If a toy suddenly falls off the tower, you can take advantage of this natural social moment by programming for joint attention. If you notice that your child is looking for a toy and you happen to have it nearby, you can use the opportunity to hold up the toy and pause to program for a request.

Create New Opportunities

You can also create your own programming opportunities. For example, you might strategically take a silly or unexpected step in the routine to evoke joint attention and socially share the moment. Or you could purposefully place some pieces of a toy out of the child's reach to evoke a request. Although these occasions may be prearranged, you should keep them natural as you embed them in the routine.

13.2.4 How Often Should You Program?

Programming is not a strategy that you use all the time; rather, it is applied systematically during strategic moments to practice the child's target skills. The amount that you program is highly dependent on the child, the session, and the routine. In general, you should try to add a few programmed opportunities in every established play routine and assess from there. You may be programming *too little* if the child does not have several programmed opportunities to use his target gestures during the session, if he does not have opportunities to work on both JA and requesting skills, or if the child is not making progress toward his target gestures over time. You are programming *too often* if programming is taking over your play turn, you are losing your equal and active roles, you are frequently losing the child's engagement, or you are frequently causing dysregulation. Remember that you are playing the role of an *equal and active* play partner. For this reason, you should avoid programming on back-to-back turns, requiring the child to request for access to the toys on each turn, or allowing programming to take place instead of responding to the child's idea, as this prohibits you from being an equal and active partner.

Why not program all the time? Programming often feels like a highly effective strategy, because it yields a response from the child; however, we must recognize that this strategy can place a high demand on the child and creates a pause in the routine that can lead to diminished engagement or dysregulation. Further, programming typically results in a prompted response, rather than an initiation. While programming represents a useful set of tools that we can use to assist children to learn the mechanics of communication, it is a stop along the way to our ultimate goal of spontaneous initiations. In order to make progress toward this goal, we must be careful to maintain an equal and active role overall throughout the routine and work to fade our support and shift the balance back to initiations as well. Now that we have explained some of the features of programming, we will explain how to use this strategy within the routine.

13.3 Prepare to Program

Before you program, you should prepare the child for the programmed opportunity within an established routine. The goal is to create an expectation of communication throughout the routine and then give the child an opportunity to fulfill the expectation with a word or gesture. Follow the steps below to ensure that your programmed opportunities are successful.

13.3.1 Establish Engagement in a Routine

Use the strategies in Chapters 5–12 to engage the child in a routine. Remember, the routine is a context not only for play but also for communication. You should not expect the child to use target skills without a solid foundation of engagement and a context to communicate about. This gives the child a foundation for the new skills and ensures that the child is regulated and engaged enough to try something new and potentially difficult.

13.3.2 Model Communication Targets throughout the Routine

In order to program successfully, you should make extra effort to model the joint attention gestures and language you intend to program for throughout the routine (as described Chapter 12; see Figure 13.3). As you model, you are introducing the child to the skill you will later expect the child to use. For some children, modeling will be enough support to begin learning these skills, but most children will likely need explicit programmed opportunities to practice. Modeling familiarizes the child with the expectation and provides clear examples of the form of each gesture and words the child can say.

You can also model requesting gestures and language in preparation to program; however, this is less common and should only occur during natural moments (see Box 13.1). Modeling joint attention will typically suffice. Now that we have explained how to prepare to program, we will introduce some strategies you can use to create these clear opportunities within the routine.

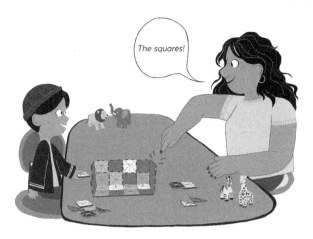

FIGURE 13.3. The adult models communication in preparation to program for joint attention later in the session.

13.3.3 Identify an Opportune Moment

If you have established a routine and modeled language and gestures, and the child still has not initiated, look for an opportune moment to program. To be successful, your programmed opportunities must be well timed and noticeable to the child. You can increase the saliency of these opportunities by modeling during moments when the child is motivated, engaged, and likely to communicate with you. This gives the child the best chance to respond with the least amount of support. In Figure 13.4, we provide some signs that indicate it is too soon or too late to program.

13.4 Introduce a Programming Opportunity

After building a clear context and expectation for communication, it is time to provide explicit programmed opportunities for the child to practice target skills. As mentioned in Section 13.2.3, you can take advantage of natural opportunities that arise, or you can create a clear opportunity for communication. Figure 13.5 provides some examples of opportunities we might use to

---

BOX 13.1. Should I Model Requesting Skills?

Modeling gestures and language primarily applies to joint attention, as there are fewer opportunities to model requests naturally within the routine. For example, you should not ask the child to help you fix something or request help to reach a toy for the purpose of modeling a request; however, you can model the request as a *response* to the child's request. For example, if the child is reaching for a baby doll, you could model a requesting point and say, "Want baby!"

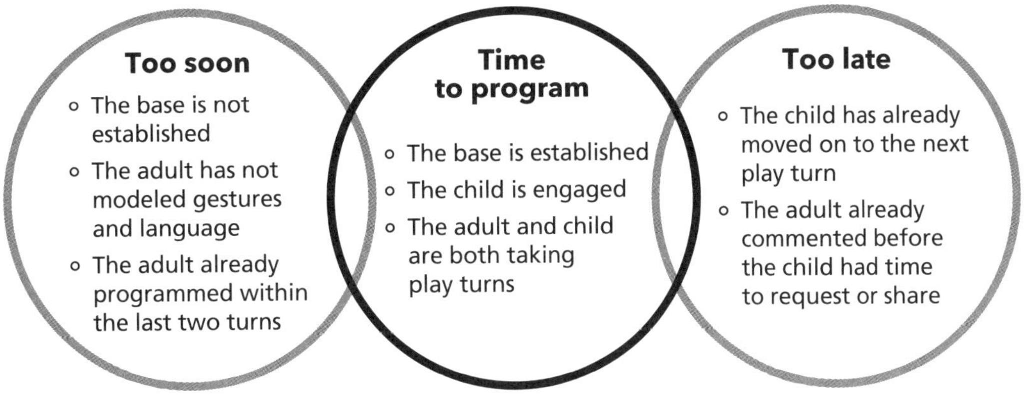

Too soon
- The base is not established
- The adult has not modeled gestures and language
- The adult already programmed within the last two turns

Time to program
- The base is established
- The child is engaged
- The adult and child are both taking play turns

Too late
- The child has already moved on to the next play turn
- The adult already commented before the child had time to request or share

FIGURE 13.4. Timing of programming.

program for joint attention or requests. This is not an exhaustive list but rather some strategies we have found to be successful to provide clear opportunities. When you use these strategies, you should pause "expectantly" in silence and look at the child with a sense of anticipation. During this time, you should not talk, prompt the child, recruit the child's attention (by gasping, using sounds effects), draw attention to objects (by tapping, shaking, or banging toys), or otherwise try to evoke these skills. You should simple wait a moment in silence. We want the child to learn to communicate under natural circumstances so that these skills transfer to other settings. If the child uses the skill, you can then use your response to reinforce the child's communication (see Section 13.5.1). If programming and pausing is not enough to evoke the skill, you can choose to include a directive prompt (see Section 13.5.2) or try again another time (see Section 13.5.3). The process of programming for joint attention and requesting varies slightly. We will address the strategies for joint attention first, followed by requesting.

OPPORTUNITIES TO PROGRAM ☑

Joint Attention
- ☐ Take advantage of unexpected moments
- ☐ Introduce an interesting expansion toy
- ☐ Introduce a silly step
- ☐ Arrange materials in a nontransparent container

Requesting
- ☐ Take advantage of natural opportunities
- ☐ Allow the child to run out of materials
- ☐ Hold up two options
- ☐ Pause before an expected step
- ☐ Allow the child to attempt something that requires assistance

FIGURE 13.5. Opportunities to program.

13.4.1 Programming for Joint Attention Skills

Choose a strategy to program for the child's target joint attention skill within the routine. The goal is to create a moment when the child is motivated to share an object or event with you. Here are some examples of strategies you could use to encourage these skills.

Take Advantage of Unexpected Moments

Capitalize on interesting and unexpected moments that happen naturally within the routine to program for a target skill. When the moment occurs, pause expectantly for the child to communicate his reaction. Here is an example:

> *You and the child create a structure out of magnetic tiles and add figures on top of it. After placing several figures on the structure, it falls apart. You pause expectantly to see if the child will communicate.*

Instead of rushing to respond in moments of surprise, you can pause expectantly and see if the child will communicate.

Introduce an Interesting Expansion Toy

Sometimes children use joint attention when they see something exciting and want to share it with you. Here is an example:

> *You and the child are attaching frosting to a cupcake toy. You model a joint attention point and say, "Frosting," as you place frosting on a cupcake. Once the base of the routine is established and you have modeled the target gesture consistently, you introduce candles into the child's sight and reach. You pause expectantly to see if the child will say anything about them.*

By pausing in silence and leaving space for the child's reaction in this moment, the child has an opportunity to share excitement.

Introduce a Silly Step

Include a silly or unexpected step during a familiar sequence to program as the child communicates his humor or surprise. For example:

> *You and the child have a familiar routine of assembling sandwiches for lunch and then eating cake. You model a silly new step by placing a slice of cake on top of the sandwich and pause expectantly to see if the child will communicate.*

Arrange Materials in a Nontransparent Container

Allow the child to open the nontransparent container and share the surprise he discovers (see Figure 13.6). This creates an opportunity to program for joint attention as you and the child take turns revealing what is inside. This works well as an expansion step when the toys can also be used as the next step in the routine. For example:

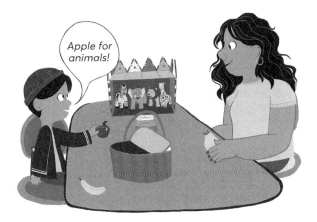

FIGURE 13.6. The adult creates an opportunity for joint attention skills by putting pretend food in a picnic basket.

> The adult <u>adds a closed picnic basket</u> full of fruit to the table and <u>pauses expectantly</u> as the child opens the basket. The child pulls his fruit out of the basket, shows her the fruit, and says, "Apple for animals!"

This is a fun way to program for joint attention, but it should not make up a large part of your routine. Choose four to six pieces, select a few moments to use this type of strategy throughout the session, and then return to the typical sequence of the routine.

13.4.2 Programming for Requesting Skills

Children are likely to communicate when they want something or have a need that they would like to be fulfilled. Use the motivation in these moments to program for the child's requesting targets. Remember to respond immediately if the child requests, as this is the primary way we reinforce the child's skills. The goal is not to frustrate the child or frequently withhold toys but rather to create a clear opportunity for the child to use targeted skills.

Take Advantage of Natural Opportunities to Program Requests

Pause during a moment in the routine when the child wants something or needs help. For example:

> <u>The door comes off a truck</u> as you and the child are placing animals inside. You <u>pause expectantly</u> to see if the child will request.

Instead of rushing to fulfill the request, you can use this moment to program.

Allow the Child to Run out of Materials

Instead of replenishing materials during the routine, allow the child to run out of materials and then pause to allow the child to request. For example:

You and the child place pegs onto a foam board. You stop moving pieces into the child's environment and allow the child to run out of pegs. On the child's next turn, she looks around the table for another peg. You pause expectantly and wait to see if she will request.

Be mindful to keep the additional pieces close to you and well out of the child's reach, so the child cannot reach out and grab them (see Box 13.2).

Hold Up Two Options

Create an opportunity for the child to request by providing a choice of toys (see Figure 13.7). Hold up two different items out of the child's reach during a moment when the child does not have other options. For example:

You and the child create a routine with magnetic tiles and animals. The child stacks the last tile in front of him. You hold up two options, a square tile in one hand and a triangle tile in the other and pause expectantly as you look at the child to see if the child will request one of the shapes.

Do not verbally prompt at this stage. Simply hold up the options and pause in silence to see if the child will request. Make sure the options are well out of the child's reach, so the child cannot reach out and grab them (as described in Box 13.2).

Pause before an Expected Step

Model the target skill during a consistent moment in the routine to build a clear example of what communication can occur on a particular step, and then pause. The goal is for the child to communicate to keep the routine going. For example:

In Figure 13.8, each time the adult places an animal in the structure, she points and says, "Animal goes in!" After modeling the communication consistently, she pauses on her next turn and looks expectantly at the child. The child says, "Add more animals!"

BOX 13.2. Manage the Toys When Programming for Requests

If you are a programming for a request during a moment when the child wants an object, keep the object well out of the child's reach so there is clear time and opportunity for the child to request. If the item is within reach, the child will likely reach out and grab it or take it from your hand. Remember that the goal in this moment is for the child to use a target skill to communicate (e.g., reach or point to request). Grabbing is not an appropriate way to communicate a request. It is not a target skill, nor a response that we would reinforce in this moment. Thus, you must be prepared to preempt this pattern by preventing the child from grabbing and instead use this as an opportunity to help the child practice verbally or nonverbally requesting in more productive, appropriate ways.

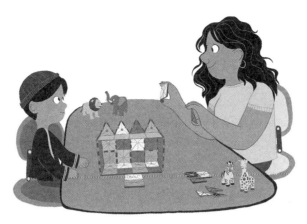

FIGURE 13.7. When the child runs out of pieces, the adult holds up two choices out of the child's reach and pauses expectantly to program for a request.

For this opportunity to work, you must model the skill consistently during a well-established and highly motivating routine. If you pause without building up the expectation, the child may not understand why you stopped.

Allow the Child to Attempt Something that Requires Assistance

These are often actions that require fine motor skills, such as placing a figure into a chair or fitting shapes into a shape sorter. For example:

> You and the child are putting clothes on babies after giving them a bath. The child has a <u>hard time putting the doll's pants on</u>, so you <u>pause expectantly</u> for the child to use a gesture or language to request for help.

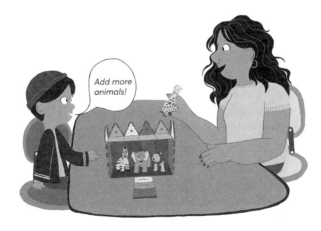

FIGURE 13.8. The adult pauses before an expected step within an established routine to program for communication.

Another way to do this is to place some preferred items in a hard-to-open container and pause for the child to request help in opening it. This strategy is particularly useful if the child has a preferred expansion to a familiar routine. For example:

The child is very interested in insects, so you establish a base of building blocks into a tree and then <u>introduce a transparent jar</u> of plastic butterflies. You allow the child to attempt to open it and <u>pause expectantly</u> for the child to request help.

13.4.3 Pause Expectantly after Each Opportunity for the Child to Respond

After you program for joint attention or requesting using the strategies and steps above, pause expectantly to give the child time to demonstrate the target skill. For example:

You and the child are building a castle for the villagers. You set a couple of dragon figures on the table within the child's reach. Rather than draw the child's attention or model, <u>you pause expectantly</u> to allow the child time to notice the dragons. The child sees the dragons and looks up at you and back to the dragons.

Pausing is an imperative part of the programming process. Remember that you should be silent and avoid prompting or recruiting the child's attention during this time. The break in the sequence helps the child to notice that something is expected of him and prepares him to respond. The amount of time you wait will vary depending on the child. Do not wait so long that the child loses engagement or becomes dysregulated.

Take a moment to complete Exercise 13.1 and see if you can identify the best way to create a programming opportunity in each scenario.

EXERCISE 13.1. Creating Programming Opportunities

Identify the most appropriate strategy to use on the next turn based on the information provided.

Scenario	Adult's action
1. You and the child give a doll a bath and dry it off. You want to create an opportunity for the child to use a requesting point.	A. Limit access by holding up the baby. B. Hold up a brush and a shirt.
2. You and the child have an established routine building a cake, putting on candles, and cutting the cake. You want to create an opportunity for the child to comment on what is happening.	A. Raise your volume each time you comment on the cake. B. Put something silly, like a piece of cheese, onto the cake.

3. You and the child are putting pieces in a puzzle. You want to create an opportunity for the child to use a requesting give.

   A. Choose a puzzle that is too hard for the child to complete on his own.

   B. Place a few of the puzzle pieces in a sealed container.

4. You and the child are putting wooden Velcro fruit pieces together. You want to create an opportunity for the child to demonstrate a JA point.

   A. Attach a piece of orange with a piece of banana.

   B. Shake a container of fruits to gain the child's attention.

5. You and the child are building a tall house. As the house gets taller, the child has a hard time placing the blocks on top. You want to create an opportunity for her to use a requesting give.

   A. Pause expectantly as she tries to reach the top.

   B. Say, "Give me the block."

13.5 Notice the Child's Response to the Opportunity

The child might respond to the programmed moment in subtle ways, so pay close attention to all signs of communication. Ideally, the child will respond with the target skill. If the child responds, reinforce the child's communication by imitating and expanding with language and gestures (following the guidelines in Chapter 12). If the child does not respond, you can add more support by prompting, or you can try again another time (particularly if the model was unclear). Here are a few examples of how this process of creating an opportunity, pausing, and noticing the child's response comes together in a flower garden routine:

- ***Programming for request.*** You and the child have built all the stems for the flower toys, and the next step in this familiar routine is to add the flower petals. You place a closed container with the petals on the table. You pause expectantly while the child tries to open the container. The child looks up at you for a moment and then gives you the container to request help. You take the container, point to it, and say, "Want flowers!" You open the container and hand it to the child (reinforcement).

- ***Programming for joint attention.*** You place a nontransparent bag containing four to six brightly colored bugs on the table in the child's reach. The child notices the bag and looks inside. You pause and look expectantly toward the child. The child pulls out a bug, inspects it for a moment, and then says, "Bug," while holding the toy out in front of his face. You gently touch the child's elbow to help extend his arm and turn the bug to face you (prompting). You point to the bug and say, "Pink bug!" (reinforcement).

See Figure 13.9 for the complete programming process, and we will explain the details of each response in the sections below.

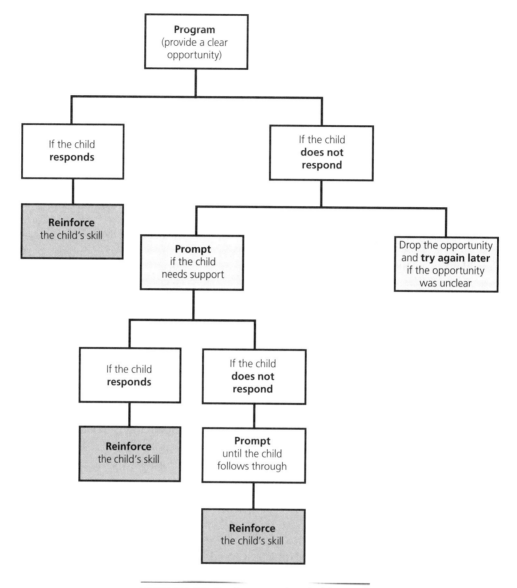

FIGURE 13.9. Programming decision tree.

13.5.1 Reinforce the Child's Communication

If the child successfully uses the target skill or makes his best attempt to communicate in this moment, you should quickly reinforce the child's communication by imitating and expanding. You should also pair this response with high, positive affect.

When you respond, you can either directly imitate the child's gesture (e.g., the child gives and then you give something back) or respond with a different gesture (e.g., the child shows and then you point, as in Figure 13.10). If the child responds with eye contact alone, you can still imitate and expand on the child's response by modeling language and a gesture. Consider the example below, where the child responds with a skill other than the target.

You are targeting a requesting point. You <u>hold up two toy choices</u>, you <u>pause</u>, and the child looks toward one of the toys. You expand the child's communication by pointing to the item, naming the object, and giving it to the child.

Even though the child did not use the target skill, the child still appropriately communicated to request through gaze. By responding with gestures and language, you show the child more skills to use during a moment of engagement.

This process of reinforcing the child's communication also applies after you provide directive prompts (see Section 13.5.2). When the child demonstrates the skill in response to your prompt, respond and expand the child's communication to reinforce the skill. During these moments when the child is working hard to learn a new skill, it is especially important to respond and reinforce the new skill he is learning.

13.5.2 Use Directive Prompts to Help the Child Use the Target Skill

If the child does not respond within a few seconds of a programmed opportunity but is still engaged, you can help him produce the target skill by using a *verbal*, *gestural*, or *physical* prompt to make the expectation clearer.

- ***Model with an expectation.*** Model again after the programmed opportunity and pause expectantly for the child to use the target gesture (e.g., model and hold a point).

- ***Gestural prompt.*** Extend your hand with your palm facing up to encourage the child to give you an object.

- ***General verbal prompt.*** Ask the child an open-ended question (e.g., "What happened?" (for joint attention) or "What do you want?" (for a request) or use a general comment (e.g., "I need some too").

- ***Specific verbal prompt.*** Instruct the child to use the target skill (e.g., "Point," "Show me," "Give me") or provide the child with words he can use (e.g., "Say, 'Want train' ").

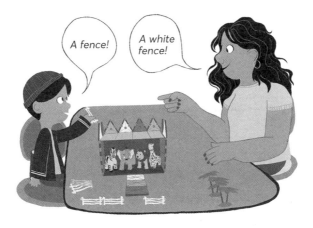

FIGURE 13.10. The adult responds to the child's communication with another gesture and language.

- **Partial physical prompt.** Gently touch the child's arm or hand as a reminder to use a gesture.
- **Full physical prompt.** Gently form the child's hand into the target gesture.

Choose the type of prompt that will allow for the most independence possible. The guidelines for these strategies are introduced in Chapter 8 and summarized below.

Guidelines for Prompting (see Chapter 8 for details)

- Start with the least intrusive form of support needed. As you get to know the child, you will be able to skip to the most appropriate prompt for the moment.
- Use each prompt one time (unless the child does not notice your prompt, in which case you can repeat it during a moment when the child is attending to you). For example, you should not say, "What do you want? What do you want, Naya? Do you want this?" If the child does not respond, repeating the prompt is not likely to be successful, and the child may learn that she is not expected to respond the first time.
- Give the child enough time to respond to the prompt, without losing the child's engagement.
- If the child does not respond to the prompt, increase the level of support to help him be successful (e.g., if you start with a general verbal prompt, you can move on to a specific verbal).
- Continue to move your way through the prompts until the child produces the target skill.
- Fade prompts quickly so the child learns to communicate independently.

Table 13.1 provides examples of how to target different joint attention skills during a specific play routine, and Table 13.2 provides examples of how to target various requesting skills.

Use Exercise 13.2 to evaluate your understanding of prompting in response to a programmed opportunity.

EXERCISE 13.2. **Prompting and Programming**

Indicate whether each statement is true or false according to JASPER guidelines.

1. You can physically prompt the child to make eye contact.	True	False
2. You do not have to prompt the target skill if the child used another form of communication.	True	False
3. You should immediately pair the programmed opportunity with a directive prompt.	True	False
4. You can increase the level of prompt to help the child follow through with the target skill.	True	False
5. Plan to fade prompting as soon as possible (even within session).	True	False
6. Try to program and prompt at least every other turn.	True	False

---

TABLE 13.1. Programming and Prompting Strategies for Joint Attention

Target skill	Create a clear opportunity	Model with an expectation	Gestural prompt	General verbal prompt	Specific verbal prompt	Partial physical prompt	Full physical prompt
Scenario: The adult and child establish a zoo routine with blocks and animals. Throughout the routine, the adult picks up various animals, shows them to the child, and tells the child what animal they have (e.g., "I have a monkey").							
JA show	Adult hands a new or favorite animal to the child.	Adult picks up a monkey, shows it to the child, and says, "I have a monkey," and then pauses expectantly.	N/A	Adult says, "What do you have?" as the child holds a monkey.	Adult says, "Show me."	Adult touches or taps the child's elbow to move his arm upward.	Adult helps the child form his hand into a show.
Scenario: The adult and child establish a birthday party routine with cake, oven, and figures. The adult models joint attention points throughout the routine, for example, pointing toward the cake and commenting, "It fell!"							
JA point	Adult drops the cake when putting it in the oven.	Adult points to the cake and pauses expectantly.	N/A	Adult says, "Wow! What happened?"	Adult says, "Point."	Adult gently touches or taps child's wrist.	Adult gently forms the child's fingers into a point.
Scenario: The adult and child establish a bathing routine with baby dolls, a bathtub, towels, soap, and hairbrushes. Throughout the routine, the adult gives the child various toys so she is able to take her turn in bathing the baby dolls.							
JA give	Adult moves the towels and brushes near the child and pauses	Adult gives the child the other hairbrush she was using, says, "Here's this brush," and then pauses expectantly.	Adult holds out her hand in a palm-up position.	Adult says, "I need a brush."	Adult says, "Give me."	Adult nudges or taps child's elbow to move her hand toward her palm.	Adult gently takes the child's hand and helps her give it to the adult.
Scenario: The adult and child establish a farm routine with farm animals, a barn, and a tractor. Throughout the routine, the adult models appropriate language to share at the child's correct language level.							
Language to share	Adult brings out dinosaur figures to add to the routine.	Adult says, "It's a dinosaur!" while showing it to the child.	N/A (unless the child uses an SGD, see Table 14.1)	Adult says, "What is this one?"	Adult says, "Say it's a dinosaur."	N/A (unless the child uses an SGD, see Table 14.1)	N/A (unless the child uses an SGD, see Table 14.1)

13.5.3 Try Again Another Time

The timing of programmed opportunities to communicate is essential, but challenging, in a fast-paced interaction. There may be times when you start an opportunity and realize that you have not selected the right time to do so. You do not have to prompt every time you start to program. Here are some signs that you may need to try again another time:

- You created the opportunity out of the child's line of sight, and the child did not notice.
- You were not quick enough to present the opportunity, and the child already moved on to something else or initiated another step in the routine.
- Your timing was off, and the child lost engagement (see Box 13.3).

TABLE 13.2. Programming and Prompting Strategies for Requesting

Target skill	Create a clear opportunity	Model with an expectation	Gestural prompt	General verbal prompt	Specific verbal prompt	Partial physical prompt	Full physical prompt
Scenario: The adult and infant have a routine tossing a balloon back and forth and then throwing it through a net. Throughout the routine, when the child gazes at a new balloon, the adult models reaching toward and labeling the balloon.							
Reach to request	Adult sticks balloons to the ceiling using static electricity.	Adult reaches to the balloon and pauses expectantly to see if the child will reach.	N/A	Adult asks, "What do you want?"	Adult says, "Reach."	Adult gently touches the child's elbow to encourage him to lift his arm.	Adult gently lifts the child's arm in the direction of the balloon.
Scenario: The adult and child have a block routine with large cardboard bricks, tiles, and bristle blocks. Throughout the routine, the adult gives the child various blocks.							
Give to request	Adult and child stack blocks into a tall tower that the child eventually cannot reach.	Adult gives the child a block.	Adult holds out her hand in a palm-up position so the child can easily hand her the block.	Adult asks, "What do you need?"	Adult says, "Give me."	Adult nudges or taps on the child's hand to encourage him to give her the block to put it on the tower.	Adult gently helps the child give her the block and then puts it on the tower.
Scenario: The adult and child have a picnic routine with food, utensils, plates, and dolls. Throughout the routine, the adult models a joint attention point. If the child starts to reach for an item, the adult models the action by pointing and says, "Want cup."							
Point to request	Adult holds a sandwich and a cup out of reach. Child reaches toward the cup.	Adult points to the cup and pauses expectantly to see if the child will point.	N/A	Adult asks, "What do you want?"	Adult says, "Point."	Adult gently touches the child's fingers to help him tuck them into his palm.	Adult gently forms the child's fingers into a point.
Scenario: The adult and child establish a spaceship routine with blocks and figures. Throughout the routine, the adult models appropriate language at the child's correct MLU.							
Language to request	Adult says, "3–2–1 . . . go" and then launches the spaceship.	Adult says, "Go" before blasting off the spaceship.	N/A (unless the child uses an SGD, see Table 14.1)	Adult asks, "What should it do?"	Adult says, "Say go."	N/A (unless the child uses an SGD, see Table 14.1)	N/A (unless the child uses an SGD, see Table 14.1)

> **BOX 13.3. Support Engagement**
>
> If the child loses engagement when you create an opportunity, stop attempting to program and instead provide support to help the child reengage. Once you have established engagement in a routine again, look for a new moment to practice the child's target skills. If the child continually loses engagement and you are unable to be successful, you may need to troubleshoot other factors using the ACT framework. Remember to consider all aspects of the intervention, as there may be other contributing factors outside of the opportunity itself (for example, the child's engagement may be fragile because he is bored and ready to expand). It should eventually be possible to program successfully during the routine.

If you realize that the opportunity you provided was not very clear, you should not force the child to follow through. Simply try again another time. For example:

> *You are targeting a joint attention point in a doggy daycare routine. A <u>dog falls off one of the kennels you built</u>, so you <u>pause</u> and look at the child, but she has already turned to take her dog to the bath station and did not seem to notice.*

Since the opportunity was not within the child's attentional focus and she is already proceeding with the next step of the routine, you can simply move on. Here is an example targeting a request:

> *You and the child are pretending to do laundry. You are taking turns adding clothes to the washing machine and the child looks around. You <u>hold up two expansion options</u>—a basket with more clothes and soap for the washer. The child then discovers another couple of pieces of clothing under her leg and starts to add them to the washer.*

Instead of getting the child's attention or prompting in this moment, you should simply imitate the child's action and try again another time. Do not be discouraged if the child does not use the target skill right away or it takes you some practice to get the timing right. You may need to repeat the process several times for the child to understand your expectations, especially in the case of joint attention.

13.6 Achieving High-Quality Programming and Prompting

Beyond learning the basic process of programming, you should practice programming in a way that will be most effective for the child. In our experience, programming is one of the most difficult strategies for new JASPER therapists to master. In the following section, we introduce some considerations to ensure you are making the most of your programming opportunities.

13.6.1 Create Clear Opportunities

Consider the clarity of your programmed opportunities and evaluate the timing, context, and frequency. Here is a summary of some of the factors you should keep in mind:

*Signs that the programmed opportunity was **clear**:*

- It took place during a motivating moment within an established routine.
- Joint attention gestures were modeled prior to programming.
- It took place within the child's line of sight.
- It was timed appropriately within the routine.
- Opportunity very clearly evoked the intended skill.
- It was followed by a silent pause.
- It was delivered with appropriate frequency.

*Signs that the programmed opportunity was **not clear**:*

- The timing was not right.
- The child did not notice.
- The child had already moved on to something else by the time you programmed.
- The adult prompts or recruits the child's attention (e.g., gasping, banging, or shaking objects)

13.6.2 Tailor Programming to the Child's Needs

Programming for gestures and language should be layered on top of all the strategies covered in the last chapters. While these moments are valuable in teaching the child new skills, they will not be meaningful unless they are balanced with other core strategies and tailored to the child's needs in the moment.

Consider Engagement and Regulation

While your main focus is to model target gestures, there will be some moments in the session where the child shows increased regulation and engagement. You can take advantage of these moments to program for the target skill. If the child is having difficulty engaging in a routine or showing early signs of dysregulation, it is not time to program. Instead, try to introduce a programming opportunity during a better moment for the child. There should always be at least a few programming opportunities in every session, even for children who have limited engagement and regulation, as this is how you work toward communication targets. Thus, it is important to monitor the child's engagement and regulation closely in order to find an ideal moment to pursue these skills.

Consider the Child's Progress

If the child has a slow-moving target, you may choose to increase opportunities for these specific targets. For example, if the child's target is a joint attention show, one of your first routine options could include the child's favorite character figures in a nontransparent container. You could then build in several opportunities to practice and prompt for joint attention shows as you take turns taking them out of the container.

Be Creative and Flexible

Arrange programming opportunities based on what is motivating to the child. For example, if the child is very motivated by building blocks, you could program for a requesting give by building cardboard blocks into a tower so tall the child eventually cannot reach. This will likely be more successful than an activity that is more frustrating to the child (e.g., creating opportunities for a requesting give using a puzzle that the child cannot fit the pieces into). It is important to think about what opportunities are more likely to be successful for the child in front of you. If the child is particularly frustrated by objects that do not open easily, you could try holding up two options as a more favorable alternative. If the child is particularly averse to being touched, you may need to rely more heavily on verbal rather than physical directive prompts.

13.6.3 Maintain an Equal and Active Role

As you begin to program opportunities, remember to continue taking your play turn and creating a fun and engaging interaction. If you program too frequently, the interaction will likely become demanding and you will not be able to maintain a robust routine. Eventually, we want the child to be able to use target communication skills in other interactions outside of intervention. When the routine gets overrun with programmed opportunities, this puts the child in the position of the responder and does not help the child move closer to the goal of initiating. Thus, we must always balance programming with the other goals of the intervention.

13.6.4 Fade Support over Time

Programming and prompting can feel like the "heavy lifters" of your strategies because they often yield a response, but it is crucial not to become too reliant on them. Our goal is not simply for the child to respond with the skill; our goal is to help the child progress from programmed and prompted responses toward spontaneous initiations. By programming and prompting, we help the child understand very clearly what is expected of him and give him opportunities to practice using the target skill. Once the child demonstrates understanding and ability to follow through, you should fade support. You can be confident that the child has a better understanding of the expectation and may need less support in order to produce the same skill next time. Through this process, the child should eventually use the target skill with less and less support, until the child is able to initiate the skill spontaneously.

13.7 Common Challenges with Programming

Programming takes a high level of awareness and coordination from the adult while simultaneously asking a lot of the child. Although this can prove a challenge, programming is an essential strategy to teach target skills. As you program, you may come across challenges, such as breaks in engagement, resistance to using a new skill, or confusion around the expectation. The following sections introduce some common questions and case examples.

13.7.1 Common Questions

In the section below, we address common questions regarding the process of programming within a JASPER routine.

What if the child uses a different skill from the one I was targeting?

Sometimes the child uses a skill that is different from the one you intended to program. For example, you might program for a joint attention gesture, and the child might respond with language. If the child responds with a different skill, you can scaffold the child's skill with your response by imitating and expanding and try programming for the target skill another time. If the child continues to use mastered skills, without ever responding with the target skill, then you most likely need to move to prompting to help the child use the target skill. Once you choose to prompt, then you must continue to add support until the child produces the specific gesture. Consider the following scenario:

> You model a joint attention point as you crash the blocks.
> The next time the <u>blocks crash</u>, you <u>pause expectantly</u> (taking advantage of a natural moment) and wait for the child to point.
> The child says, "Crash!" but does not point.
> You clearly model the joint attention point and say, "Crash blocks!" (reinforce).

Since the child did not gesture, you model the joint attention point, expand the child's language, and try again. The next time through, you add support.

> After the <u>blocks crash</u>, you <u>pause expectantly</u> (taking advantage of a natural moment) to see if the child will point.
> The child says, "Crash!" but still does not point.
> You model a joint attention point and continue to <u>pause</u> without language (model with an expectation).
> The child does not respond.
> You tap the child's elbow (partial physical) to remind him to point.
> Once the child points, you imitate and expand by pointing and saying, "They crashed!" (reinforce).

This may sound like a lot of steps, but this can happen quickly with little wait time in between. The goal is to show the child with your pauses that something is expected and then help the child follow through.

What if the child responds only to directive prompting?

If you find that you are repeatedly using several prompts before the child uses a target skill, then you may need to reconsider the timing and clarity of the opportunity. Perhaps the child did not notice the opportunity, or it did not make sense within the context of the routine. It is also possible that you should target a different skill, and the child is not developmentally ready for the skill you originally chose.

What if the child gets dysregulated?

Sometimes children are resistant to this process and become dysregulated when you program or prompt. When this happens, remain calm and in control and try not to let the child's response affect your emotional state. Use the strategies in Chapter 16 to help the child return to a regulated state, reestablish engagement in the routine, establish the base, and then try prompting again. Keep trying, even if it is difficult and even when you face resistance. All of the strategies we have introduced so far create the context for the child to learn these communication skills. It is a wasted opportunity to go through the work of establishing routines, modeling, and so on, without ever helping the child follow through to learn these target skills.

13.7.2 Case Examples

The following section provides fictional case examples addressing challenges with programming for gesture and language.

Point of No Return

Dear JASPER,

I'm a new trainee, and I have just started practicing programming within my sessions. One of the kids I work with has mastered reaching to request, so we are working on targeting a point to request. It feels so productive when I program, because he points pretty much every time I hold up two choices. Our most successful programming routine is with a shape sorter. I hold up two different shapes before each of his turns, and he now knows to point to it to get a piece. This has been going really well, but in our last few sessions, he seems less interested in the shapes. He will ask for a couple of shapes, but then he seems to get frustrated. Am I doing something wrong?

Thanks,

Point of No Return

Dear *Point of No Return,*

It sounds as if you have set a developmentally appropriate target to progress from reaching to pointing to request. That's great! However, based on your description of the child's increasing dysregulation, it appears that the programming opportunities are happening too frequently. Remember that you need to maintain an equal and active role as a play partner. Programming should not replace your play turn. For example, if you are holding up a choice before each turn, the child's play becomes somewhat prompt dependent and turns into a task. Your programmed opportunities should occur sporadically during extra motivating moments rather than a requirement in order to access the materials to play. Plan to reduce the rate of your programming and ensure you are consistently and immediately imitating the child's productive play acts on your turn. This will support the child's engagement and also provide the child opportunities to gesture spontaneously on his turn. When you do choose to program, try to mix up the opportunities and keep them as natural as possible. For example, move some toys out of reach rather than holding up two options to see if he will request for those objects.

You've got this!

JASPER

Sharing Is Caring

Dear JASPER,

The child I am working with has been communicating so much during our last few sessions! She points for new toys that I put on the shelf, gives me blocks when she can't reach the top of the tower, and has started to pair words with these gestures. The problem is that I am not seeing an increase in her joint attention skills. She will occasionally use coordinated joint eye contact when she's really excited about something, but no gestures or words. What is the best way to help her use more joint attention?

Thanks,

Sharing Is Caring

Dear *Sharing Is Caring,*

It's fantastic to hear that your child is communicating more frequently! Take a moment to assess your joint attention target skills. Since the child uses coordinated joint looks to share, her target will be showing to share and single-word comments. Try to plan moments to both expand and program for these skills. First, when she shares with her gaze, respond by modeling a gesture and language. Second, try consistently modeling the target skills throughout the session. Third, plan opportunities to program for joint attention shows. For example, children will sometimes show to share after noticing an interesting toy. You could try setting out some animal figures in an opaque container and then pause expectantly when the child pulls one out to look at it. You can also use a physical or partial physical prompt to encourage her to show you the animal she has in her hand before her play turn.

Keep it up!

JASPER

13.8 Conclusion

Programming and prompting are essential steps to work toward the child's target communication skills. As we have discussed throughout the chapter, we must be careful not to program too much and lose the equal and active roles in the routine; however, it is also important not to program too little either. In many ways, programming is the pinnacle of our communication strategies and the final level of support (along with prompting), so it is important to layer this strategy in balance with the others in order to help the child learn new target skills.

The core strategies we have discussed here and in previous chapters lay the foundation for communication—you will support the child's engagement, provide a play context for the conversation, imitate and expand the child's communication, and model communication. Then through programming, you take advantage of key moments in the interaction to give the child explicit practice to use the new skill. By programming within the context of the routine, you put the child in the best position to understand the expectations, become an active participant in the social interaction, and ultimately learn new ways to communicate. Once you are successful at programming and the child uses the new skill, you should celebrate this as a meaningful step in the child's progress! As you repeat this process, you should begin to fade the level of support until the child is able to initiate the skill spontaneously. Review Chapter 13 strategies in Figure 13.11.

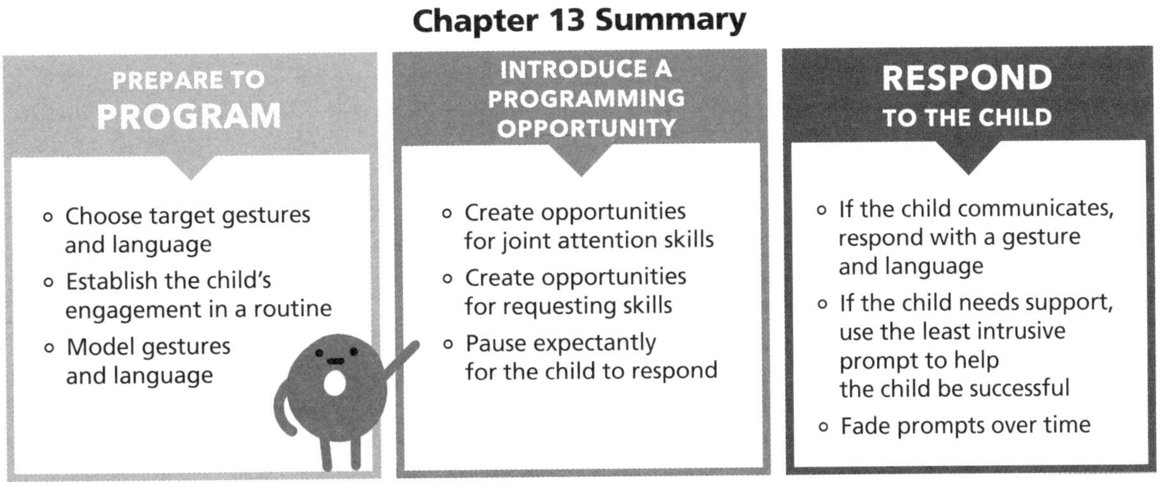

Chapter 13 Summary

PREPARE TO PROGRAM	INTRODUCE A PROGRAMMING OPPORTUNITY	RESPOND TO THE CHILD
o Choose target gestures and language o Establish the child's engagement in a routine o Model gestures and language	o Create opportunities for joint attention skills o Create opportunities for requesting skills o Pause expectantly for the child to respond	o If the child communicates, respond with a gesture and language o If the child needs support, use the least intrusive prompt to help the child be successful o Fade prompts over time

FIGURE 13.11. Chapter 13 summary.

Incorporating a Speech-Generating Device

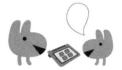

14.1 Introduction

If the child has minimal spoken language, you can incorporate an augmentative and alternative communication (AAC) system in your session to make it easier for the child to request or share with you. There are many types of AAC, including unaided systems (i.e., using only your own body, such as sign language) and aided systems (i.e., using a tool in addition to your body, such as pictures or electronics). AAC can also be low tech (e.g., picture communication systems) or high tech (e.g., speech-generating devices; Beukelman & Mirenda, 2013; Romski, Sevcik, Barton-Hulsey, & Whitmore, 2015). All of these forms of AAC can be included in JASPER. In this chapter, we will focus specifically on speech-generating devices (SGDs), which have been included within JASPER research trials and linked to gains in both augmented and spoken language (Kasari et al., 2014a); however, many of the guidelines in this chapter apply to other modes of AAC as well. The goal is to learn the system, make sure it is clear to the child, and then respond clearly with both augmented and spoken words. If the child has a speech–language pathologist (SLP), you can work together to develop a plan that is tailored to the child and the AAC system. In the sections that follow, we will explain how to set up the device, as well as how to use the communication strategies in Chapters 12 and 13 to imitate, expand, model, and program communication using an SGD.

14.2 Prepare a Communication Device

There are many considerations when preparing an SGD for your session. The goal is to make the device as easy as possible for the child to use in the routine, both in the way you set it up and in the words you choose to include.

14.2.1 Set Up Navigation

Plan additional time to prepare the SGD, as you may need to set up a new device or coordinate using an existing device with the child's caregiver, SLP, and other clinicians. You will need to navigate the device throughout the session, so familiarize yourself with the device, its current organization, and the child's use of the device prior to the session.

Established SGD Users

Get to know the child's existing system and his current familiarity and success with it. Pay close attention to relevant icons that the child is already using. Notice if the child is combining words or creating phrases and sentences. Further, notice if and how the child is navigating the pages by scrolling within pages, or moving among pages or folders, and whether the child is able to program the device to add new icons. Consider how the existing setup is compatible with your JASPER sessions. You may choose to add more relevant icons to the existing setup (e.g., add icons of toys and actions common to your routines). In some cases, it may be better to create a new folder specifically for JASPER sessions so you have more flexibility in organization.

New SGD Users

For many early communicators, you will start by setting up a few icons and increase the number over time. The number of icons on each page can range from a few icons to dozens. Most new users can start with a field of four icons and increase from there. If you start with too many icons, this can be overwhelming and distracting for the child. You may choose to implement an icon discrimination task to evaluate the child's ability to move between icons. For example, you could measure the child's success identifying a known object in a field of four photos, in an array of nine photos, in an array of 16 photos, and so on. This will assist in deciding how many icons you should use per page or screen.

Categorizing Icons

Create folders to organize the icons so they are easy to navigate in the routine (see Figure 14.1). You can have one page or several pages (e.g., one for each routine) to reduce confusion in navigation.

Within each folder, you should have a mixture of words relevant to the routine. For new uses, you may choose to create one page and select a small number of high-frequency nouns and verbs that may occur across routines (see Figure 14.2). You can then expand the number of icons as the

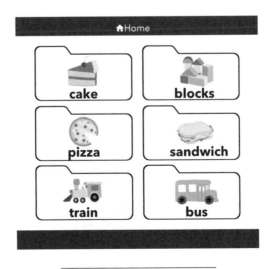

FIGURE 14.1. SGD folders.

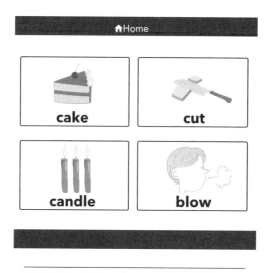

FIGURE 14.2. Example of an SGD page.

child begins to use these first icons. Another option is to create multiple pages (e.g., one for each routine) and organize these within a folder in order to keep only a small number of words on each page.

The number of icons and the specific arrangement of nouns and verbs with SGDs is an ongoing area of research. In JASPER research trials, we have remained flexible in the exact organization of icons. If your child has an SLP, you should collaborate when determining this arrangement.

Physical Access

Consider the size of each icon. In many applications, the icons are often 2 by 2 inches by default. For children with fine motor difficulties, it may be difficult to touch a small icon and much easier to activate icons that are larger in size. Choose the size that is appropriate for your child's needs.

14.2.2 Select Clear Icons

Before each session, update the application with relevant words and icons to the routine. Pick a combination of nouns and verbs that are related to the objects and actions you anticipate communicating about. Select words that can be clearly represented by visuals, either photos or picture symbols. For example, in Figure 14.2, we show an example of a page that uses symbols for a birthday cake routine. We chose a variety of words that best match the steps of the routine (cake, candle, cut, and blow).

Iconicity of Symbols

If you are setting up the device for a new user, consider the iconicity of symbols. Icons can be extremely concrete (like photos of real objects) or abstract (like a drawing). In choosing whether to use photos or symbols for the icons, you will need to assess the child's ability to differentiate among the symbols and understand that a certain symbol or drawing represents an actual object or action. If a child is not able to do so, then taking photos of the actual toys or actions will help the child understand what the icons represent. Figure 14.3 shows different styles of iconicity: a cartoon drawing of a block, a black-and-white line drawing of a block, and a photo of real blocks. Make sure the child is able to understand the level of abstraction you choose.

Language Complexity

Just like spoken language, choose icons that match the child's language level. If the child communicates with one-word utterances, then the icons should reflect single words like simple nouns and verbs. If the child uses two-word combinations, you may consider buttons that speak two words with a single touch, or you can press two buttons in sequence to combine words together. For more sophisticated communicators, you may also consider other aspects of grammar and language complexity (e.g., pronouns, plurals, articles).

Diversity of Words

Consider a mix of nouns and verbs that you frequently use within each routine. For example, in a dollhouse routine, you might choose icons such as doll, bed, sleep, and snore. It is crucial to provide a variety of icon options so your communication remains diverse and interesting.

Function of Language

Provide icons the child can use to both comment (e.g., "Build") and request (e.g., "More"). This requires thinking ahead. Consider what the child is motivated by and might want to communicate with you throughout the session and then provide appropriate icons to accommodate those needs.

14.2.3 Limit Distractions

If the child is easily distracted by other features of the device (e.g., scrolling through icons, using the keyboard, and accessing other applications), then reduce these possible distractions by restricting access to other functions in the settings before introducing the SGD to your session.

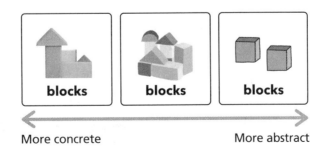

FIGURE 14.3. Different styles of icons require different levels of abstraction.

Remove Access to Other Functions

Some tablets allow you to customize access to applications. You may be able to create a user log-in for the child, limit the child's access to other applications, or require a password to exit out of the AAC application. You may also choose to remove other motivating functions (e.g., games, entertainment applications, internet browsers), so that the purpose of the device is solely for communication. Some applications provide options for editing, access to keyboard, home buttons, scrolling, and so forth. You may choose to disable these functions during the session as well. Some children get distracted by a device's scrolling function. If the device does not allow you to disable the scrolling function, you can arrange icons in folders to reduce scrolling, as illustrated in Figure 14.1, or limit the icons to fit on one page.

14.2.4 Update Vocabulary

Keep the device updated with new words as your routines grow and change across sessions. Revising and adding in new icons is helpful not only for expanding a child's vocabulary but also for children who are not yet initiating language, as it gives them more access to a variety of words. Add more complex word combinations, longer phrases, and number of icons per page as the child's language increases. Remove words and phrases that are typically not used. For example, you might begin the sandwich routine with four to six icons. After several repetitions of the routine across sessions, your page might grow to include a dozen or more words, depending on the child's rate of communication and length of utterance. See Figure 14.4.

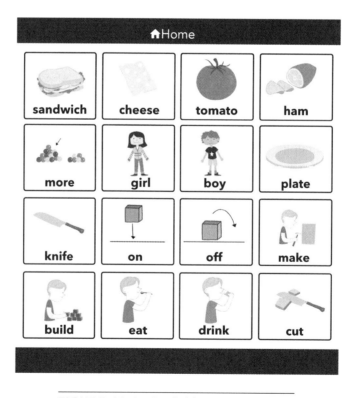

FIGURE 14.4. Sandwich routine SGD page.

14.3 Incorporate the SGD in Session

The same JASPER guidelines for environment and communication apply when using an SGD. Set up the SGD in the environment and use the strategies covered in previous chapters to encourage more communication from the child in the routine.

14.3.1 Environmental Considerations

By incorporating an SGD, you have added a critical component to your physical environment. What used to be a three-part interaction with you, the child, and the toys has now become a four-part interaction with the addition of the SGD. Keep the device easily accessible to the child without disrupting the routine.

Place the SGD within the Child's Reach

Just like the toys, the SGD should be in between you and the child. The screen should be oriented toward the child, not toward you (see Figure 14.5). For children who have difficulty shifting their eyes and bodies, try to make the device even more available to the child. For example, you can prop it up on a small table, chair, or box, or use a case or stand that props the device up toward the child. As you and the child move around the physical space, bring the device with you so it is consistently within the child's reach.

Select the Page Relevant to the Routine

Keep the application updated to the current routine. If you change routines or if you have multiple pages on the SGD, change the page to reflect the current steps.

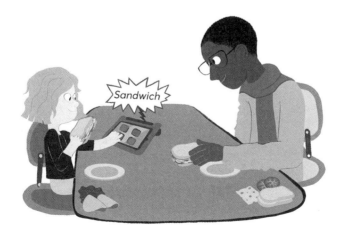

FIGURE 14.5. The SGD device is readily available during the food routine.

14.3.2 Pair Spoken and Augmented Language

Follow the communication guidelines in Chapter 12. As with verbal communication, you should model communication on your turn and leave space for the child to practice communicating on his turn. When you communicate, whether you are modeling language or responding, you will pair your spoken language with the SGD. For example, if you and the child are establishing a base stacking pieces of ice cream, you should use your turn to add a piece to the stack, verbally say "Ice cream," *and* press *ice cream* on the SGD. There is no prescribed order of either pressing the SGD icon or verbally saying a word first, as long as they are modeled closely together. Try to keep the process natural and capitalize on moments when the child is already motivated to communicate with you.

Leave Room for the Child to Communicate

Do not talk or use the SGD on the child's turn; instead, watch carefully to see what she does. In Figure 14.5, the child uses the device on her turn and the adult is prepared to respond. Allow the child time to scan the array of icons on the SGD. We do not want the child to become object engaged with the device, but it is understandable if the child needs more space to decide what she wants to say or to find the correct icon.

Imitate and Expand the Child's Communication

If the child communicates with the device, respond with imitation and a language expansion on your turn. When you are communicating with an SGD, use the device in conjunction with spoken language. You are essentially demonstrating the same word in two different forms, spoken and AAC. For example, in Figure 14.6, the adult responds to and expands on the child's initiation from Figure 14.5 by saying, "Eat the sandwich!" and pressing the *eat* and *sandwich* icons on the SGD. Do not forget to take your play turn as well.

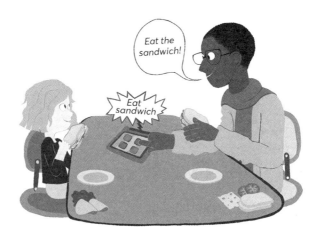

FIGURE 14.6. The adult imitates and expands the child's communication using both spoken and augmented language.

Model Spoken and Augmented Language

If the child does not communicate, model spoken and augmented language on your turn. For example, if the child pretends to take a bite of food, you could pretend to take a bite of food, say, "Eat," and then press the *eat* icon on the SGD.

Use Gestures

Use gestures as you normally would along with your play act. Essentially, you are showing the child up to three forms of communication on your play turn: spoken language, AAC, and a gesture. For example, you can point to the cheese, verbalize "Cheese," and press the *cheese* icon on the SGD. This requires some practice and coordination to perform fluidly. Your hands may feel very busy at first. Remember that you do not have to gesture every turn. Choose moments when the child is most engaged.

   Before learning about programming and prompting with an SGD, test your knowledge on the basic strategies of incorporating an SGD in session using Exercise 14.1.

EXERCISE 14.1. Incorporating a Speech-Generating Device

Identify whether the following statements are true or false.

1. You are only allowed to use words that are programmed into the device during session.	True	False
2. You should set up your device to include nouns, verbs, and parts of speech appropriate to the child's language level.	True	False
3. If a child is distracted by the SGD, you should remove it and no longer attempt using an SGD during session.	True	False
4. When setting up a device, consider the child's understanding of symbols and choose icons the child will understand.	True	False
5. If you use the SGD to imitate or expand language, there is no need to use verbal language or gestures in addition.	True	False
6. Throughout your session, you should move the device so it is facing and in reach of the child.	True	False

---

14.3.3 Programming and Prompting with an SGD

If the child is not starting to use the SGD following your models, you may choose select moments to program and prompt for language and gestures with an SGD, using the same guidelines from Chapter 13. For example, if the child cannot find a toy and does not know how to ask for it, you can pause to help the child use the device to request what he wants. If the child does not communicate, you can increase the support with a prompt. The following are some examples of how to prompt with the SGD. Begin by creating a clear opportunity. For example, the child is looking for a toy, so you move the SGD into the child's sight and reach and pause expectantly. Then, choose an appropriate prompt:

- **Environmental prompt.** Hold up the device as a visual cue for the child to use it or move the device closer to the child.
- **Model.** Show the child how to use the device by activating the icon(s) on your turn.
- **General verbal prompt.** Ask the child what he wants in simple language: "What do you want?" or "What happened?"
- **Specific verbal prompt.** Provide the child with words he can use (e.g., "Say 'block'").
- **Gestural prompt.** Hover your index finger over the icon(s) you intend for the child to use and wait.
- **Partial physical prompt.** Gently touch the child's arm or hand as a reminder to use the device.
- **Full physical prompt.** Physically help the child touch the icon(s) with his index finger.

As always, you will choose the least intrusive prompt to help the child be successful. You may also need to pair prompts. For example, it might be helpful to pair the specific verbal prompt "Say 'block'" with a model of pressing the *block* icon. See Table 14.1 for specific examples of prompting target skills using an SGD.

TABLE 14.1. Programming and Prompting with a Speech-Generating Device (SGD)

Target skill	Create a clear opportunity	Environmental prompt	Model and wait	Gestural prompt	General verbal prompt	Specific verbal prompt	Partial physical prompt	Full physical prompt
Scenario: The adult and child establish a safari routine with figures, wild animals, and a safari truck. Throughout the routine, the adult verbalizes and presses various animal icons on the SGD (e.g., lion, zebra, elephant).								
Language to share	Adult adds the child's favorite dragon figure into the environment next to the various wild animals and pauses.	Adult moves the SGD closer to the child.	Adult models pressing the *dragon* icon on the SGD and pauses.	Adult hovers her index finger over the *dragon* icon.	Adult asks the child, "What do you see?"	Adult instructs the child to "say 'dragon.'"	Adult gently taps on the child's hand or wrist.	Adult gently helps the child press the *dragon* icon with his index finger.
Scenario: The adult and child establish a block routine with magnetic blocks of different shapes. Throughout the routine, the adult verbalizes and presses block on the SGD when it is his turn to add a block.								
Language to request	Adult holds back a block instead of handing it to the child and pauses.	Adult moves the SGD in front of the child.	Adult models pressing the *block* icon on the SGD and pauses.	Adult hovers his index finger over the *block* icon.	Adult asks the child, "What do you want?"	Adult instructs the child to "say 'block.'"	Adult gently taps on the child's hand or wrist.	Adult gently helps the child press the *block* icon with her index finger.

14.4 Common Challenges Incorporating an SGD

As you become familiar with using an SGD in your session, you may encounter some challenges. We have addressed some common questions and case examples below to help your troubleshooting process.

14.4.1 Common Questions

In this section, we address some common questions regarding the SGD.

Can I only use words that are on the SGD?

You are not restricted to the words on the device. If you want to use a word that is not on the device, say the word verbally. It is more important to communicate naturally than to rigidly stick to the prepared icons. If a word continues to be relevant to the routine, you can quickly add the new word as an icon on your page or add it after session.

What if the child presses icons without intentionally communicating?

When first introducing the SGD, the child may need some time to explore and become familiar with it by pressing different icons. This is expected! You should allow the child some time to explore, notice which icons the child tries, and respond by pairing the icon with a relevant toy or action. For example, if the child presses the *cake* icon, you should take your turn to JA show the child the cake; model an action with the cake; verbally say, "Cake!"; and press *cake* on the SGD. While this might sound like a lot of time, it can happen quickly and naturally in the moment. By responding to the icons that the child presses, you show that the SGD is related to specific meaningful actions and consequences. However, if the SGD continues to be distracting throughout sessions, you may need to establish an engaging routine first before you introduce the device. As the child learns its purpose, you should work toward keeping it available for the entire session.

What if the child already uses a communication system other than an SGD?

If a child is already effectively using a different AAC system, such as the Picture Exchange Communication System (PECS; Frost, 2002), manual sign, or picture communication symbols, you can include this method in your JASPER sessions. You should collaborate with the child's other providers (e.g., speech–language pathologist) to apply the child's current system in your sessions. You can then use our core communication strategies, such as imitating, modeling, and expanding communication, with the child's existing AAC system.

14.4.2 Case Examples

The following fictional case examples address challenges with using an SGD specific to a child.

Lost in Translation

Dear JASPER,

The student I am working with is very interested in toys, and she has many great ideas that she adds to our routines. However, she doesn't have very much language, which results in a ton of frustration (for the both of us!). She often looks around the room for something to add to our routine, but because I can't figure out what she needs, she becomes upset and cries. Our great routines are ruined because I'm not able to understand her well. How can I help her express her ideas?

Best,

Lost in Translation

Dear *Lost in Translation,*

We know this can be frustrating, but the great news is that you've assessed the situation and appear to have identified the reason behind this behavior. Although it must be very frustrating for the child to have ideas to share and not have the message understood, we appreciate that she is continuing to try. First, let's assess the environment. Are there ways that you can organize the environment so the toys are more easily accessible? Try placing toys on a shelf within the child's reach or in clear containers to help the child see the options available. We also suggest incorporating an AAC device in your session to help provide access to more vocabulary. This will give her another way to share her ideas and request for toys. Try to include icons for the toys and actions you use most often in your routines as well as language for some novel steps. When the child uses the AAC, continue expanding spoken words to comment and request as well . For example, if she presses the icon for *car,* respond verbally by saying, "Green car!"; model pressing the buttons *green* and *car*; and give her the car.

Keep it up!

JASPER

Stressed with the SGD

Dear JASPER,

I am working with a child who has minimal spoken language, and I think he could really benefit from using an SGD. I have set up a folder for our session with icons for the toys that we use. I also try to have it easily accessible to him during session, but it just sits there and the child doesn't use it to communicate. If anything, he seems to get distracted by looking at the SGD screen. How can I better support his learning with the SGD?

Stressed with the SGD

Dear *Stressed with the SGD,*

You are doing great at having the SGD set up and present in your session! It can be common for children to want to explore something new, especially something technology related. First, since this is a new form of communication and may be distracting, start with just a few icons that match the toys you are playing with. Next, model how to use the SGD to comment and request, for example, press the corresponding icon and also say the word on your play turn. This will provide the child with opportunities to imitate your models. If he does not start to imitate, you may choose to introduce programming opportunities and directive prompts (e.g., a physical prompt) to show him how to use the SGD. Remember to keep the SGD within sight and reach of the child throughout the session and open to icons that are relevant to the routine you're working on. This can be easy to forget when you are focused on the other JASPER strategies; however, it is critical to provide consistent opportunities to practice using the SGD.

Good luck!

JASPER

14.5 Conclusion

Incorporating an SGD is helpful in providing the child with consistent language models and an additional modality to communicate. Prepare the SGD ahead of time and keep it available throughout session, so it is easy for the child to use. Review the strategies checklist in Figure 14.7.

This concludes Part V. Now that we have introduced the strategies for play and communication, we will move on to Part VI, which covers challenges with engagement, regulation, and restricted and repetitive patterns of behavior (RRBs).

Chapter 14 Summary

PREPARE A SPEECH-GENERATING DEVICE	USE AN SGD DURING SESSION
○ Choose an SGD	○ Keep the SGD in sight and reach
○ Match the number and type of icons to the child's language level	○ Use SGD and spoken language on your turn to model or respond
○ Organize the icons	○ Keep your language natural
○ Reduce distractions and other functions	○ Program for communication with the SGD
○ Keep vocabulary up to date	

FIGURE 14.7. Chapter 14 summary.

PART VI

TROUBLESHOOTING

In this section, you will learn how to use core and conditional strategies to troubleshoot the child's engagement, regulation, and productive play.

Goals

✓ Increase time spent engaged and regulated

✓ Increase quality of interactions

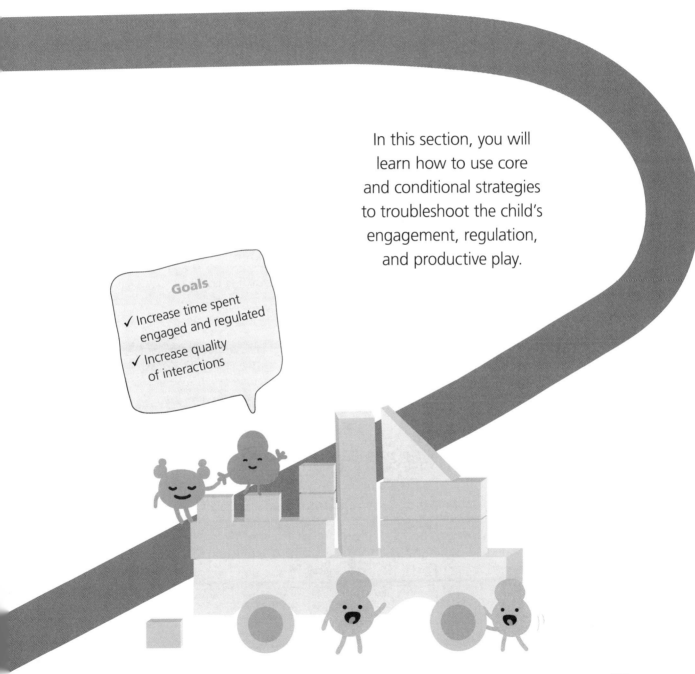

Supporting Engagement

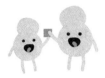

15.1 Introduction

In this chapter, we return to the concept of engagement. As we discussed in Chapter 2, children with ASD spend less time jointly engaged than their typically developing peers. Without support, they might show a variety of challenges with engagement, such as wandering, difficulty choosing a toy, jumping from toy to toy, or difficulty staying in one routine. Children with ASD also spend more time in the lower states of engagement, such as unengaged and object engaged, with reduced instances of play and communication initiations. Our goal is to help children transition out of the lower states of engagement and into joint engagement, which provides a crucial context for learning. It is in this joint engaged state, attending to objects and people, that we can best address the many targets and goals of JASPER. This requires active participation and support from the adult. After all, a state of joint engagement cannot occur without your participation too. We have already set the foundation for supporting engagement in Chapter 8. Now, we will apply the ACT troubleshooting framework to the domain of engagement to increase quality and duration of the child's engagement across session (see Figure 15.1).

We will first explain how to assess engagement in the moment, noticing signs of joint engagement and diminishing engagement. Then we will explain how to create a plan using the core and conditional strategies. The *core* strategies from Chapters 5–14 make up the bulk of our approach

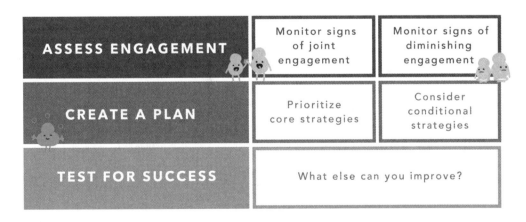

ASSESS ENGAGEMENT	Monitor signs of joint engagement	Monitor signs of diminishing engagement
CREATE A PLAN	Prioritize core strategies	Consider conditional strategies
TEST FOR SUCCESS	What else can you improve?	

FIGURE 15.1. ACT on engagement.

257

to engagement. They foster engagement and provide our first line of support when engagement declines. The *conditional* strategies can be applied in select cases when the child needs additional support to improve engagement. We will intersperse some case examples throughout to help illustrate the strategies and provide some guidelines for how to blend these strategies together. At the end of the chapter, we will use common questions and a case vignette to show how you can test for success. We do not attempt to provide all the information necessary to address challenges with engagement in this chapter but rather offer a introduction to our approach. Additional information and feedback are provided during training. In training, you will learn how to individualize your approach to the child, choose the right strategy for the moment, blend the core and conditional strategies together, and fade support over time.

15.2 Assess Engagement

In JASPER, we monitor the child's engagement throughout the routine. We try to get a sense of the child's baseline engagement from the SPACE assessment and the first few sessions, and then pay close attention to changes in engagement. Figure 15.2 shows common signs that indicate more and less engagement. Most children will not be able to spend the entire interaction jointly engaged (and some children may spend very little time at first). As you learn more about the child's indicators of joint engagement, you can provide support responsive to the child's needs.

15.2.1 Assess the Level of Interference

Notice the degree to which engagement has decreased.

- ***Mildly diminished engagement.*** The child is still playing, but the quality of the social interaction is diminished or inconsistent. This may include a slight decrease in social communication,

SIGNS OF JOINT ENGAGEMENT	SIGNS OF DIMINISHING ENGAGEMENT
○ Increased shared attention marked by eye contact ○ Use of joint attention gestures and language ○ Use of requesting gestures and language ○ Social, interactive, and cooperative play ○ Acknowledgment of interaction partner ○ Increased shared affect	○ Shift in attention (e.g., looking around the room) ○ Shift in body position or moving away from the interaction ○ Decrease in social communication ○ Intense focus on toys ○ Increase in RRBs ○ Increase in dysregulation ○ Change in pace ○ Change in affect

FIGURE 15.2. Signs of engagement.

pace, or affect. The child might take longer than usual to take play turns and occasionally glance around the room.

• **Moderately diminished engagement.** The child is still attending to the routine but has noticeably slowed down and has shifted to moments of object engagement or onlooking. There is a noticeable decrease in communication, attention, and affect (see Figure 15.3). The pace may have slowed or increased considerably. The child might watch you take turns, fiddle with the toys, become restless, and look for something else to do.

• **Significantly diminished engagement.** The child is *unengaged or object engaged* and no longer attending to the play routine. The child might leave the play space and become agitated, upset, or dysregulated. The child may actively reject or stop your turns. Or he might stay in place without attending to anything and become so focused on the object or toy that he is no longer aware of the social partner or interaction.

When the challenges are mild to moderate, you can typically respond with the core strategies. When challenges are moderate to significant, the child may need a mix of core and conditional strategies, as illustrated in Figure 15.4.

15.3 Create a Plan to Increase Engagement

In this section, we will discuss the core and conditional strategies we use to support engagement throughout the routine. These serve as a "toolbox" of supports, which can be applied based on the individual needs of the child and the difficulty of the situation. When the challenges are mild to moderate, the core strategies typically suffice. When challenges are moderate to significant, the child may need a mix of core and conditional strategies. In general, we try to notice the child's patterns of behavior over time and use these strategies to provide support *before* the child becomes unengaged. Figure 15.5 illustrates the distinctions between core and conditional strategies for engagement.

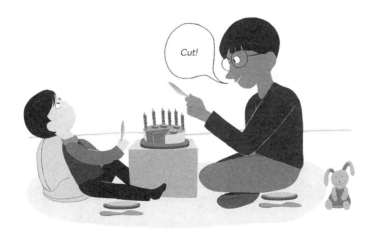

FIGURE 15.3. The child shows signs that he's losing engagement by gazing toward the ceiling.

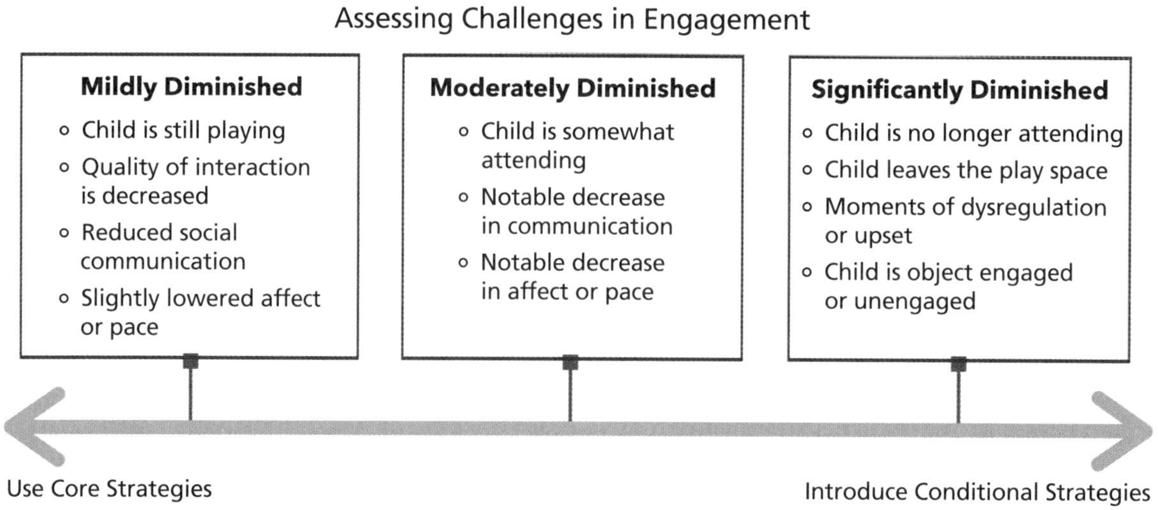

Assessing Challenges in Engagement

Mildly Diminished
- Child is still playing
- Quality of interaction is decreased
- Reduced social communication
- Slightly lowered affect or pace

Moderately Diminished
- Child is somewhat attending
- Notable decrease in communication
- Notable decrease in affect or pace

Significantly Diminished
- Child is no longer attending
- Child leaves the play space
- Moments of dysregulation or upset
- Child is object engaged or unengaged

Use Core Strategies   Introduce Conditional Strategies

FIGURE 15.4. Monitor the severity of the child's engagement in order to effectively respond.

15.3.1 Core Strategies for Engagement

When troubleshooting engagement, begin by evaluating your use of core strategies. Many of the strategies we introduced in Chapters 5–14 also improve engagement. By choosing toys, setting up the environment, building routines, and fostering communication, you are also facilitating engagement! In Figure 15.6, the adult facilitates each aspect of the interaction to encourage joint engagement in the routine. In this section, we will explain how these familiar strategies (italicized in the text below) can be applied specifically toward engagement, both to set the child up for success and to respond to moments of diminishing engagement. Then we will introduce some case examples to illustrate specifically how this works.

STRATEGIES TO SUPPORT ENGAGEMENT ☑

Core Strategies
- ☐ Manage the environment
- ☐ Be an equal and active play partner
- ☐ Promote productive and flexible play
- ☐ Establish and expand routines
- ☐ Respond to communication

Conditional Strategies
- ☐ Use person engagement to reconnect
- ☐ Introduce a well-mastered routine

FIGURE 15.5. Strategies to support engagement.

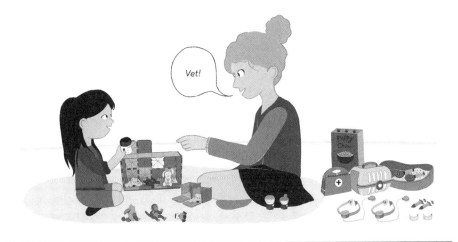

FIGURE 15.6. The adult responds to the child's initiation of showing the vet character.

Manage the Environment

Set up the environment to maximize engagement and minimize distractions. Make sure the child always has *developmentally appropriate toy choices available,* and *modify the number of toys* as you go. There should be enough choices to maintain the child's engagement, but not so many that it leads to distraction. Ensure you are in an *optimal position* with the toys in between you and the child. Move along with the child, so you can monitor engagement and respond to any social bids. Throughout the session, be sure to *add options for expansions* into the environment to extend the child's engagement in each routine. If challenges arise, *reorganize the environment* to provide support. Declutter the play space, consider moving to the table or floor, and reevaluate your choice of toys. See more in Chapter 7.

Be an Equal and Active Player

Show the child what it looks like to engage with a social partner by *playing and communicating during the routine.* Avoid passively facilitating or overly directing the play as these roles make it harder for the child to engage. Ensure you are providing a balance in your role and *leaving room for the child to initiate* play and communication throughout. If the child begins playing too slowly or too quickly, help *modulate the pace* of the routine so you are both connected and playing together. If the child's affect is too high or low, *modulate your own affect* to support an appropriate state. See more in Chapters 5, 8, and 10.

Promote Productive and Flexible Play

Roadblocks in play can create significant challenges reaching joint engagement. *Avoid toys and actions that are too distracting,* that is, toys that lead to interfering actions and periods of object engagement. Follow the child's play ideas as much as possible, using *consistent and immediate imitation* to acknowledge and respond to the child's efforts to engage. If the child starts to lose engagement or play becomes less productive, *model* an appropriate play act (see also Chapter 17).

You may also need to remove interfering toys for a time and try incorporating them again at a later time. See more in Chapters 6 and 9.

Establish and Expand Routines

Establish the base of the routine to provide a foundation for the child's engagement. If the sequence of the routine becomes too difficult or loses direction, you could *return to an earlier step* or *restart the routine* to ensure a clear direction in the routine. Incorporate a combination of *horizontal and vertical expansions* to increase motivation and lengthen the routine. Consider *bridging* established routines together to increase the child's duration of engagement throughout session. Support the child to stay in the routine as long as you can. *Transition to a new routine* when the child shows interest in a new toy or activity or when the current routine is no longer productive or engaging. See more in Chapters 5, 10, and 11.

Respond to Communication

Leave plenty of room for the child to communicate and *respond to the child's social communication bids.* This shows the child that you are interested in what he has to say and builds on this moment of engagement. If the child is not communicating, *model appropriate language* to show the child what it looks like to be an engaged social partner and help invite the child into a higher state of engagement. See more in Chapter 12.

Use Exercise 15.1 to practice matching the JASPER strategies we have already covered to four scenarios.

EXERCISE 15.1. **Supporting Engagement**

Match each scenario with the most appropriate strategy to support engagement.

Description of the interaction	Potential strategies
1. During the SPACE, the child is able to build a house with blocks, put the puzzle animals in the house, brush the dolls, and mix cookies in a bowl. You start the session with a peg board and nesting boxes. The child looks around the room, reluctantly places a peg in the board, and then turns away from you.	A. Choose developmentally appropriate toy choices B. Leave room on the child's turn C. Move in front of the child
2. You and the child have each taken 10 turns putting toppings into a tummy stuffer. You notice the child slow down his turn taking and lessen his communication even though you are imitating putting the toppings in.	A. Use consistent and immediate imitation B. Maintain the routine with expansions C. Model appropriate language

3. You and the child are putting pretend food into a blender. This routine used to launch into a breakfast and packing for school routine, but now the routine is not progressing past the base. Even though you are playing at the child's level and have tried to model several different expansions, she is becoming increasingly less engaged and is showing signs of early dysregulation.

   A. Transition to a new routine

   B. Establish the base

   C. Move in front of the child

4. You want to see the child's idea for a new routine, so you watch as he puts people into a rocket. You talk about what he is doing, but he does not seem to notice you are there.

   A. Use consistent and immediate imitation

   B. Remove interfering toys

   C. Modulate your affect

15.3.2 Conditional Strategies for Engagement

Whereas the core strategies are used throughout the sessions, the conditional strategies are only necessary in select cases to prevent or respond to lower states of engagement. When the child's behaviors become moderately or significantly interfering, you can use the conditional strategies to build social connection and reestablish engagement before returning to the normal demands of the routine once again. We will explain the basic guidelines of each strategy below and then provide some case examples to illustrate them in action.

Use Person Engagement to Reconnect

Use periods of person engagement to transition from lowers states of engagement (such as unengaged, onlooking, or object engaged) into a higher state of engagement (supported or coordinated joint engaged). This moment of person engagement could be a song or a simple activity, for example:

- **Children's songs:** The alphabet song, "Itsy Bitsy Spider," "Row, Row, Row Your Boat"
- **Simple games:** Peek-a-boo (for very young kids), tickle games, clapping games (e.g., Patty Cake)
- **Big action games:** Swinging, jumping

As you use person engagement, continue to use the JASPER communication strategies. Respond to the child's communication, model language and gestures, and maintain an equal and active role. Once you are connected with the child and in a rich state of person engagement, add the toys back in to move into a state of joint engagement. This strategy can be used at various points in the session, depending on the child's needs. You can also use person engagement as a segue into the routine at the beginning of the session, in between routines, after a period of dysregulation, or as a fun motivating step in the routine (see Figure 15.7). Here are some examples:

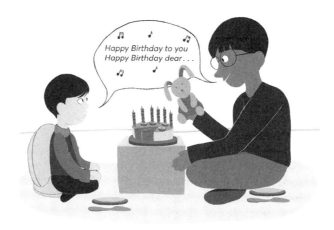

FIGURE 15.7. The adult sings "Happy Birthday" to include person engagement into a cake routine.

- Around 30 minutes into the session, the child usually becomes tired and dysregulated. To get in front of this, prepare a song or activity ahead of time that you can pair with one of the routines, then introduce this step before the child becomes dysregulated to help the child stay motivated and engaged.

- After the child has been crying and dysregulated, she begins to calm down but has not yet shown interest in toys. Sing "Wheels on the Bus," put people on the bus as you sing, and stop singing the song once the child is playing along.

Introduce a Well-Mastered Routine

Prepare a routine at the mastered play level (or one step below) for moments when the child has lower engagement. This could be a familiar routine, a highly motivating routine, or a well-mastered routine that you prepared in Chapter 6, Section 6.2.1. Here are some examples:

- For a child who plays at a general combination level, put shape figures into a shape sorter to establish engagement (presentation combination); then take turns stacking the nesting boxes (general combination) and putting figures into the open nesting boxes (child as agent).
- For a child who plays at the symbolic level, you could first build a dungeon for the dragons (physical combination) to establish engagement and then dress up dolls as heroes who will charge the dungeon (doll as agent).

Once the child's engagement increases, you can transition back to a routine at the child's developmental level.

Take a moment to practice using these conditional strategies to respond to a child's fragile engagement in Exercise 15.2.

EXERCISE 15.2. **Responding to Fragile Engagement**

Identify the best way(s) to support the child's fragile engagement using core or conditional strategies.

1. At the beginning of the session, you try to establish a routine at the child's mastered play level with a base step of putting pieces of cake onto plates, but the child is onlooking and does not take any turns. How could you alter your routine to increase engagement?

    A. Physically prompt the child to take her turn so she is an active participant in the play.

    B. Start the routine with a lower-level combination of sticking candles on the cake.

    C. Use person engagement by singing "Happy Birthday" before beginning to put the cake onto plates.

    D. Either B or C

2. The child takes one to two turns with a toy before moving on to another toy, making it difficult to engage him long enough to establish a base routine. What should you do?

    A. Always follow the child's lead so you are imitating each action.

    B. Limit other toy choices in the environment until the base is established.

    C. Tap or call attention to the toy that the child is supposed play with.

    D. Allow the child to explore each toy for the first half of the session and then narrow down his choices.

3. The child initiates building a block structure, so you begin handing her pieces to facilitate her idea. You try commenting on what she is doing but notice she has become object engaged and is visually inspecting the blocks. How can you help her to reach joint engagement?

    A. Withhold each piece so that the child has to look at you and request for more blocks to put on the tower.

    B. Quickly take away the blocks and introduce a different toy instead.

    C. Add the verbal prompt "look at me" before each turn so she will notice you.

    D. Pair your comments with your turn so you have an equal and active role.

4. Throughout the session, you have struggled to successfully establish a routine despite using environmental strategies, taking an equal and active role, and modeling fun new steps. You almost had a routine started at the child's play level, but he kept turning away and losing engagement. What change could you try to help the child engage?

    A. Switch to playing with only sensory toys since he is having an off day.

    B. Introduce tangible reinforcers, like gummy bears, whenever he takes a turn.

    C. Offer a well-mastered routine and then build up to target-level routines.

    D. Add verbal prompts on each of his turns to help him learn the routine.

15.4 Test Your Plan for Engagement

After implementing your plan, you will likely notice more ways you can improve upon it. As you reflect, consider what changes you can make to support the child more proactively. There is almost always something more you can do to set the child up for success and to improve your response. In the sections below, we explain how to improve your approach over time and answer some common questions about this process. Last, we provide a vignette that shows how an interventionist uses the ACT framework throughout session to balance core strategies and conditional strategies.

15.4.1 Plan for the Future

As the intervention progresses, remain responsive to changes in the child's motivation and engagement. Make sure to update the environment, toys, and supports as necessary to support the child's needs. As you get to know the child, you should get more efficient at responding. This typically results in less time in lower states of engagement and fewer conditional strategies.

Get Ahead of Patterns of Unengagement

Over time and with familiarity, you may begin to notice certain patterns of unengagement. Instead of responding when challenges arise, you should begin to spot the pattern earlier and provide support before it is too late. As you get to know the strategies that work best for the child, you should also become more successful and recover more quickly after a period of unengagement.

Fade Support

It is important to continually update your approach as the child progresses. After several sessions, think about where the child started in terms of engagement and where you are now. Are the strategies you initially used still relevant? In most cases, you should be able to fade support, so you are relying less and less on the conditional strategies and more on the core strategies. You should expect changes in the child's capacity to engage; adjust your expectations and level of support accordingly.

As you support engagement, look at the bigger picture and broader goals of the session. If you become overly reliant on the conditional strategies, the overall progress of the session will stagnate. While some aspects of engagement might improve in the moment (e.g., child moves from unengaged to person engaged), using primarily conditional strategies can also limit opportunities to be jointly engaged and work toward new skills. Thus, the conditional strategies should only serve as a transitional period to help support the child back into higher states of joint engagement.

15.4.2 Common Questions

In this section, we address some common questions regarding engagement strategies.

How do I recover from periods of low engagement more efficiently?

When the child becomes unengaged, it can be difficult to return quickly to a higher state. This can be frustrating when you are trying to spend as much time as possible jointly engaged in routines. Here are some tips to respond quickly and efficiently:

- Increase support at the first signs of diminishing engagement, *before* the child becomes too object engaged or loses engagement entirely.

- Keep the conditional strategies brief. There is no need to continue these strategies once the child is engaged.

- Once the child connects with you, try to return to a high-quality routine. This may be as simple as restarting the base, moving a toy forward, or modeling an action in the current routine, or it may require starting over with a new routine.

- Troubleshoot other aspects of the interaction if the child's engagement remains lower than you expect it to be. Perhaps the play level is off, the child needs more environmental structure, or you need to spend more time establishing the base before you expand. You should not have to rely heavily on the conditional strategies to keep the child engaged.

- Get ahead of recurring patterns. If you know a particular aspect of the session or routine is difficult for the child, provide extra support leading up to this moment.

- Build the child's endurance for engagement over time. You should see an increase in the child's capacity to engage.

How do I determine what strategy to choose?

The answer is highly dependent on the child, the degree of difficulty, the challenge itself, and also whether this is an isolated challenge or a recurring pattern. In general, start with the least amount of support necessary to help the child reengage and increase support from there. As you gain training and experience, you will improve in your approach, choosing the right strategy from your toolbox of supports to help the child return to a state of joint engagement.

What if the child is not interested in the routine?

Sometimes routines come to a natural end, or the child will lose motivation to play with certain toys despite your efforts to maintain engagement. As long as this is not happening so frequently that you rarely establish a solid routine, it is often appropriate to follow the child's interest and transition to a new routine (see more considerations in Chapter 11, Figure 11.11). This is similar to the process covered in Chapter 8 of starting the session. To begin a new routine, start by adding new choices into the environment while leaving the current routine available. If the child starts playing with one of the new choices on his own, follow him to the new toy and imitate his first play acts to establish the base. If the child needs support to start a new routine, you can help the child make a choice by holding up two different options. For example, you can ask if the child wants the current toy or a new toy. If the child seems interested in a toy but does not initiate a play act, you can model the first step.

What if I get stuck in person engagement?

If you are getting "stuck" in longer periods of person engagement, assess when person engagement is occurring. If the child is receiving fun periods of person engagement, and thus avoiding or escaping challenging play with objects, then you may see routines becomes shorter. To support more time in play routines, you may try a "first, then" verbal statement or visual to help the child understand that you heard her request for person engagement but will play before the person engagement routine. You may also be able to incorporate person engagement as a single step within a routine.

Why does engagement seem so different across routines?

There are many reasons a child's engagement might vary across routines. The most obvious cases are when the child is not motivated by the steps, the steps of the routine are at the wrong play level, or the child has grown tired of the same thing. You may also see less engagement at the beginning or end of the session. Another common explanation is the complexity of the routine. Sometimes engagement and regulation look different depending on the skills you are targeting and the level of demand in a routine. If the child has mastered physical combinations, he may have higher engagement, longer routines, and more initiations, because these steps are comfortable and familiar. Contrast this with a routine involving agents, in which the majority of the steps in the routine are less familiar to the child. Understandably, the child will have less engagement, shorter routines, and fewer initiations when the routine is more complex. Different routines progress at different paces. It is good to have a mix to support different skills. The goal is to see an upward trajectory in engagement within each of these routines, even if it varies across routines.

15.4.3 Case Examples

In the following cases examples, we illustrate how these core and conditional strategies can be incorporated to respond to challenges that may arise during the session.

Fizzling Out

Dear JASPER,

At the start of our session, the child is ready to go. She makes a choice from the routines I've set up and has recently started initiating expansions once we establish the base. It feels as if we've added about 20 expansions beyond our base. For example, we have a castle routine where we build the castle, royalty comes riding in on horses, pirates storm the castle, and sometimes our moat even overflows and the people have to climb the castle tower. But after a while she just doesn't seem interested in the routine anymore. I keep trying to add new steps, but she starts to fidget a lot, which usually leads to her shoes coming off so she can play with the laces. At this point, I clear away the old toys and bring out new ones, but she doesn't make a choice easily as in the beginning. I'm not sure how to keep her interested anymore. Where do I go from here?

Thanks for your help!

Fizzling Out

Dear *Fizzling Out,*

It's great that you have developed creative, complex routines. Even if you have a really robust routine, children might get bored with the toys and story after some time. This is expected, so your job is to notice when the child is beginning to lose interest and provide some new toy options before she loses engagement. You have done a good job assessing your routines and noticing that you need to add expansions. We'd like to offer a few more strategies. Within the pirate routine, you could try to mix up the steps to create a new base and different story with the same materials. Another option is to start the same base of the pirate routine and then offer opportunities to bridge to other routines. For example, if you were playing with princesses and knights in a castle, you could bring out food toys to bridge with a baking routine, and then you could hold a feast. However, if these materials seem less interesting at this point, another option is to offer different routine choices at the start of your session and put the pirates aside for a little bit. You may find a natural moment to bring the pirates back into another routine as an expansion or bridge.

Keep playing!

JASPER

I Want It All

Dear JASPER,

I am supporting a child who is brand new to JASPER. His play skills are just emerging, and I am excited to support advancement in his play. At this point, we tend to have shorter routines with more periods of person engagement, because he isn't particularly motivated by the toys. When I notice he's starting to fade in a routine (e.g., starts to turn away or no longer reaches for toys), I'll start a song or tickle game. But I notice we're spending less and less time with toys. I want to be able to have more toy-based routines, but I'm not sure how to build on them without relying so heavily on person engagement. How do I incorporate more toy-based play and joint engagement in our routines?

Thanks,

I Want It All

Dear *I Want It All,*

You're on the right track aiming to add more toy-based routines to your sessions. For some children, person engagement can help ease them into JASPER sessions. It is also appropriate for this child to have periods of person engagement, since he is just starting to learn to play with toys; however, we want to be careful not to use person engagement after play has become challenging or dysregulation has begun, because this reinforces the child's desire to escape the demand. Instead of waiting until the child loses engagement, try adding a song and increasing your affect earlier in the routine to help the child maintain motivation.

Keep it up!

JASPER

Patty Cake

Dear JASPER,

I am pretty confident that my child plays at a symbolic level. During the SPACE, he pretended that the cookies were hot and sang the "Happy Birthday" song to the baby doll. This is my second session with him, and I am struggling to keep him engaged. I introduced fun food routines (a kitchen set, the birthday cake with the oven mitts, and baby dolls with a bath set), but he seemed unimpressed. I feel as if I am modeling play acts all the time, and he's not following along! What am I doing wrong?

Sincerely,
Patty Cake

Dear *Patty Cake,*

It's great that you are trying to keep up with the child's highest play level, but with only two acts, he has not yet mastered symbolic play. It may be too challenging right now for the child to stay engaged with play at this level. Review the child's SPACE data and create a plan to introduce routines with base steps at the child's mastered presymbolic level. It sounds as if he likes food routines, so you can bring those out again for your next session. Try conventional combination play by building the cake and putting it in the oven or cutting the slices and putting them on plates. If he is engaged with this base routine, you can expand horizontally by adding utensils or setting the table. One you have momentum in the base, then you can work your way up to singing "Happy Birthday" and feeding dolls, but don't rush it. And remember, if you vertically expand to feeding the dolls and you think he is losing interest, you can move back to presymbolic play by extending the cake to yourself (pretend self) or restarting the routine.

You're doing great!
JASPER

15.4.4 ACT in Action

The following vignette shows how you can use the ACT framework to troubleshoot as you encounter challenges in engagement throughout the session.

> *The child and adult are establishing a veterinarian routine where they build a pet hospital and put animals inside. The child is motivated by the routine, and they have several fun steps right from the start. The adult decides to restart the routine to make sure the child is comfortable with these steps, as she notices that the child keeps fidgeting. On the third time through, the child abruptly stands up and disengages from the routine (see Figure 15.8). Once the child is unengaged, the adult has a difficult time reengaging her in the routine, and a lot of time is spent trying to reestablish the base. The adult assesses the situation in the moment and creates a plan to try restarting earlier, thinking the child might need more support to establish the base. When this does not work, she decides that maybe an expansion is what the child needs. She tries this in the moment and sees some improvement but is not yet confident in this approach. Feeling uncertain of how to proceed, the adult decides to fill out the ACT framework at the end of the session to look closer at what might be going on.*

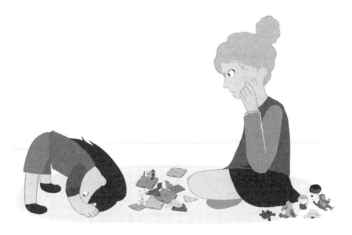

FIGURE 15.8. The child becomes unengaged during the restart of the routine.

See Figure 15.9 for an example of her filled-out form, as well as below for a discussion of her thought process.

- ***Assess the situation.*** The adult notices a few key changes in the routine and the child's behavior. First, she realizes the challenges seem to arise near the end of the base, surrounding the moments when they restart the routine. She also notices that the child fidgets with the toys and seems less interested in playing as the routine progresses. She realized she had been introducing the expansion too late! This makes sense given that the child is becoming increasingly comfortable with the routine and is likely ready to expand sooner than she used to be. The adult now has a clear basis for plan.

- ***Create a plan.*** The adult decides that she has been restarting the routine too frequently and that she should make the expansion options available earlier. She also realizes that she has not been updating the expansion options and prepares a few new steps that she thinks will be motivating. She considers a brief person engagement song she could include as a conditional support if the child does lose engagement to reduce the amount of time she spends wandering and unengaged.

- ***Test for success.*** In the next session, the adult tests her plan. She monitors the child closely throughout the routine. After the second time through the base, the child starts fidgeting, so the adult puts the expansion materials out in the environment. The child turns away. The adult realizes she is still too late; the child is already standing up and turning away from the toys. So, the adult uses a moment of person engagement to reengage the child. The next time through, the adult introduces the expansion options into the environment much sooner. The child initiates a new step. The adult imitates, and they expand the routine!

After the session, the adult reflects on what she did well and where she could improve. She makes note to expand sooner and have person engagement in her back pocket as an option to help the child stay engaged. These steps are a success, and she is pleased that she no longer loses the child's engagement as frequently as before. In thinking ahead, the adult suspects that the child will not need person engagement to restart the routine for long and plans to be quick and efficient in resetting the environment so the child is less reliant on the song. She even has a creative

ACT: Assess the situation, Create a plan, and Test for success

Child: _S. S._ Adult: _W. S._ Date: _September 08_

Assess the situation: What happened? What challenges occurred in the routine or in the child's behavior?

Check the routine	Check the child's behavior
—Was able to establish the base —Restarted the base three times —Child started having difficulty restarting	—Child loses engagement —Fidgets with toys —Seems less interested in play Try using the "Check the Child's Behavior" Form!

Create a plan: What can I do to help? How can I use core strategies and conditional strategies to produce change?

Change the environment	Change your own actions	Respond to the function of the child's behavior
—Increase variety of expansions available **Core Strategies**	—Increase pacing of expansions —Monitor signs the child is ready to move on —Choose to expand instead of restart **Conditional Strategies** —Add in person engagement	N/A

Prioritize core strategies
- Arrange the environment
- Imitate and model
- Establish play routines
- Expand play routines
- Use communication strategies
- Program for gestures and language
- Support engagement and regulation
- Support productive play

Consider conditional strategies
- Incorporate visual supports
- Use directive prompts
- Use conditional strategies for engagement and regulation
- Prepare for fading

Test for success: Did my plan have the intended effect? Is there anything I can improve in the future?

Note what worked	Plan for the future

—Person engagement was effective!
—It worked well to expand sooner in the routine
	—Have expansions prepared as soon as the base is established
	—Fade person engagement
	—Pre-build part of the structure to quicken the restart
	—Prepare more routines that we could bridge together
	   —go to the park
	   —make and eat food
	   —go home
	
	Prepare to fade support!

FIGURE 15.9. Filled-out example of the ACT framework form (Form 8.1 in Chapter 8).

idea to prebuild part of the vet structure, so they do not have to start over from the very beginning each time they restart, thus supporting a quicker transition back into the routine. Last, she thinks about the different routines they have established over the last few weeks and brainstorms ways to bridge each one together to extend the child's engagement.

15.5 Conclusion

Over time, as you provide support, there should be a growing momentum in the child's engagement and improvement toward the child's goals. You should be able to increase the amount of time in routines and increase the child's ability to coordinate the interaction, marked by more initiations of play and communication. Where you may have lost the child's engagement before, you are able to maintain engagement for longer periods of time. This process often takes time. You must continue to monitor the child's engagement and choose the right level of support in your response. We provide additional information and feedback in training to help you individualize your approach to the child and balance these strategies along with our other goals. Before moving on, review strategies to support engagement in Figure 15.10.

Chapter 15 Summary

ASSESS ENGAGEMENT	CREATE A PLAN TO INCREASE ENGAGEMENT	TEST YOUR PLAN FOR ENGAGEMENT
○ Look for signs of engagement ○ Look for signs of diminishing engagement ○ Assess the severity of diminished engagement	○ Use core strategies 　▪ Promote engagement 　▪ Respond to mild to moderate challenges 　▪ Use strategies from Ch. 5–14 ○ Consider adding conditional strategies 　▪ Use person engagement 　▪ Introduce a well-mastered routine	○ Plan strategies to support the child in the future ○ Be proactive and get ahead of patterns of behavior ○ Fade support

FIGURE 15.10. Chapter 15 summary.

Supporting Regulation

16.1 Introduction

In this chapter, we will return to the concept of regulation. As discussed in Chapter 2, children with ASD may experience episodes of dysregulation that are greater in type and degree than typically developing peers (Sofronoff et al., 2007). As a JASPER interventionist, it is your responsibility to support regulation through the routine. When moments of dysregulation arise, our goal is to help the child return to a regulated state and reduce the frequency and intensity of future episodes of dysregulation. We recognize that this can be a difficult process and an individualized approach is necessary to address each child's unique needs. In Chapter 8, we set the groundwork to promote the child's regulation. Here, we will follow the ACT troubleshooting framework to increase periods of regulation and respond to dysregulation (see Figure 16.1).

We will begin this chapter explaining how to assess the child's regulation in the moment, notice early signs of dysregulation, and create a hypothesis regarding the function of the behavior. Next, we will explain how to create a plan. Similar to engagement, there are two levels of support for regulation: core strategies and conditional strategies. The core strategies in Chapters 5–15 can be used to promote regulation and respond to dysregulation. The conditional strategies provide a second level of support and can be used in select moments, responsive to the function of the child's behavior. Finally, we will explain how to test the plan for success and reflect on areas for improvement. We do not attempt to provide all the information necessary to address dysregulation in this

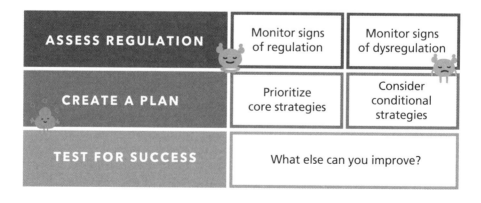

FIGURE 16.1. ACT on regulation.

chapter but rather offer a brief introduction to our approach along with some common strategies we use. Additional information and feedback are provided in training. There you will learn how to individualize your approach to the child and balance these strategies along with our other goals.

16.2 Assess Regulation

To support regulation, you must actively monitor the child throughout the session. Use your experience from the SPACE and early sessions to learn the signs that indicate the child is regulated and the cues of dysregulation (see Figure 16.2).

16.2.1 Assess the Level of Interference

Dysregulation can affect the child and the interaction in varying degrees.

- *Mildly interfering.* You are able to continue in a routine, and the child may or may not require additional support. The child may be slightly fussy, display a less pleasant affect, or begin to exhibit more repetitive behaviors.

- *Moderately interfering.* You are able to continue in a routine, but the child requires your support to do so. The child may take fewer play turns, disrupt the environment (e.g., swipe toys off of the table), or seem antsy and uncomfortable in his body.

- *Significantly interfering.* You are no longer able to play, and the child needs help to return to a regulated state. The child may refuse to play, move about the space, communicate inappropriately (e.g., screaming) or show some signs of aggression. (The most severe forms of dysregulation include aggressive or injurious behaviors toward self or others.)

Children often display early signs of diminishing regulation before significantly interfering behaviors occur. If the child is unable to regulate or the behaviors go unaddressed, the child's

SIGNS OF REGULATION	SIGNS OF DYSREGULATION
○ Calm, attentive, and ready to learn	○ Emotional responses disproportionate to the situation (e.g., crying, screaming)
○ Emotions are appropriate for the social context	○ Incongruent affect (e.g., level of excitement is not matched to the situation)
○ Flexible and adaptive to the changing environment	○ Interfering behaviors (e.g., throwing or banging toys, protesting)
○ Absence of dysregulation and challenging behaviors	○ Aggressive behaviors (e.g., self-injurious or injurious to others)
○ More joint attention, engagement, and play skills	○ Difficulty engaging in the session
	○ Increased RRBs (e.g., repetitive singing, visual inspection, repetitive actions)
	○ Change in demeanor (e.g., change in pace)

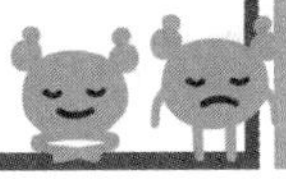

FIGURE 16.2. Signs of regulation.

dysregulation may quickly escalate from mildly interfering to significantly interfering. Prevention is the best approach. Try to learn the child's subtle signs of dysregulation so you can increase support before the child becomes dysregulated.

When the challenges are mild to moderate, you can typically respond with the core strategies. When challenges are moderate to significant, the child may need a mix of core and conditional strategies, as illustrated in Figure 16.3.

16.2.2 Assess the Function of the Behavior

When dysregulation is reoccurring or more significantly interfering, JASPER draws from the principles of applied behavior analysis (ABA) in considering the four common functions of interfering behaviors: social attention, escape/avoidance, access, and automatic/sensory (Fisher et al., 2011; Cooper et al., 2017). The function hypothesizes why the behavior might be happening in order to provide an appropriate response. The four functions are illustrated in Figure 16.4 and described briefly below.

Social Attention

When a behavior serves the purpose of social attention, the child will often repeat the behaviors that get her the most attention and the strongest response. Therefore, a child might seek out a reward or reprimand through appropriate or less appropriate behaviors. In Figure 16.4, a girl puts toys on her head and makes silly faces at the adult to gain attention.

Escape/Avoidance

Some behaviors are used for escape or avoidance. The child might want to stop a certain routine, or a step in the routine, or avoid a demand, a toy, the room itself, or even interacting with a particular person, such as a new interventionist. You might notice an increase in avoidance behaviors when you add more difficult steps such as programming or vertical expansions, press for flexibility,

Assessing Challenges in Regulation

Mildly Interfering	**Moderately Interfering**	**Significantly Interfering**
○ Able to continue playing ○ Small moments of dysregulation ○ Child might need some support	○ Able to continue playing ○ Consistent episodes of dysregulation ○ Child requires more support	○ Not able to continue playing ○ Child requires significant support

Use Core Strategies   Introduce Conditional Strategies

FIGURE 16.3. Monitor the severity of the child's regulation to provide appropriate support.

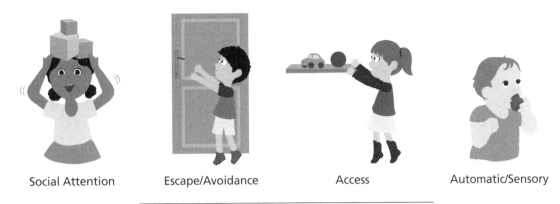

Social Attention   Escape/Avoidance   Access   Automatic/Sensory

FIGURE 16.4. The four common functions of behavior.

or transition to or from an activity. For example, in Figure 16.4, a boy reaches for the door to escape the demand of session.

Access

Some behaviors may be an attempt to obtain something. This could be something within the current routine, a different routine, or something outside of the session. It could be a particular item, a person (mom or dad), or an event (going home). If the child's request is not acknowledged or fulfilled, this can lead to frustration and dysregulation. In Figure 16.4, a girl reaches up to a high shelf to gain access to a favorite toy.

Automatic/Sensory

Some children demonstrate atypical sensory behaviors, such as repetitive hand or body movements, tensing, attraction or aversion to touch or texture, and unusual visual exploration. When we see behaviors like these, we often consider the other functions first, as some of these behaviors manifest in conjunction with or as the result of attention (e.g., licking a toy to get a negative response), avoidance (e.g., rocking to avoid engaging with the toys), or access (e.g., banging toys as an unclear form of communication instead of a verbal request). If we cannot identify another possible function, then we consider the behavior to be *automatic*, meaning something about the experience is immediately and inherently rewarding to the child. In other words, the child is not engaging in the behavior to get something (attention or access) or to avoid something (avoidance) but is engaging in the behavior for its own inherent reward. For example, the child inspects a toy because he likes the visual appearance, bangs the blocks on the table because he likes the feeling in his hands, or chews on his shirt because he likes the feeling in his mouth. In Figure 16.4, the baby puts a rubber ducky in his mouth to gain sensory input.

16.2.3 Understanding the Behavior

As you notice signs of dysregulation, it is often necessary to consider what happens before and after the dysregulation to understand the function of the child's behavior. In some cases, the cause of dysregulation may be clear, for example, the child is screaming and reaching for a toy (access).

In other cases, however, the child's behavior may feel unexpected or unclear. You might not know in the moment why the behavior occurred, what triggered it, or how to respond. There are many ways to learn about behaviors, but the most common practice is to use an antecedent–behavior–consequence—or "ABC"—chart, similar to Form 16.1 (see p. 295), to track the child's behaviors over time. Describe the behavior, and then consider what occurred directly before and immediately following the behavior. This information can help you develop a hypothesis regarding the function so you are better able to respond. Use this form in conjunction with Form 8.1 (ACT: Assess the Situation, Create a Plan, and Test for Success).

16.3 Create a Plan to Increase Regulation

In this section, we will discuss the core and conditional strategies to support the child's regulation throughout session. These serve as a toolbox of supports, which can be applied based on the individual needs of the child and the degree to which the behavior interferes with the child's engagement. When the challenges are mildly to moderately interfering, the core strategies typically suffice. When challenges are moderately to significantly interfering, you may need to assess the function of behavior and use a mix of core and conditional strategies to respond. If the behaviors put the child or others at risk, then you may need to work with a specialist to develop a behavior plan. Figure 16.5 provides an overview of core and conditional strategies to support regulation.

16.3.1 Core Strategies

The strategies from Chapters 5–15 support regulation. In the sections below, we will explain how you can use the core strategies (italicized below) to promote regulation and respond to early signs of dysregulation. Then we will provide some case examples that demonstrate these strategies in action within a routine.

Set Up the Environment

Often, children become dysregulated when the physical space or the routines are unclear. *Structure the environment* to clarify expectations for the children. Clearly define a place for the child to

---

STRATEGIES TO SUPPORT REGULATION ☑

Core Strategies	Conditional Strategies
☐ Set up the environment	☐ Require appropriate requests
☐ Help the child understand expectations	☐ Redirect
☐ Be a balanced play partner	☐ Follow through on expectations
☐ Foster communication	☐ Actively ignore attention-seeking behavior
☐ Support engagement	

FIGURE 16.5. Strategies to support regulation.

sit. Use physical barriers such as space dividers or bookshelves to help create a smaller and clearer play space. Provide choices to *play at the child's developmental level* so the play is not too challenging or too boring (see Figure 16.6). Once you start playing, you may find that certain toys become distracting and lead to dysregulation. You may need to *remove distractions* from the session and then reassess at a later time to decide if they should be reintroduced (see Chapter 17).

Help the Child Understand Expectations

Dysregulation can occur when a child is unsure what is expected. When setting an expectation, *use clear and developmentally appropriate directions.* In addition, provide a *visual support* to help the child understand if helpful (see Figure 16.7). Make sure you also *start and end the session on a positive note.* Be *clear, confident, and consistent* during moments of dysregulation. The more you panic and talk, the more you may further dysregulate a child. If you are not sure what to do, it is better to take a moment to think about it than to continue rushing ahead. This moment might actually help the child to self-regulate independently, and if not, it gives you time to assess the situation and make an informed judgment as to what to do. Transitioning into or out of a session can sometimes lead to dysregulation as well. Build a consistent plan at the beginning and end of session to *support transitions* so that the child knows what is coming. See more in Chapter 8.

Be a Balanced Play Partner

There are many aspects of the routine and your own actions that you can adjust during moments of dysregulation. If the child is feeling overwhelmed by the demands of the routine, you can adjust the level of demand by *returning to the base* or *restarting the routine.* Constantly pushing children to perform at their target play or communication level can be taxing and lead to dysregulation. In these moments, the child may need you to *provide time and space* to make a request or initiate an idea. Adjust the *pace* of your play or communication.

Dysregulation is not always a sign that the routine is too hard; in some cases, it may be a

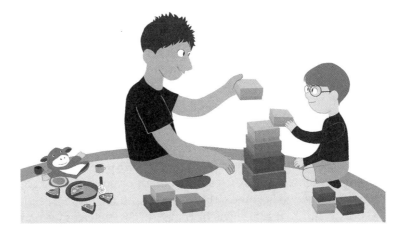

FIGURE 16.6. The adult uses information from the child's SPACE assessment to promote regulation.

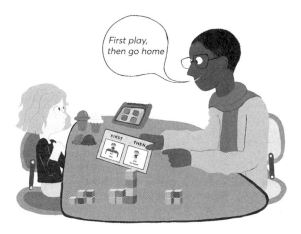

FIGURE 16.7. The adult shows the child a visual schedule to set expectations for the session.

clue that the child is bored and ready for something new. In this case, you should actually increase the level of demand. Provide a mixture of *horizontal expansions* and *vertical expansions* to avoid making the routine overly challenging and frustrating, or too easy and boring. Model appropriate *affect* and modulate as necessary to help the child display emotions effectively while staying connected to a play partner. See more in Chapters 8–11.

Foster Communication

Help the child communicate appropriately to reduce moments of frustration. *Program for requesting and joint attention gestures* to help the child express thoughts and needs and to help the child to use the SGD (if applicable). For many children, dysregulation has been an effective way to communicate. Similarly, dysregulation may be a result of not being understood or receiving a response. We want to make sure all children can have a way to appropriately and effectively communicate. If a child makes a request you cannot immediately fulfill, *respond* to the request and clearly state when or how it will be fulfilled in a developmentally appropriate way. See more in Chapters 12–14.

Support Engagement

Often, loss of engagement and dysregulation occur together. Engagement may begin to fade, which could lead to an increase in dysregulation or vice versa. Notice how this pattern applies for each child, so you can read the signs and respond sooner. After responding to dysregulation, help the child calm down and reconnect by *supporting engagement*. If necessary, use a short time of *person engagement*, introduce an *easier routine*, or provide a short *alternative activity* after a period of dysregulation to help the child reconnect and reengage. See more in Chapter 15.

Use Exercise 16.1 to practice matching the JASPER strategies we have already covered to different scenarios.

EXERCISE 16.1. **Supporting Regulation**

Match each scenario with the most appropriate strategy to support regulation.

Description of the interaction	Potential strategies
1. The child has many ideas during routines, but her communication is difficult to understand. She becomes frustrated when you do not participate in her ideas, but you cannot understand what she is trying to convey.	A. Try adding an SGD B. Add more structure to the environment C. Support transitions
2. You and the child have built a routine with a solid base and several vertical expansions. You model a step that is at the child's target level and notice that he begins singing loudly to himself and stops taking turns.	A. Return to the base B. Balance horizontal and vertical expansions C. Either A or B
3. While doing sessions in the child's preschool classroom, the child often whines and wanders to different areas of the class.	A. Add more structure and supports to the environment B. Provide the child time and space C. Increase your affect
4. After putting all the shapes in a shape sorter, you notice the child becomes wiggly in his chair and turns his body away from you. The child stops taking his turns and looks toward the wall.	A. Program for communication B. Consider your pacing of the routine C. Provide clear, confident directions

16.3.2 Conditional Strategies

Moderate to significant episodes of dysregulation often require more support in addition to the core strategies from Chapters 5–15 outlined above. In these cases, the following conditional strategies may be necessary: Require appropriate requests, redirect the child, help the child follow through on expectations, and actively ignore inappropriate attention-seeking behaviors. These strategies will not apply to every behavior or situation; rather, you must assess the function of the behavior and choose from among them to provide a response that addresses the challenge at hand. In this process, the goal is not to stifle or punish children for dysregulation but rather to equip children to communicate their experiences in more appropriate and effective ways while helping them engage in the routine. We will explain the basic guidelines of each strategy and then provide some case examples to show how they fit alongside the core strategies.

Require Appropriate Requests

During moments of dysregulation, children might not be able to communicate or may use suboptimal strategies to request, such as screaming or crying. If we are inconsistent in requiring the child to use developmentally appropriate communication, it proves that these behaviors are effective. Instead, try to view this as an opportunity to change the child's pattern of behavior and teach a new expectation, skill, or way to communicate. In these moments, require the child to use an appropriate skill (preferably one that is already mastered). Set an expectation and help the child follow through with an appropriate response. Here is an example:

> The child screams because she wants access to a toy, so you help her form an appropriate request. You first model, saying "More" (or pressing the button more on the SGD). The next time the child screams, you hold up the blocks and pause. If the child does not respond, you provide a verbal prompt, such as "Want more?" If the child still does not respond, you move on to a specific verbal prompt, "Say, 'more,'" or help her press the button on the SGD.

In the short-term, this process may lead to more dysregulation, so ensure you are setting clear expectations and following through on prompts to help the child be successful. If you cannot fulfill the request, you can try the next two strategies: *redirect the child* and then help the child *follow through on expectations.*

Redirect

Redirect the child away from the source of distraction or dysregulation and toward a more appropriate and productive choice. Redirection can take many forms. Try to start with suggestive prompts such as moving a toy forward or modeling a new action. Depending on the function and level of interference, you may need to use a directive prompt to give a clear instruction or incorporate a visual support (see Chapter 8 for more on visual supports and setting clear expectations). It may also be helpful to redirect the child using a brief moment of person engagement to help the child connect; however, be careful that the moment of person engagement is not reinforcing the child's dysregulation, especially in the case of escape or attention-seeking behaviors. If the child continues to want access to a toy or activity that is no longer productive, then you may need to swiftly remove that item before providing other choices. Here are some examples:

- A toddler has a very difficult time separating from her caregiver, but the caregiver prefers not to be in session. You support the transition into the session by calmly singing her favorite song and then showing her a few exciting toys.
- The child increasingly asks for his favorite doll, but you know it will not lead to productive play. You let the child know it is not available right now and then model a fun new action to build on your current routine.

Follow Through on Expectations

In Chapter 8, we provided a set of strategies to establish the expectations of the intervention. When moments of dysregulation arise, follow through on the expectations and directions you provide. When the child is upset, it may be harder to process information, so it is important to be clear and consistent in your directions in these moments. State what exactly you want the child to do (e.g., "Sit down" or "It's time to play"). Try to use the same words and short phrases; use a calm, direct tone of voice; and follow the same general plan each time. Choose the instructions carefully, and only set demands you are willing to carry out, as you may need to help the child follow through using prompts. Here are some examples:

- As you are nearing the end of session, the child becomes frustrated over a missing piece of a toy set and escalates to crying on the floor while screaming, "Go home!" After she begins to calm down, you set up two choices of well-mastered routines and calmly state, "Five more minutes of play." You help her engage in the familiar routine and support engagement and regulation by keeping the environment clean, setting out choices, and modeling so you can end session on a positive note.

- The child throws all the toys on the floor and repeats, "All done! All done!" You respond by showing him a visual schedule of "First play, then all done," while calmly reading out the words. You then help him reengage in the play using core strategies such as environmental arrangement, imitation, and modeling.

Actively Ignore Attention-Seeking Behavior

Active ignoring is a strategy where you purposely withhold your response to social attention-seeking behavior. For example, if the child throws a toy, repeatedly swipes the toys, or whines while checking your reaction, ignore the behavior and withdraw your attention from the child (see Figure 16.8). There are varying degrees of active ignoring. You can limit your response using the following strategies: Avert your gaze by casting your eyes down, position your body away from the child, stop responding to communication and remain silent, or reduce your affect to a neutral state. Be careful not to be too overt in how you actively ignore. If you make a big deal out of ignoring, it might be so noticeable that it actually provides a response. In most cases, it is sufficient to gaze down or slightly turn your body away. While some behaviors should not be ignored due to safety concerns, it is still important to consider how your eye contact and tone of voice can be reduced to avoid reinforcing attention-seeking behaviors.

Here are some examples of actively ignoring an interfering behavior:

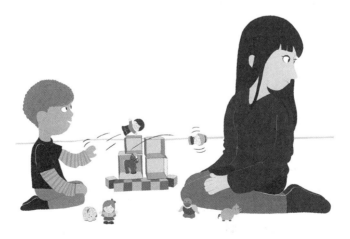

FIGURE 16.8. The adult actively ignores the child's attention-seeking behavior.

- The child whines through an activity and looks up to see your reaction. You ignore the whining and redirect by modeling quickly and handing her a piece.

- The child pretends to have the animal figures eat the people. You start out imitating but quickly hypothesize that this is reinforcing attention-seeking behaviors, as the child continues this action repeatedly while laughing, looking at you, and escalating his affect. Instead of continuing to imitate, you actively ignore this behavior and instead model an appropriate and exciting expansion such as having the animals go to the circus.

Additional support beyond these strategies may be necessary in select cases when dysregulation is severely and persistently interfering. See Box 16.1 for more information. See Table 16.1 for signs, examples, and potential responses for each function of behavior, and use Exercise 16.2 to practice balancing core and conditional strategies to respond to dysregulation.

EXERCISE 16.2. Responding to Dysregulation

Choose the best strategy to respond to the child's dysregulation.

1. The child drops the toys off of the table, so you say, "Keep the toys on the table. Let's play!" and increase your affect to make the routine more fun. The child continues to drop toys onto the floor while looking at you and smiling. What should you do next?

    A. Ignore the child's dropping and model a new step of the routine.
    B. Help the child pick up all the toys off the floor.
    C. Use person engagement to sing "Happy Birthday."
    D. Tell the child again to stop the behavior.

2. You decide to remove a toy pirate ship from the room because the child is very object engaged. You say, "All done with ship on three"; count to three; say, "All done ship"; and quickly remove the ship out of view. The child continues to ask for the ship throughout session, sometimes screaming and crying with her request. How should you respond?

    A. Ignore the child's request and continue playing.
    B. Try redirecting first, but bring the pirate ship back if the child gets upset.
    C. Tell the child "first play, then ship" with a visual schedule and redirect her to new options.
    D. Lower the play level so she is not frustrated.

3. Five minutes into the session, the child slouches out of his chair to hide underneath the table. How should you respond?

    A. Accept that the child does not want to play, end the session, and try to lengthen the session more and more over time.
    B. Teach the child to say, "All done" and help him make a new toy choice.
    C. Use a visual schedule to remind the child "First play, then break."
    D. Either B or C

BOX 16.1. Severely and Persistently Interfering Behaviors

When dysregulation is severely and persistently interfering, you may need to create a temporary plan to help the child regulate and engage. This is most commonly at the start of the session, the end of the session, or after moments of significantly interfering episodes of dysregulation (e.g., lasting several minutes). To reduce the frequency and severity of dysregulation, additional supports may be necessary for a time and then faded as the child becomes more comfortable in the session. For example, we might prepare a token board to help reinforce positive behavior. We might plan an *alternative activity* to help the child transition. In this case, we would remove the demands of play while still maintaining the other elements of the intervention. For example, model joint attention as you show the child a book at the child's language level. We might also prepare to incorporate a planned break in the middle of the session. These strategies are exceptions to our general rules and should only be implemented for a short time in very select cases. For example, the child cries for 10 minutes at the beginning of the session. You read a book to help the child connect and calm down. You spend 3 minutes reading in the first session, 2 minutes the second session, and 1 minute the third session, and then start with a well-mastered routine during the fourth session. This type of response must be highly individualized to the child and is thus beyond the scope of this book. Additional information is available in training.

TABLE 16.1. Functions of Behavior

Signs by Function	Examples	Potential Response
Social Attention • Looking directly at someone while engaging in the behavior • Smiling and laughing during or after the behavior • Behavior happens more when it gets a response	Child puts the pizza toppings in his mouth, rather than on the pizza. Child looks up at you and smiles while he does so. Child swats at your hand after you model a new step during the routine and then looks to you for your response.	➜ Reduce affect and calmly block the child from putting pizza toppings in his mouth, transition to a new routine with large pieces that do not fit in the child's mouth to avoid the choking hazard. ➜ Actively ignore by keeping your hand out of the child's reach, model a new step.
Escape/Avoidance • Physically trying to escape the area (e.g., running away) • Behavior stops suddenly when the demand stops • Behavior increases or escalates when the demand remains	Child hides under the table. Child closes his eyes and "disappears." Child moves to another toy when the adult models a new way to use the current toy.	➜ Adjust the environment to increase structure. ➜ Increase pacing and affect to support engagement and build a routine. ➜ Modulate the level of demand within the child's developmentally appropriate range.
Access • Requesting or searching for an object • Behavior stops when the child receives the object • Behavior escalates when the object is withheld	Child walks around the room looking for his tablet to watch cartoons. Child repeatedly requests until she has all the red blocks.	➜ Add a "first play, then cartoons" visual. ➜ Adjust the environment to include different color blocks. ➜ Redirect to a new routine if you are unable to build a routine together.
Automatic • Displaying repetitive sensory behavior: pushing on chin, visibly uncomfortable, visually inspecting, hitting, banging, mouthing objects	Child visually inspects the wheels of the car while he spins them. Child rocks back and forth in his seat as he is playing.	➜ Reconsider toy choice and remove toys with wheels from the session. ➜ Support engagement and continue the routine.

16.4 Test Your Plan for Regulation

After implementing your plan, assess what worked well and what you can improve upon. Troubleshooting is an ongoing process, and there is always room for improvement. In the next sections, we explain how to reconnect with the child after a period of dysregulation and improve your approach over time. We then answer some common questions and illustrate this process with a vignette.

16.4.1 Reconnect and Reengage

Have a plan to support the child's regulation and engagement after a period of dysregulation; otherwise the child might quickly become dysregulated again.

Reinforce Positive Behavior

As soon as the child begins to calm down and do something productive, you should quickly reinforce the child's appropriate behaviors. In general, we offer natural reinforcement through positive affect and imitation. In some cases, it may be necessary to provide verbal praise as added reinforcement after a bout of dysregulation. This is an exception to our general approach and should only occur once the child starts showing appropriate behaviors after a period of dysregulation.

Transition Back to the Routine

As the child becomes more regulated, you can begin to reengage the child (using strategies from Chapter 15), and return to the routine (using imitation strategies from Chapter 9 and strategies to support the base from Chapter 10). You may need to incorporate strategies to increase engagement to help the child reconnect with you before returning to the routine (see Chapter 15, Section 15.3.2).

16.4.2 Plan for the Future

As the intervention progresses, you should see improvement in the child's ability to regulate with fewer instances of dysregulation, of less intensity, lasting shorter periods of time. Use the strategies below to continue improving upon your approach.

Prevent Patterns of Dysregulation

As you get to know the child, you may start to notice certain patterns of behavior. Instead of responding only when dysregulation occurs, create a plan to promote regulation prior to the challenging situation. Revisit Chapter 8 strategies to make sure you have supports you need, and think about how to improve the routine and your own actions. Then notice the result of your response. Ensure that you are not reinforcing interfering behaviors.

Fade Support

Evaluate your plan, not only in the moment, but also over time. As you implement your plan consistently, it should become easier for the child to understand the expectations, and the child may no longer need the same level of support as before. Consider ways to fade support, so the child is less reliant on these extra measures to regulate. Ideally, we want to help children to learn new patterns of behavior, so they are able to interact successfully outside of the intervention setting, where added supports may not be available.

Keep in mind the broader goals of the session as well. You may notice that dysregulation increases when you add more difficult steps such as programming or vertical expansions, when you press for flexibility, or when you transition. Try to choose moments when the child is more likely to be successful to work toward these more challenging goals. For example, it is often more effective to program during moments of increased motivation, rather than moments when the child is struggling to engage. While there is much you can do to support the child, you may not always be able to prevent dysregulation. Sometimes it is necessary to work through dysregulation in order to achieve other goals.

16.4.3 Common Questions

In this section, we answer some common questions that may arise as you support regulation.

How do I respond more efficiently when the child becomes dysregulated?

Respond immediately and efficiently to signs of dysregulation, so you do not spend significant time away from routines. Consider the following tips:

- Identify and respond to the first signs of diminishing engagement. Do not wait for the child to become dysregulated. The longer you wait, the harder it may be to respond.
- Reinforce the child's successes. It is crucial to respond quickly once the child stops an unwanted behavior or returns to a wanted behavior.
- Do not reinforce unwanted behaviors.
- Once the child has calmed down, help the child return to the routine. In some cases, you may need to use strategies to support engagement, such as a brief moment of person engagement to aid the transition. (Be careful not to reinforce unwanted behaviors with these engagement strategies. You do not want to get stuck in a cycle of dysregulation and easy engagement activities that take time away from routines.)
- If the child is more dysregulated than you would expect, troubleshoot other aspects of the interaction.

How do I avoid reinforcing unwanted behaviors?

Be mindful that you may inadvertently be reinforcing a child's challenging behavior in subtle ways. For example, you might reprimand the child for flickering the lights off and on, which could grow into a game with inappropriate attention-seeking behavior. Similarly, you might offer the child hugs or a new set of toys each time she whines, which could inadvertently reinforce escape behavior. Notice the result of your response. Does your response increase or decrease the behavior *over time*? Some strategies may stop dysregulation in the moment but lead to longer-term challenges. Thus, ensure that your response works toward both your immediate and future goals.

If the child's behavior gets worse, does that mean I did something wrong?

At times, it may feel as if your response is increasing the child's dysregulation, instead of decreasing it. This does not necessarily mean you are doing something wrong. As children have new demands put on them that aim to decrease challenging behaviors, the behaviors can sometimes get worse before they get better (in ABA, this is called an *extinction burst*).

16.4.4 Case Examples

Here are some examples of how the core and conditional strategies can be used to increase regulation.

Is It Escape?

Dear JASPER,

I'm working with an awesome 6-year-old. We have a great time with food toys where we stack scoops of ice cream and make salad bowls together. I notice that when I try to add in dolls or animals to our food routines, she asks to go to the bathroom. This doesn't happen when we're building the food toys. When I take her to the bathroom, she does not have to go, so I'm thinking she's more interested in trying to escape the change in our routine than go to the bathroom. We waste so much time going on these bathroom trips. Last session, I tried ignoring one of her requests since she had already gone, but then she just screamed and dropped to the floor. How do I help her stick with me?

Regards,

Is It Escape?

Dear *Is It Escape?*

You've done some good detective work! From your assessment, it sounds as if she is asking to go to the bathroom after a new step at a higher presymbolic level as a means of escape. When creating a plan to address this, perhaps you could consider other combination steps to add to your food routine to keep the play level more manageable. For example, you could try including conventional combination steps such as scooping the ice cream onto a spoon. You could also consider pretend-self steps such as extending the spoon with the ice cream to yourselves. You might also look into characters or figures that might be more motivating to engage. If she still requests to use the bathroom, use clear language and follow through with the expectation that it's time to play. Try to establish a pattern where you take her to the bathroom before session, you play, and then you can take her again after if she needs. A visual schedule might help her learn this pattern. After showing her the visual schedule, reengage her with the routine and continue trying to expand. It might take some time, but stick with it!

Best,

JASPER

What's with the Whine?

Dear JASPER,

The child I'm currently working with tends to whine throughout our sessions and is constantly requesting for toys other than what I have out on the table. I try to get him to keep playing with the toy I have available, but he just keeps asking for new things. When I bring out the new toy, he doesn't really do much with it either. I'm not sure what to do because it seems as though he does not want to play with anything. It is very difficult to get into a solid play routine with him. Please help!

What's with the Whine?

Dear *What's with the Whine?*

It seems the child may be whining and using his requesting skills to try to escape the demands of playing in session. Now that we have a guess based on our hypothesis about the function of the behavior (a combination of access and escape), we can try some strategies to help him regulate and engage in a routine. In order to address this behavior, it will be helpful to focus on your core strategies. In regard to environment, start with a few choices of toys that are motivating and developmentally appropriate. Once the child has some clear options at the table, limit how many toys you have in the room. You may need to put some toys away (try solid containers) so he does not see all the toy options available. To prevent him from choosing one toy and then requesting for another, you will need to be quick and fun in modeling a step and encouraging him to take his turn (e.g., hand him a piece) to get a routine going. You should follow through in playing with the toy that he selected so he understands that once he chooses a toy you will play with it for a few minutes.

Good luck!

JASPER

All Work and No Play

Dear JASPER,

I just began seeing a child who has had quite a bit of intervention in the past. Transitioning into a JASPER session is sometimes a struggle. He has minimal spoken language, but he has learned certain phrases from his prior intervention experience. Throughout the session, if he gets tired or doesn't want to play, he will cry and say, "No play! No play!" At first, I thought I was reinforcing his appropriate communication by giving him a break at these times, but now it's happening so frequently we can barely get a base routine going. How do I show him that his request is understood without completely abandoning the goals of our session? Am I supposed to just ignore him and forge on?

Thanks,

All Work and No Play

Dear *All Work and No Play,*

It's great that you're assessing his behavior and noticing that something is off. We definitely want to acknowledge his functional communication in these instances. It sounds as if you've been doing such a good job acknowledging his requests that you've been inadvertently reinforcing some escape behaviors. JASPER may be very different from his other intervention, so the demand to play and engage for an entire session may be an adjustment for him. Here are some strategies you can use to set clear expectations and help him engage throughout the session: At first, respond verbally to him, so he knows your hear him (e.g., "Play for a few minutes") and then model returning back to the routine to redirect him. If he continues to say, "No play," calmly show him a visual schedule to make the expectations of the session clearer. Rather than stopping the session to give him a big response to his request (which may continue to reinforce escape), briefly show him the schedule and then redirect him to the routine. Also, avoid switching out the toys or offering a person engagement break too frequently, because this could contribute to his escape behaviors. Instead, try adding more expansion toys so there are new options available for productive play before an escape behavior occurs.

Keep it up!

JASPER

Raining Cats and Dogs

Dear JASPER,

I am working with a young child who is just under 3 years old, and I have been having a hard time the last few sessions. We start out great, but after the first few minutes she becomes dysregulated when I try to add expansions to our base routines. For example, when we were building a structure of magnetic tiles, tried to put some dog and cat figures inside. She started to scream really loud while looking at me and then started to throw the animals across the room. I thought she was trying to escape from the harder task of using the animals, so I told her no and made her go get up and pick the animals from the floor. But as soon as I tried to expand again, the same thing happened. What can I do to help reduce these interfering behaviors?

Thanks,

Raining Cats and Dogs

Dear *Raining Cats and Dogs,*

Good question! First, think about the play level of the expansion step. Often we see increased dysregulation behaviors like throwing if the child does not know what to do with the toy or how to use it in a productive way. She may not be ready to move up to child-as-agent level expansions. Perhaps working on her building skills to the physical combination level could be another way to expand vertically and play to her strengths. It may also help to think about the function of the behavior (yelling and throwing figures). This behavior might be a means for attention, in addition to escape. Next time, try actively ignoring her throwing and avert your gaze. Then you can model putting a figure inside again. You can clarify the expectation and reduce the demand by clearing the environment and handing her one figure. It may also help to use a verbal statement to clearly state expectations (e.g., "First dog, then new toys") and provide appropriate support to follow through. For example, you could require her to put one figure in before ending that step of the routine and moving to another toy. Thus, you are not providing reinforcement for negative attention-seeking behavior and are following through with the expectation you have set.

You can do it!

JASPER

16.4.5 Vignette

Here is an example of how the strategies you have learned so far come together with the ACT framework to support regulation.

> *The adult and child build a base routine nesting the boxes, dumping the boxes out, and then stacking the boxes up into a tower. The child loves to knock over the boxes and giggles loudly before yelling, "Crash it!" The adult smiles and pushes the boxes saying, "Crash it down!" The adult models stacking up the boxes again, and a similar pattern repeats with the boy getting even more excited this time. The adult laughs with him as they knock down the boxes and determines the boy's enthusiasm is a sign that the base is established. The next time through, the adult puts out figures and other building materials for expansions. The adult tries to support the child to expand the routine. He puts the figures between them and waits to see what the child will do. As he waits, the boy begins giggling and tapping the boxes already on the tower. The adult tries modeling by adding a figure onto the tower. The child knocks over the boxes and then begins throwing toys around the room while laughing and looking at the adult (see Figure 16.9). The adult tries modeling again, and the child continues throwing boxes and mixing up the toys in front of him.*

The adult thought the routine was off to a great start with the high positive affect but then realizes they have gotten off track somewhere along the way. He quickly thinks through the ACT framework to figure out what might have gone wrong and to create a plan to adjust. He does not have time to fill out the ACT form (Form 8.1) in the moment but quickly thinks through the troubleshooting framework. His thought process is as follows:

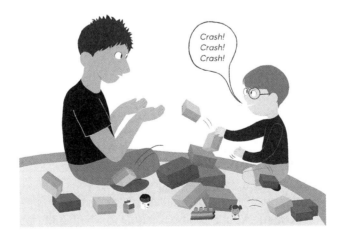

FIGURE 16.9. The child becomes overly excited and dysregulated knocking down the boxes.

- ***Assess the situation.*** The adult noticed that the child started acting silly when they knocked down the boxes. This response seemed to grow until the child became dysregulated, showed overly escalated affect, and started throwing toys. The adult suspects this occurred as an attention-seeking behavior, since the child was looking up and laughing while throwing the toys. He recalls that these behaviors peaked when he tried to model adding figures to the boxes, so he also suspects that the child might be attempting to avoid expanding the routine. The adult wonders what would have happened if he had attempted the expansion earlier, before the child's dysregulation escalated.

- ***Create a plan.*** Since the primary function of the behavior appears to be attention seeking, the adult actively ignores the child's crashing and throwing. Instead of mirroring the child's high energy, he decides to reduce his affect to a more neutral state next time. To address the function of escape, he plans to introduce more expansion options, to look for motivating next steps, and to introduce these materials earlier in the routine.

- ***Test for success.*** The adult quickly cleans up the environment and moves the mess of materials out of the child's reach to prevent throwing. He keeps his affect very calm while they begin to establish the base. To prepare to expand, he adds people, animals, shapes, and Lego blocks into the environment. The child looks at them and then begins giggling and throwing again. The adult ignores his behavior and decides he needs to make the expectation clearer. The adult realizes the child is trying to escape the harder demand of expanding and makes a plan to add extra support around this step. He decides to begin with a horizontal expansion (e.g., adding more blocks to the building) before adding in figures. He also decides to increase his pace. The adult moves the expansion materials forward just long enough for the child to notice them, and then quickly models and hands the child a piece before the child has the opportunity to knock down the boxes. The child adds a block and the adult increases his affect as he comments and takes his play turn. They have made it past the first expansion, and the adult continues to monitor his own pace and affect to support the child.

After session, the adult decides to record his thinking using the ACT form (Form 8.1) so that he has a record of the challenges and can be more proactive next time (see Figure 16.10). In thinking ahead, he decides he wants to be quicker to get ahead of the child's attention-seeking and avoidance behaviors. He plans to incorporate more programming opportunities so the child learns skills to appropriately share with him. He also decides to bring in more types of toys that cannot be so easily crashed in the future. By having more types of combination materials, such as food toys and interlocking blocks, he hopes he will be able to fade support and reduce the amount of modeling, so the child has more opportunities to initiate.

16.5 Conclusion

Supporting regulation is a process of continual evaluation and refinement. It is important to proactively support the child's regulation needs using core JASPER strategies and employ the ACT framework to troubleshoot when challenges arise. As you get to know the child, you may begin to recognize what regulation and dysregulation looks like for this particular child and when these behaviors start to emerge. Your response is central to whether the interfering behavior will increase or decrease. Although some actions may stop the behavior in the moment (e.g., giving the child what he is screaming for might help the child immediately calm down), they can contribute to

ACT: Assess the situation, Create a plan, and Test for success

Child: __C. K.__   Adult: __A. G.__   Date: __January 17__

Assess the situation: What happened? What challenges occurred in the routine or in the child's behavior?

Check the routine	Check the child's behavior
—Able to establish a base —Not able to expand the routine	—C. K. is becoming dysregulated —Showing inappropriate affect —Throwing toys —Maybe attention seeking? (looking up, smiling) —Maybe avoiding expanding? *Try using the "Check the Child's Behavior" Form!*

Create a plan: What can I do to help? How can I use core strategies and conditional strategies to produce change?

Change the environment	Change your own actions	Respond to the function of the child's behavior
—Add expansion options	—Modulate affect —Increase pacing of expansions	—Ignore attention seeking behavior when C.K. crashes and throws

Core Strategies

Conditional Strategies

Prioritize core strategies
- Arrange the environment
- Imitate and model
- Establish play routines
- Expand play routines
- Use communication strategies
- Program for gestures and language
- Support engagement and regulation
- Support productive play

Consider conditional strategies
- Incorporate visual supports
- Use directive prompts
- Use conditional strategies for engagement and regulation
- Prepare for fading

Test for success: Did my plan have the intended effect? Is there anything I can improve in the future?

Note what worked	Plan for the future
—Keep calm affect to balance out the child —Add more horizontal expansions —Increase my pace and support during expansions —Increase affect during productive behaviors	—Create more opportunities to program for JA gestures and language so C.K. can gain attention more appropriately —Plan materials and routines that cannot crash so easily to support productive initiations —Reduce my pace of modeling over time *Prepare to fade support!*

FIGURE 16.10. Example of a filled-out ACT framework form (Form 8.1 in Chapter 8).

more problems down the road by reinforcing a less socially accepted behavior (e.g., teaching the child that screaming is a good way to get what he wants). It is up to you to break this cycle, set clear expectations for the child's behavior, and help the child return to the routine. Over time, this should lead to more time regulated, less time dysregulated, and overall improvement in the child's ability to stay engaged in the routine. Take a minute to review strategies to support regulation in Figure 16.11. In the next chapter, we will continue to troubleshoot interfering behaviors, focusing specifically on repetitive behaviors.

Chapter 16 Summary

ASSESS REGULATION	**CREATE A PLAN** TO INCREASE REGULATION	**TEST YOUR PLAN** FOR REGULATION

○ Look for signs of regulation
○ Look for signs of dysregulation
○ Assess the severity
○ Assess the function
  ▪ Social attention
  ▪ Avoidance/escape
  ▪ Access
  ▪ Automatic/sensory
	○ Use core strategies
	  ▪ Promote regulation
	  ▪ Respond to mild to moderate challenges
	  ▪ Use strategies from Ch. 5–15
	○ Add conditional strategies
	  ▪ Require appropriate requests
	  ▪ Redirect
	  ▪ Follow through on expectations
	  ▪ Actively ignore attention-seeking behaviors
		○ Reconnect and reengage
		○ Plan for the future
		○ Get ahead of patterns of behavior
		○ Fade support

FIGURE 16.11. Chapter 16 summary.

FORM 16.1. **Check the Child's Behavior**

Child: _____   Adult: _____

	Describe the behavior(s)	What happened immediately before?	What happened immediately after?	Possible function of the behavior
Session #: Date:				
Session #: Date:				
Session #: Date:				
Session #: Date:				
Session #: Date:				
Session #: Date:				
Session #: Date:				
Session #: Date:				

295

Supporting Productive Play in the Context of RRBs

17.1 Introduction

In this chapter, we will explain how to promote productive play within the context of restricted and repetitive behaviors (RRBs), interests, or activities. As you may recall from Chapter 6, productive play is developmentally appropriate, flexible, diverse, and creative, and it allows the child to remain jointly engaged; this is contrasted against actions that are *interfering* and may interrupt joint engagement. One of the challenges faced in productive play is the presence of RRBs. As we described in Chapter 2, this includes a variety of atypical behaviors core to ASD, such as rigidity, restricted interests, repetitive behaviors, and sensory behaviors. There is still much we do not know about RRBs—when and why they occur, whether they present in times of stress, or whether they help the child remain calm. When faced with these behaviors, our goal is to increase the productivity, flexibility, and overall quality of the actions and the routine. Similar to challenges with engagement and regulation, we do not attempt to provide a comprehensive guide to RRBs in this book; this level of troubleshooting is highly specific to the child, and your response may vary greatly. Instead, we provide a basic outline of our approach following the ACT framework (see Figure 17.1).

We start by monitoring the child, the interference of the behaviors, and the possible context in which they occur. Then we provide strategies to respond in cases when the child needs support. Our response relies on both core and conditional strategies. We use core strategies such as

ASSESS THE QUALITY OF PLAY	Monitor the interference of behaviors	Hypothesize why the behaviors occur
CREATE A PLAN Consider the specific RRB	Prioritize core strategies	Consider conditional strategies
TEST FOR SUCCESS	What else can you improve?	

FIGURE 17.1. ACT to promote productive play.

environment arrangement and modeling to address most challenges. When the child needs more support, conditional strategies may be used in addition to the core strategies to help the child play productively. Like the previous chapters, we include case examples to demonstrate how these strategies layer and interact. Additional information and feedback are provided in training. Before we move on, take a moment to review in Figure 17.2 the strategies we have covered so far in this book.

17.2 Assess the Quality of Play

As we discussed in Chapter 2, RRBs can manifest in many ways and may affect the quality of your play interaction. In this chapter, we talk about four common categories: rigidity, restricted interests, repetitive behaviors, and sensory behaviors. When RRBs are interfering, they are often actions at lower play levels (indiscriminate and discriminant acts), rigid and repetitive rather than flexible, and not socially motivated. Monitor the child for signs of RRBs and interfering actions throughout the routine. See Chapter 2, Box 2.3, for signs of RRBs and Chapter 6, Section 6.2.3, for signs of productive and interfering play acts. The goal is to notice when these behaviors occur, why they occur, and how intrusive they are to the interaction so that you are prepared to respond.

17.2.1 Assess the Interference of the Behaviors

RRBs may lead to increases in object engagement, less social play, and lower-quality routines, or they might occur in the background and possibly improve the child's regulation. Notice the degree to which the behavior interferes with the session in order to decide if you should add support or continue to monitor the behavior.

- ***Not interfering or mildly interfering.*** You and the child are still engaged in a routine. The behavior is occurring in the background and not interfering or only mildly interfering. For example, the child briefly visually inspects each block before placing it on the tower.

- ***Moderately interfering.*** You are able to keep playing, but the child may have periods of

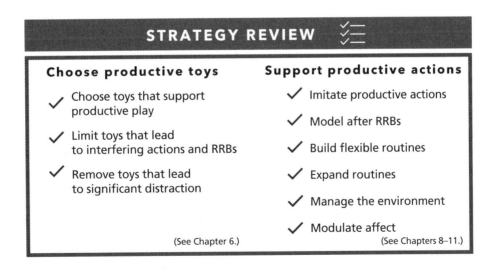

FIGURE 17.2. Strategy review.

object engagement and may require occasional modeling to play productively, remain engaged, and expand the routine.

• *Significantly interfering.* You are no longer able to play productively. The child may be exclusively object engaged, rigidly insistent on his own ideas, or dysregulated. You may not be able to take a turn or build a routine.

Figure 17.3 shows how your level of support increases as the child's behaviors become more interfering to the session's goals. When the behaviors are not interfering or mildly interfering, you can typically continue to monitor the child; you may also consider using core strategies to prevent the behaviors from increasing in frequency or severity. If the behaviors are moderately interfering, provide support to help the child play more productively. You can try shaping or scaffolding the child's idea to be more productive, instead of completely abandoning it or using a more directive strategy. When challenges are severely interfering, consider removing distractions, switching toy choices, and using a mix of core and conditional strategies to support the child's engagement and regulation and work toward productive play.

We are not aiming to stop all RRBs from occurring. Our goal is to facilitate an interaction in which children can engage and learn to the best of their ability, not only with the interventionist in session, but also with peers in social settings and everyday life. In some cases, this may require support to engage; in other cases, the child may need help to learn a new way to play.

17.2.2 Hypothesize Why the Behaviors Occur

If a behavior significantly or repeatedly interferes with the session, try to hypothesize what might cause the behavior.

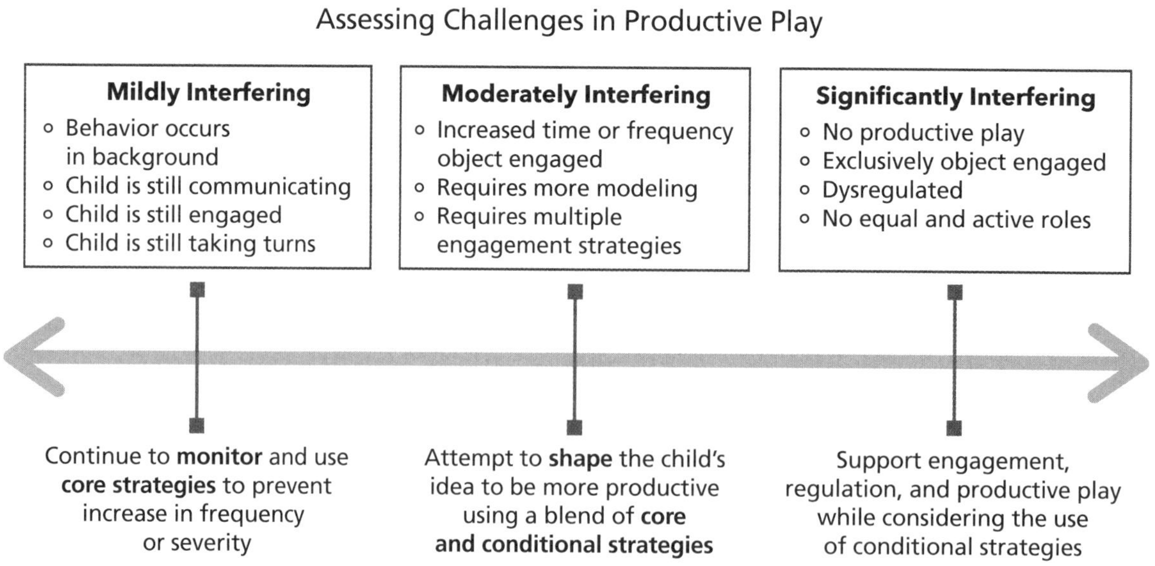

Assessing Challenges in Productive Play

Mildly Interfering
- Behavior occurs in background
- Child is still communicating
- Child is still engaged
- Child is still taking turns

Moderately Interfering
- Increased time or frequency object engaged
- Requires more modeling
- Requires multiple engagement strategies

Significantly Interfering
- No productive play
- Exclusively object engaged
- Dysregulated
- No equal and active roles

Continue to **monitor** and use **core strategies** to prevent increase in frequency or severity

Attempt to **shape** the child's idea to be more productive using a blend of **core and conditional strategies**

Support engagement, regulation, and productive play while considering the use of conditional strategies

FIGURE 17.3. Assess the severity of the child's RRBs to determine how and when to respond.

Assess Regulation

RRBs can be a sign that the child is dysregulated. In this case, you may need to consider the other functions of behavior (see Chapter 16) or use Form 16.1 (Check the Child's Behavior) to gather more information. Pay close attention to what happens before the repetitive behavior occurs. For example, does the child's scripted singing become louder and more intense each time you try to expand the play or when your pacing becomes too slow? Once you learn more about the behavior, you can get better at responding to the child and "get ahead of it" next time.

Assess Additional Factors

Outside factors, such as getting a bad night's sleep or having bad allergies, can affect the child's ability to play productively. Speak with the child's family or teacher before the session and note how the child transitions into session. Based on this information, you should choose how much to target flexibility in a certain session.

Use Exercise 17.1 to practice determining whether to continue monitoring the child or to provide support.

EXERCISE 17.1. **Determining When to Respond**

Identify whether the adult should continue monitoring or provide more support in the following scenarios to promote productive play.

1. The child is verbally scripting lines from a TV show under her breath but continues to take turns.   Continue monitoring   Provide support

2. The child holds a peg in one hand through the routine but continues to take his turn.   Continue monitoring   Provide support

3. The child rolls a car back and forth while staring at the wheels for several minutes.   Continue monitoring   Provide support

4. The child refuses to stack the boxes, pushes your hand away each time you try to model building, and then proceeds to nest the boxes together.   Continue monitoring   Provide support

5. The child occasionally stops to point at the ceiling lights while smiling at you during session.   Continue monitoring   Provide support

---

17.3 Create a Plan to Increase Productive Play

Figure 17.4 lists some examples of strategies you can use for each of the four categories of RRBs. We have organized suggested responses by each category of RRB; however, these strategies should be used flexibly and often overlap. This is not an exclusive list and should be used creatively. There are often multiple RRBs occurring at the same time, and you will often use several strategies simultaneously to respond. As with the other domains, you should always start with core strategies (specifically environmental strategies) before moving on to conditional and more directive strategies.

In the following sections we will introduce the different types of RRBs, strategies to respond, and case examples.

17.4 Addressing Rigidity

One common form of RRBs is *rigidity*. Rigidity can manifest in many ways, including inflexibility, insistence on "sameness," adherence to patterns, or difficulty transitioning from one activity to another (American Psychiatric Association, 2013). Within the context of a JASPER session, rigidity leads to less time jointly engaged, less flexible and diverse play, and increases in dysregulation when asked to interact more flexibly. Here are some common examples:

• **Insistence on a pattern or sequence.** The child prefers to follow a particular pattern or sequence in the routine and resists attempts that deviate from the preferred way of playing (e.g., all shapes go into the shape sorter in the same order).

STRATEGIES TO INCREASE PRODUCTIVE PLAY ☑

Ideas for Rigidity

☐ Preempt the pattern

☐ Incorporate varied materials

☐ Reset the materials differently when you restart

☐ Practice similar steps with different toys

☐ Manage the number of pieces available

☐ Change a familiar sequence of steps

☐ Hold your piece on

☐ Model 2-3 times to build momentum

☐ Work toward equal and active roles

☐ Use parallel play

Ideas for Restricted Interests

☐ Choose strategic moments to incorporate a preferred toy

☐ Prepare the environment to keep the routine going

☐ Find other ways to incorporate the interest

☐ Remove a toy for now

☐ Set clear expectations

Ideas for Repetitive Behaviors

☐ Select toys that prevent repetitive behaviors

☐ Allow the child to explore the toy

☐ Use environmental prompts

☐ Return to a more successful step in the routine

Ideas for Sensory Behaviors

☐ Evaluate sensory input in the environment

☐ Capitalize on moments of attention

☐ Support the pace of the routine

FIGURE 17.4. Strategies to increase productive play.

- *Insistence on completion.* The child becomes dysregulated when a toy is not "completed" (e.g., pieces in a puzzle or cookies fit evenly on a tray) and may have difficulty with any steps that "undo" the finished item.
- *Insistence on a role.* The child resists equal and active participation from the adult when it interferes with the child's vision for the routine.

Rigidity can become a significant barrier to joint engagement. The child might refuse your expansions and models, outwardly reject your participation (e.g., push your hand away or tell you "No!"), or become dysregulated if you attempt to interrupt the rigid behavior. Altogether, rigid behaviors make it difficult to make progress toward the child's goals.

17.4.1 Use Core Environmental Strategies to Support Flexibility

When a child is playing rigidly, our primary goal is to increase the flexibility of the child's play. We use core strategies, especially environmental strategies, to address rigidity and promote new and creative ways of interacting with toys. As you start to notice patterns in the child's behavior, use these strategies more proactively to encourage the child to play productively.

Preempt the Pattern

Set up the environment and plan materials to provide visual cues of new ways to use a toy. Table 17.1 provides some examples of ways to do this before the child begins the usual pattern. Try to prevent unnecessary frustration to the child. The goal is not to stop the child from her preferred way to play but rather to support more flexible actions.

Incorporate Varied Materials

In addition to preempting the pattern, you can also add variations to the toys and flexibility to the actions by intentionally mixing materials. For example, if you are playing with Lego blocks, add foam blocks or magnetic blocks of different shapes and sizes as horizontal expansions. If you normally have people figures, try the same routine with a slightly different toy instead, such as using

TABLE 17.1. Strategies to Preempt the Pattern

Child's preferred pattern		Possible solution to increase flexibility
Prefers to play with only fire trucks	➜	Set out different types of cars and remove the fire trucks before the session
Prefers to add figures in matched pairs	➜	Remove duplicates so there are not any identical pairs
Prefers to assemble the blocks in the exact same way every time you build	➜	Set up the routine with a different base structure prebuilt
Prefers to keep toys complete	➜	Remove extra pieces from sets so that the perfect completion is not possible (e.g., missing a couple of pizza pieces, not enough figures to fill the seats in the car)
Prefers to bring toys up to the table, even when you set up bigger play stations on the floor	➜	Try playing at a larger table to increase the surface of the play space

animals or mixing the animals and people together. (See Chapter 11, Section 11.7.1, for additional examples.)

Reset the Materials Differently When You Restart

When you restart the routine, reset the materials in a way that promotes flexibility. For example, if the child prefers to stack blocks vertically, prebuild a different structure such as building a big square foundation (see Figure 17.5). This shows the child a different way to play before the child can begin re-creating the preferred layout. You can also change the order in which you present the expansions or provide access to new expansions after you restart to lead the routine in a flexible new direction.

Practice Similar Steps with Different Toys

Try the same routine with a different toy that is similar in function to give the child exposure to something slightly new. For example, try a pop-up toy with animals instead of *Sesame Street* characters, or a sandwich routine instead of a pizza routine.

Manage the Number of Pieces Available

A child may immediately launch into a familiar pattern if given all the pieces to complete that idea. You can prevent getting caught in rigid patterns like these by providing only a few pieces and then being ready with expansion options to continue the routine. This allows the child to engage in his preferred pattern briefly while incorporating flexibility. For example, a child may prefer to arrange pegs in a pegboard in a specific order. To increase flexibility, you could provide just a few pegs and then quickly introduce blocks that stack on top of the pegs to keep the routine moving forward.

Change a Familiar Sequence of Steps

Add new steps to the routine or change the order of the familiar steps. For example, in a "getting ready for bed" routine, you could brush teeth last instead of first; add a new step, such as rocking the dolls to sleep; or sing a different lullaby each time you do the routine. You could also add something unexpected (e.g., having only one bed available for the figures instead of two) or something the child might find silly (e.g., adding a toilet). These small changes promote flexibility and help break rigid patterns without undoing the familiar and motivating parts that the child enjoys.

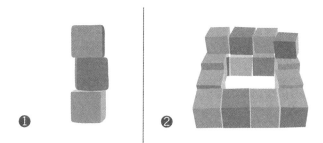

FIGURE 17.5. Quickly rearrange and prebuild the materials differently when you restart the routine.

17.4.2 Consider Conditional Strategies to Support Flexibility

When a child is still playing rigidly after implementing core strategies, or the rigidity begins to interfere with establishing and expanding a routine, incorporate some conditional strategies to target specific moments of flexibility.

Hold Your Piece in Place

If your child has a tendency to remove the pieces you add or undo your turn, hold your piece in place after your turn. This encourages the child to take her turn instead of rejecting yours. To help the child continue with her turn, you can also move the new pieces even closer or hand the child a piece as you hold your piece on.

Model Two to Three Times to Build Momentum

If the child is resistant to your models or expansions, you can show the child how the step works by modeling your action two to three times in quick succession. This creates a new visual pattern for the next step, rather than creating a singular disturbance to the current completed pattern. If you model one time, the child may see this toy or step as a disruption, whereas two to three models helps the child visualize a new pattern. As you do this, ensure there are pieces available for the child to participate in this new step.

Work toward Equal and Active Roles

If the child is consistently directing your role, you can find ways to add flexibility to the child's pattern. For example, if the child says, "Stand over there and order a lemonade," the adult could respond, "Actually, I'll order an Icee" in an effort to add flexibility. For higher-level players who may soon have goals to play with peers, it may be helpful to introduce the concept of sharing roles in the play through a social story (see Chapter 8). For example, you might start session with a short story about two friends sharing their ideas with each other.

Use Parallel Play

In some cases, it may be very difficult to play flexibly with the child, especially as you are first establishing this expectation. If the child becomes increasingly dysregulated and distressed when you attempt to participate in the routine, you may need to set up a parallel play routine next to the child to begin. For example, you can build your structure next to the child's structure. This allows you to continue the routine without disrupting the child's ways of building. After a few turns have passed, you can then create opportunities to merge the two structures into the same routine. For example, connect the gap between your two structures by building a bridge or a road, or try building the same structure together after you restart. This strategy should only be used as a last resort. If you do incorporate parallel play, transition back to playing together as soon as possible.

17.4.3 Case Examples about Rigidity

The following case examples show how you can use these strategies to respond to rigidity.

Perplexed Passenger

Dear JASPER,

My child and I built an awesome vehicle routine where we drive all around the city. Over time, I've started to realize we always do the same thing. First, we go straight on Broadway, then we turn right on Main Street, and then we go three blocks and turn right again on Sixth Avenue. He's so smart, and he knows how to get to many of his favorite places. I have tried to build on these driving plans by adding new characters for the vehicles, different destinations and routes, and even different ways to drive (e.g., fast, slow, bumpy, under the tunnel), but it's still very hard for me to take a turn. Often when I introduce something new, he gets upset, takes all the vehicles, and turns away from me. How can I be a part of this routine? I want to follow his interests, but I'm not sure what else to try. Should I give up on this routine and try something else?

Thanks,

Perplexed Passenger

Dear *Perplexed Passenger,*

You've clearly made some great efforts to expand this vehicle routine! Make sure to assess the overall level of play in your routines. It may feel as if the play acts are at a high play level given the child's language level, but driving a car back and forth is a discriminate act. If the majority of the routine is below his developmental level, then you may need to establish a different, higher-level routine. But if you can maintain periods of joint engagement with steps at his mastered and target play levels, this is a good place to keep working toward flexibility. You could try adding changes as you restart the routine. For example, you could make the restart fun by pretending Godzilla is coming to knock over the city and then quickly reset the materials so the streets and buildings cannot go in the exact same order. Try adding in small changes, such as adding a stoplight that is "broken," and then introduce tools and characters to fix it. If you are experiencing some success in expanding, then it might be a matter of balancing a little of the child's way and a little bit of your way, some old steps and some new. You could also bring in some new modes of transportation (e.g., boats or planes) to add more small changes into your routine.

Best of luck,

JASPER

Playing All Alone

Dear JASPER,

I support a girl who is great at presentation combination play! She loves to play with the cupcakes. We put them in the tray and dump them. She can do that routine all day long, but I feel as if she would probably keep doing that even if I was not there. I sit across from her and use positive affect to make my turn more noticeable and fun, but when I try to join, she becomes upset and pushes my hand away. It often becomes a battle between us. What can I do to help her want to play with me?

Thanks for your help,

Playing All Alone

Dear *Playing All Alone,*

You are already doing a good job with your affect and body position. Here you might want to assess the quality of engagement when putting the cupcakes in the tray. It seems she is object engaged and may need a plan to support joint engagement. Since you have already tried many strategies to play together, you may need to begin with a short time of parallel play next to one another. For example, bring in a second set of cupcakes and tray next to the child's tray and try modeling some new steps on your cupcakes next to her. This will allow her to watch your model before she needs to participate or allow a change with her cupcake. You can also assess the appropriateness of the toy. While the toy may have been an appropriate choice to get her started, it could have become too interfering. Try adding some fun surprises (e.g., feed cupcakes to the tummy stuffer) or use a novel play act (e.g., place some ice cream on top of the cupcakes) to see if you can get her to reengage with you. If she continues to be object focused and stuck on the same action, then it may be time to set the cupcakes aside for a little while. You can try them again once the child has established routines with other toys.

Good work!

JASPER

17.5 Responding to Restricted Interests

Restricted interests are another common form of RRBs that you may encounter in the context of JASPER sessions. Restricted interests are characterized by an intense focus on, or preoccupation with, a particular object or theme (American Psychiatric Association, 2013). In session, this can make it difficult to reach a jointly engaged state as the child is overly interested in a particular toy or routine. Here are some common examples:

- **Singular focus on a theme.** The child is concentrated on one idea or object and is resistant to expanding the interest.

- **Nonproductive actions.** The child may be enthusiastic about his interest but not have the play skills to take productive play actions with it (e.g., child is at an early combination play level but is interested in dolls and figures).

Restricted interests can be useful because they motivate the child, but this often comes at the cost of engagement and high-quality play routines. If the child has a restricted interest, you will need to determine when to include that interest in your play routines and when to move on.

17.5.1 Use Core Strategies to Diversify the Child's Interests

If the child is able to engage with the interest productively most of the time, we can show the child more creative and flexible ways to incorporate restricted interests using core strategies.

Choose Strategic Moments to Incorporate the Preferred Toy

If the child is more engaged and flexible early in the session, introduce the preferred toy early when the child is likely to play productively and socially with it. Alternatively, some children may be more flexible and engaged later in the session once you have established the expectations, in which case you should introduce the preferred toy later. Either way, make sure to introduce the preferred toy within an already-established routine so you have some momentum and a clear plan for the toy. For example, if the child is interested in vehicles, you could put figures in a house, have the figures build a road, and finally put the figures into vehicles to go somewhere else.

Prepare the Environment to Keep the Routine Going

Make sure there is a clear next step in the routine once the preferred toy is introduced. If you give the child his favorite Disney character without a plan, he may just want to hold it or perform a favorite play act with it (e.g., chasing another character).

Find Other Ways to Incorporate the Interest

If it is too difficult for the child to be jointly engaged while playing with the preferred toy, you may be able to find other ways to incorporate the child's interest. Instead of providing the child's preferred item, you can build the item or use a substitution. For example, in Figure 17.6, the adult and child build an airplane, rather than giving the child her favorite airplane toy. This strategy is most successful for children with presymbolic and symbolic play skills, who can understand you are building something representational.

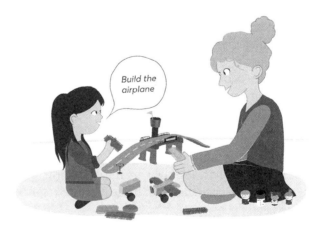

FIGURE 17.6. The adult uses a physical combination of building an airplane to include the child's interest of flying.

17.5.2 Consider Conditional Strategies to Diversify the Child's Interest

When a behavior interferes to the point that you cannot establish a routine or reach a state of joint engagement, you may need to assume a more active and directive role for a short time to create expectations for playing together or achieve a new idea in the routine.

Remove a Toy for Now

Certain toys (or features of toys) may be so motivating that it becomes difficult to accomplish anything in the session. If some of these steps do not work, it is okay to remove the toy. This is typically done as a last resort. Be prepared to use behavioral strategies and visual supports before and after removing a preferred item. Remember to stay calm in the moment and follow through with your decision. For future sessions, you may choose not to include the preferred toy while the child builds other skills. If the child arrives at session with the toy, you can create a transition routine of putting the toy in a special cubby or place before session.

Set Clear Expectations

Verbal children may request for their preferred toy or routine or protest your participation altogether. Be prepared with visual supports, clear directions, and reminders of the expectations.

17.5.3 Case Examples about Restricted Interests

The following case examples show how you can use these strategies to respond to restricted interests.

Perpetually Pyramids

Dear JASPER,

I am playing with a little girl who has some awesome symbolic play skills, can use short sentences, and is an expert in ancient Egypt. I've learned a lot about the pharaohs from her, but I'm worried she's not learning many new skills from me in our sessions. Every routine we do turns into something from Egypt. Each block gets turned into a pyramid, and every girl figure is Cleopatra. We have a solid routine around building the pyramids and then finding treasure inside. She initiates many of the steps and uses joint attention gestures to show me all the treasure, but I want her to try playing with some other themes so she'll be more successful with peers at school. I've tried swapping out the toys and bringing in new materials, but then she uses substitutions and we end up back in Egypt. How can I bring us somewhere new?

Thank you,

Perpetually Pyramids

Dear *Perpetually Pyramids,*

Your child has some really great skills, and it's great that you want to help connect these skills to other themes as well! Your pyramid routine is a great start and can help her get engaged and stay motivated. Create a plan to introduce materials with a theme that is different from, but still compatible with, the pyramid routine. For example, you could add figures that have clear roles, such as astronauts, policemen, or pirates. You can also add premade play structures (rather than just blocks) to set up a new story (e.g., an island or tree house). You can then use these materials to model steps that build on your current pyramid routine. For example, after finding treasure in the pyramid, you could build on her interest by burying the treasure somewhere new and then add a step where pirates to come steal the treasure. By adding in new variations to the theme, you can help expand her interest and build more creative and flexible routines over time.

Best,

JASPER

Picky with Piglet

Dear JASPER,

I am working with a toddler who absolutely loves Piglet from Winnie the Pooh. Her mom suggested bringing some Piglet stuffed animals into our session to help motivate her and increase her interest in playing with me. This little girl has mastered physical combination, and her target play level is child as agent, so it makes sense to include figures in the expansions of our routines. We have a great physical combination routine going where we build a giant castle out of nesting boxes. Over the past couple weeks, I've brought the Piglet stuffed animals into our session and modeled putting them into the castle. I thought she would love it—but instead the child holds a Piglet character in each hand and refuses to take a turn. She won't let go of them and quickly becomes object engaged—she turns her back to me and starts looking at the Piglet in her hands. How do I get her to reengage with me and to incorporate Piglet into our play? Help!

Thanks for your thoughts,

Picky with Piglet

Dear *Picky with Piglet,*

You are doing a great job thinking through how to motivate this little one. Although the child is motivated by Piglet, it sounds as if she has preferences about holding the stuffed animals and maintaining control over them. You may need to have a few sessions in which you do not bring the Piglet toys into the room. During this time, you can focus on establishing a solid routine with other figures first and work toward the child spontaneously adding other stuffed animals to the castle. As she more consistently uses these animals in a productive way, you can reincorporate the Piglets into your routines in an attempt to have her use them productively. You can also work on programming for a joint attention give during the initial sessions without the Piglet stuffed animals. Within the context of some of her more confident routines, model a joint attention give and then program for the child to give back. (For example, hand the child your figure;

then put your hand out. If the child gives you a figure, imitate the gesture and give her one back immediately.) Once you have introduced Piglet back into the session and have more fluid turn taking, you can practice the joint attention give with her. Since Piglet is preferred, she may be more reluctant to share, so this will likely require a bit more support.

Great work!

JASPER

17.6   Responding to Repetitive Behaviors

Repetitive behaviors involve recurring play acts, vocalizations, or motor movements (American Psychiatric Association, 2013). Sometimes a child may be able to maintain joint engagement while also displaying repetitive behaviors. However, repetitive behaviors can also interfere with establishing a successful routine, lend themselves to object engagement, and interfere with learning. The behaviors can manifest in different ways, including but not limited to the following:

- Stereotyped or repetitive movements of the body
  - Hand flapping
  - Body rocking or tensing
  - Spinning in circles
- Interfering use of toys or objects
  - Lining up, spinning, or sorting toys
  - Preoccupations with parts of toys (e.g., opening and closing the doors of a bus)
  - Turning on and off a light switch
- Abnormal speech patterns
  - Echolalia (e.g., immediately repeating words, scripting)
  - Repetitive vocalizations (e.g., humming, singing)
  - Idiosyncratic phrases (e.g., saying "To infinity and beyond" each time the child wants to go somewhere)

All children engage in repetitive play at times. It is important to distinguish whether this play is productive or interfering. The child's play level, flexibility, and level of engagement can help make this determination. If the child is jointly engaged and the action is developmentally appropriate, it can be productive, such as a simple level player taking turns with a partner to roll cars down a ramp. However, if the child is object engaged, inflexible, or far below play level, such as a presymbolic player pushing the car back and forth while watching the wheels, this is likely a repetitive behavior and requires a different response. When the behavior is not productive, you should find ways to help the child engage in play.

17.6.1   Use Core Strategies to Increase Productive Actions

When a child shows repetitive behaviors that are beginning to interfere with engagement, use core strategies to encourage more productive play actions.

Select Toys that Prevent Repetitive Behaviors

If the child demonstrates repetitive behaviors, consider toys that are less compatible with those behaviors. You might consider using bigger pieces (that the child cannot spin), different types of blocks (that are less interesting for visual inspection), or structures without hinges (to avoid repeated opening and closing).

Allow the Child to Explore the Toy

Some children may inspect a favorite color, number, or subject on a toy for a moment but are then able take their turn. Before you jump to supporting the child, give the child some space to explore the toy. During this moment, you can pause expectantly as you monitor the child. This can also serve as a good opportunity to share in the child's interest, model a gesture, and comment about the object. For example, if the child is looking at a picture of a cow printed on a nesting box, you could point and say, "Cow." If the child continues to explore the toy for a long period of time, you may need to model to return to the play routine.

Use Environmental Prompts

Use environmental prompts to show the child a more productive way to play. Move another toy closer, hand the child a new piece, or trade the child pieces. For example, if you are cutting a pizza and the child starts repetitively spinning the knife, you can move the pizza forward and then trade the child his knife for a piece of the sandwich, as is illustrated in Figure 17.7.

You could also trade the child his knife for your knife and then immediately model to show him what to do. This helps the child notice your model before he goes back to the repetitive behavior.

Return to a More Successful Step in the Routine

For example, if the child begins lining up figures after putting them down the slide, you could return to an earlier step in the routine such as building a park. When you do this, quickly offer new materials and model expansions (e.g., add ladders and swings to the park) to avoid returning to

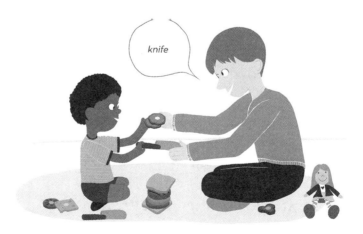

FIGURE 17.7. The adult offers the child a knife in exchange for the distracting sandwich piece.

the repetitive behavior. Resetting also provides you with an easy opportunity to transition out any materials that the child was previously getting stuck on.

17.6.2 Case Examples about Repetitive Behaviors

The following case examples show how you can use these strategies to respond to repetitive behaviors.

Counting on You

Dear JASPER,

I'm working with a child who gets very dysregulated at the start of our session. I've tried using a "first, then" schedule for the transition, having a fun affect, and singing songs to no avail. The one thing that helps him calm down is counting numbers on the different toys we have. For instance, I offer him a piggy bank with numbers on each of the coins as one of his initial choices, and he points to them and looks at me to count with him. When we do this, he immediately starts taking big deep breaths and calms down. I'm glad this is working, but I don't want to be reinforcing a repetitive behavior where he counts everything he sees. It's starting to feel as if he won't learn anything new if all we're doing is counting. How do I keep him calm but still teach him new things?

Many thanks,
Counting on You

Dear *Counting on You,*

He sounds like a super smart guy who knows just what he needs to settle down. It's great that you were able to pick up on his communication and use counting to help him regulate and settle into session. However, you're right in assessing that he's not going to learn many new play or communication skills if you continue the pattern of counting everything. Now that he's getting more comfortable in your sessions, you can slowly fade out numbered toys from each of your routines. For example, you could start with counting the coins and putting them in the piggy bank and then expand with other materials that don't have numbers, such as cookies that still fit in the piggy bank. As time goes on, you can introduce more novel toys without numbers. Just as you are currently pointing and labeling the numbers on the coins, you can point to and label different toys that you are sharing together. This way, you can model joint attention gestures and new words for him to use to share with you.

Keep up the good work!
JASPER

Healthy People

Dear JASPER,

The child I'm working with likes to script various lines that he has heard from his favorite TV show and often becomes fixated on saying, "The people are sick and need to go to the doctor." He can play at a multi-scheme symbolic play level and is quite intelligent for his age, so I thought this was a great idea at first. However, I think this is a script, as he keeps repeating this phrase and finds any chance he can to say this. Since we are playing with figures and his idea is productive, I go with it; however, I feel we are not making progress in our sessions as we keep going back to this doctor routine. How can I address this?

Sincerely,

Healthy People

Dear *Healthy People,*

Sounds like a tricky situation! You are right in that it will be difficult to improve flexibility and diversity of play if you keep repeating the same step. You may need to have other fun expansion options ready and available. You might also need to initiate these expansions earlier in the routine, before he is able to say that the people need to go to the doctor. If you have your environment set up and increase your pace, but he still suggests this doctor idea, then you might need to simply tell him you do not have the doctor toys or suggest the people do something else (e.g., "The people feel good; they want to go to the carnival!"). With children who are cognitively high functioning, ignoring their ideas or requests can be dysregulating to them and going along with all of their repetitive ideas does not work on your play targets. Therefore, simply telling them what you expect can often be the best strategy. At first, he might become upset that you do not want to follow his idea again; however, over time he will understand the expectations. Just be sure to follow through on what you say.

All the best,

JASPER

17.7 Addressing Sensory Behaviors

Sensory behaviors are a category of behaviors that encompass both hyper- and hyporeactivity toward sensory input such as sounds and touch. This hyper- and hyposensitivity can often lead to interests in sensory aspects of the environment and behaviors such as excessive smelling or touching of objects, visual fascination with lights or movement, and adverse responses to specific sounds or textures (American Psychiatric Association, 2013). In a JASPER session, this might include the following:

• *Seeking sensory stimulation.* Some children may choose toys or arrange toys in a specific way to gain input from them. For example, the child might closely look at a figure as she pushes it down a slide, tap toys together to hear a sound, or mouth toys for the sensation.

• *Avoiding sensory input.* Some children may become dysregulated from certain stimuli, such as loud noises or touch. For example, a child may become upset when materials clang loudly on the table or if the adult uses a physical prompt.

When children are seeking sensory input, they may engage solely with the object that is the focus of their sensory interest (i.e., become object engaged). This can often lead to decreases in joint engagement or can prevent children from reaching a jointly engaged state altogether. This in turn can lead to fewer opportunities to practice new types of play and communication.

17.7.1 Use Core Strategies to Increase Joint Engagement

When children show sensory behaviors, they may need additional support to engage with others. In JASPER, we do not necessarily try to "stop" or "fix" these behaviors. Our goal is simply to increase the child's engagement in the moment. If the behaviors do not interfere, we closely monitor the child for early signs of dysregulation and continue modeling productive language and play actions. If the behaviors do interfere, we provide support in the environment.

Evaluate Sensory Input in the Environment

Use materials that provide the right amount of sensory input to maintain productive play. As an example, if the child enjoys tactile input (feeling surfaces or objects of different textures), replace normal hard blocks with soft or squishy ones.

Examples to INCREASE Sensory Input

- Use textured blocks to provide input when the child stacks them together (e.g., Bristle Blocks)
- Add songs with big motor actions as a step in the routine (e.g., "The Wheels on the Bus")
- Use big materials to allow for movement (e.g., stacking large blocks)

Examples to Limit Sensory Input

- Remove toys with visually or physically distracting features (e.g., shine, reflection, holes to stick fingers through)
- Use some soft toys (e.g., foam blocks) to reduce noise for children who are sensitive to sound
- Place a towel on a hard surface or play on carpet to reduce noise of material

Capitalize on Moments of Attention

When children have a lot of sensory behaviors, they may have a difficult time noticing your turn because they are distracted by the sensory aspects of the toy. If the child is not attending to you, the support you provide will go unnoticed. Therefore, it is crucial to maximize your placement within the environment. Stay face-to-face at the child's eye level with the toys in between. Move around the room with the child, adjusting your body and your eye line to stay in the optimal position. When you take your turn or model a new action, notice where the child's attention is focused. Capitalize on moments when the child briefly looks up at you or at the toys in between you. Try to model and take your turn when you have the child's attention, however brief.

Support the Pace of the Routine

When sensory behaviors become more severe, it is challenging to build momentum. You may need to use a suggestive prompt to help maintain an appropriate pace in the routine. For example, if the child is visually examining or looking at a toy out of the corner of her eye before each turn, move a toy forward or hand the child a piece to keep the play moving. This also helps the child notice your participation and encourages engagement. Do not prompt the child on every turn or rapidly control the pace. Instead, the goal is to provide enough support so the sensory behavior does not lead to prolonged periods of object engagement.

17.7.2 Case Examples about Sensory Behaviors

The following case examples respond to sensory behaviors.

Eye Need Help

Dear JASPER,

The child I'm working with likes to visually inspect different types of toys during session, and this happens so much that it makes it difficult to get into a joint engaged state with her. She is at a presymbolic play level and has demonstrated that she can play with figures, yet every time I bring out the figures she will pick them up and closely examine them instead of taking her turn. When we build structures, she will also visually inspect the blocks that are put together. Help! How do I get this behavior to decrease so we can be more jointly engaged?

From,

Eye Need Help

Dear *Eye Need Help,*

It can be quite difficult to get into a jointly engaged state when the child is visually distracted and motivated by so many different things. Start by evaluating the types of toys you are using in session. For instance, if she becomes visually distracted by colorful figures, try swapping them out for figures with less detail (e.g., simple wooden figures). Choose other toys with simple designs as well. Since you know she will likely visually inspect when different blocks are put together, you should be prepared with strategies to keep the routine going. For example, you could increase the pace on your turn, have the environment set up for the child's turn, be ready to model, or hand her another block *before* she begins to visually inspect the object.

Hope this helps!

JASPER

Fill out Exercise 17.2 to practice implementing these strategies.

EXERCISE 17.2. **Responding to RRBs**

Choose the best strategy to respond in the scenarios below.

Scenario	Possible solutions
1. You are playing with a child with a lot of language and play ideas but never get a chance to take a turn. You've tried varying the routine, slowing down the pace by giving him a few pieces at a time, and holding your piece down after your turn, but each of these strategies cause increasing dysregulation.	A. Lower the play level B. Use a behavioral statement to set expectations C. Speed up your pace
2. You and the child have established a base sticking Velcro cake pieces together. You try to add cake toppings, but she immediately rips it off, takes the cake apart, and then begins to put the cake pieces back together. You try a few different expansions and the same pattern occurs.	A. Hold your piece on B. Model two to three times to build momentum C. Either A or B
3. You and the child have a base routine of driving different cars into a garage. He is initially engaged and sometimes shows you his car and comments on the color before taking his turn. But once the car is in the garage, he starts rolling the car in and out of the doorway. You model driving them all the way out, but he doesn't even notice and continues rolling the car until you take it away.	A. Prepare a clear next step to keep the routine going B. Increase your volume and affect to gain the child's attention C. Use a verbal prompt to tell the child to stop rolling the car

---

17.8 Test Your Plan for Productive Play

When you begin to work on flexibility and productive play, it may feel as if you are making little progress at first. Remember from Chapter 11 that even small changes in the routine are significant toward building diversity and complexity of play. Things will improve as you gain experience assessing the child's signs of RRBs and creating plans to get ahead of these behaviors.

17.8.1 Considerations over Time

As the intervention progresses, the goal is to have more flexibility, productive play, and periods of joint engagement within the routine. This should become easier as you get to know the child and improve your response.

Manage Dysregulation

Be prepared to manage dysregulation that may arise surrounding the preferred toy. Dysregulation may occur because you are trying to incorporate the toy or interest in a new way, or you are disrupting the child's typical method of play. The child might also become upset if you need to move on from the toy or remove it entirely. Often, we can be flexible and work with the child's interest or find a different approach; however, sometimes, it is valuable to push through resistance in order to advance play and see progress within the session.

Weigh the Benefits and Drawbacks of Using a Directive Prompt

After using the strategies from Sections 17.3–17.7, it may be appropriate to use a directive prompt to introduce a new idea. For instance, if the child is repetitively playing through a school routine, the adult might use a verbal prompt such as "Let's go to the pool!" to keep the routine flexible and moving forward. There may also be some instances where a slight physical prompt helps the child reengage in play. Consider how using a directive prompt benefits the child's targets and how it might impede them. Directive prompts help the child move beyond RRBs, practice new play steps, and build momentum in the routine; however, they also limit the child's chances to initiate and may cause prompt dependence or dysregulation. When using a directive prompt, keep the goal of child initiations in mind and plan to fade support quickly.

Try to Reintegrate the Interest

As the child's play becomes more flexible and productive, plan to reintroduce the challenging toys. For example, you could introduce the toy back into the routine once the child is engaged. By bringing back the interfering toy at another time, you can show the child more meaningful ways to include it as a step in the established routine.

17.9 Conclusion

By building flexibility and working through rigidity, we help to strengthen the child's ability to generalize these skills outside of the JASPER sessions and into other settings. As you continue using the strategies in this chapter, you should see improvement in the flexibility in your routines. See Figure 17.8 for a review of the strategies discussed.

This chapter concludes Part VI. Continue to support the child's engagement, regulation, and productive play throughout the session. This puts the child in the best position to learn and will gradually reduce the time you spend on nonproductive and interfering behaviors. In the concluding section, Part VII, we will provide information regarding tracking, training, and next steps.

Chapter 17 Summary

ASSESS THE QUALITY OF PLAY	CREATE A PLAN TO INCREASE PRODUCTIVE PLAY	TEST YOUR PLAN FOR PRODUCTIVE PLAY
o Assess the interference of behaviors o Determine whether monitoring or increase support o Hypothesize why the behaviors occur	o Consider the specific type of challenge o Prioritize core strategies o Consider conditional strategies	o Manage dysregulation o Consider the benefits and drawbacks for directive prompts o Try to reintegrate the interest

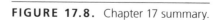

FIGURE 17.8. Chapter 17 summary.

PART VII

CONCLUSION

In this section, you will learn how to find the right balance of strategies and track progress over time.

Goals

✓ Integrate all of the JASPER strategies

✓ Track the child's progress over time

✓ Continue your JASPER training!

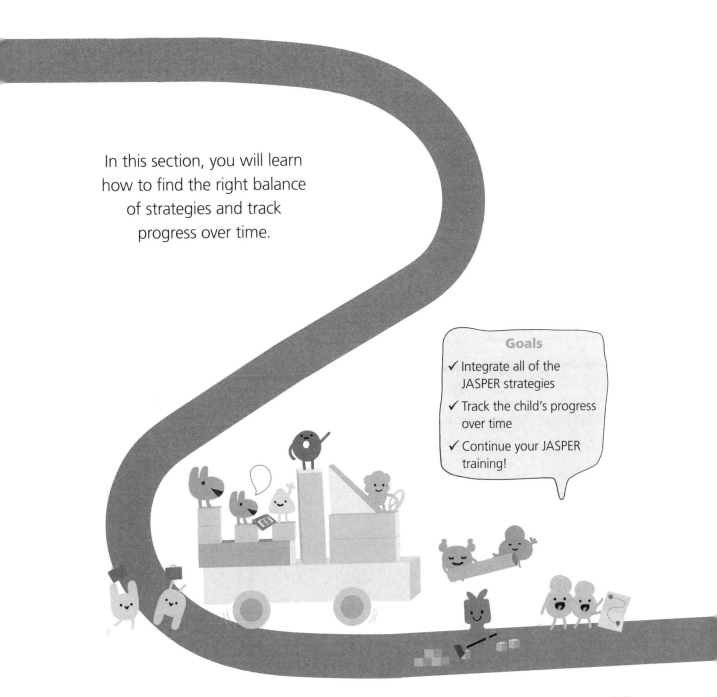

Putting It All Together

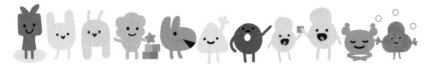

18.1 Introduction

We have reached the end of the book, and how far we have come! You now have all the information needed to assess the child and set targets to meet your goals. You have the tools to prepare the environment and the child for the session, establish and expand play routines, and support communication, engagement, regulation, and productive play. With each of these individual pieces in mind, the next step is to put them all together into an effective, holistic intervention. This involves tracking the child's progress, tailoring your own approach to the child across the course of the intervention, and of course—training! You will also evaluate what is working, what is not working, and how to improve as an interventionist to ensure the child is given every opportunity to succeed.

18.2 Integrating the Strategies

Although the information in this book is introduced sequentially, the strategies come together simultaneously in the session to meet the child's targets and goals. As illustrated in Figure 18.1, you will use your whole toolbox of strategies to support the child. As you can imagine, this requires a great deal of effort and balance on the part of the interventionist. This may look and feel overwhelming at first, and that is okay! It takes time to learn the individual components of the intervention and practice to blend them together. As you gain more experience, many of the strategies will become second nature. You will find yourself playing and communicating more naturally with less effort focused on the individual parts, and a greater focus on the interaction as a whole. When challenges arise, you will draw your attention to the bigger picture and quickly identify where to add support.

18.3 Track the Child's Progress

In order to monitor improvement, you will track the child's progress across time. There are many ways to do this. Our research results are based on meticulous data collection methods, which are

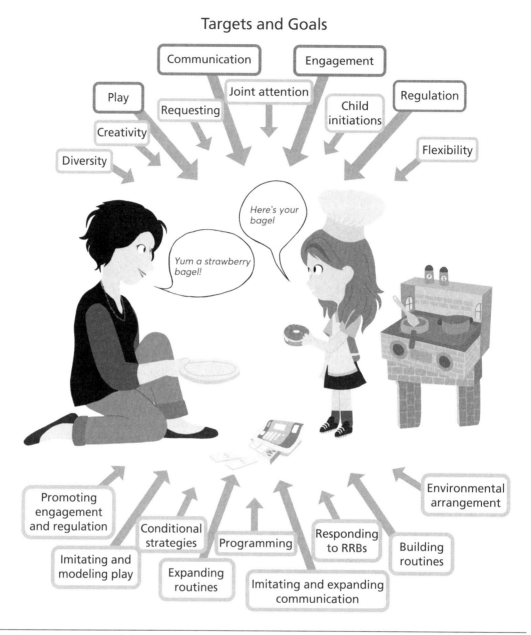

FIGURE 18.1. The adult balances all the strategies and goals of JASPER within the context of the routine.

gathered through video-recording and highly detailed coding and analysis; however, this level of detail is not necessary for clinical purposes. Instead, we recommend that interventionists use a method familiar to them to focus on examining the core domains targeted in the intervention. We provide a couple examples of ways to gather information about the child in the forms located at the end of the chapter. Form 18.1 is a qualitative intervention log, where you can track challenges, signs of progress, and new targets. Form 18.2 is a quantitative data collection sheet, where you can track individual skills. You can use something similar or add JASPER goals to your current data collection approach.

18.3.1 Video-Record the Session

In addition to video-recording the child's SPACE assessments, we also recommend video-recording every session or every few sessions (with permission from the child's caregiver). Video-recording is helpful for reviewing the child's progress and for planning future sessions. Signs of change are easy to miss in person. Not only do they happen quickly, but they are also often subtle. Video-recording is imperative for assessing and improving your skills and troubleshooting challenges. It allows you to notice moments you may have missed and to build on them during the next session. It also allows you to receive feedback from other JASPER interventionists (with permission from the child's caregiver) and brainstorm ways to improve. This is especially helpful if you see multiple children, as it may be difficult to recall the details of each session.

18.3.2 Record Skills

After the session, record the child's skills using one of the tracking methods above or a similar method of your own. Assess each aspect of the session with an eye for change. In what areas is the child progressing, and in what areas is the child slow to change? Focus on the big picture highlights or challenges of the session, such as meaningful signs of progress, challenging behaviors, necessary modifications, and so on. This does not have to be an exhaustive process in which you record every individual skill. Rather, focus on information that is most meaningful and relevant to each child.

While tracking progress is an important part of JASPER, it should never interfere with the session. You should avoid taking notes or recording skills during the session, as this distracts from your play together and interferes with engagement. Instead, write down what you can recall after the fact, and review the video-recording of your session for added detail. As you get to know the child, salient moments of progress become quite clear and memorable and are easy to recall after the fact. Figure 18.2 provides an example of data recording.

18.3.3 Set New Targets

If the child consistently demonstrates a skill in a variety of routines and settings, this means he has *mastered* the skill and is ready for a new target. You will continue to update the child's targets on the Intervention Log (Form 18.1). Change the target for the next session and add any changes you

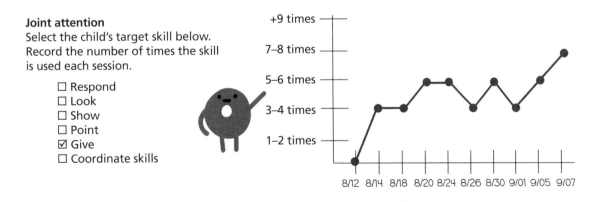

FIGURE 18.2. Example of a child's joint attention progress across sessions.

may need to make to your routines. In addition, formally reassess the child every 2 to 3 months using the SPACE.

18.3.4 Notice Small Signs of Progress

Progress is not always linear. Some children show little progress at first and may need several sessions of support to establish expectations and show signs of improvement. It is also common to experience ups and downs across sessions, with some days better than others. If you feel as though you are seeing little to no progress, remember to look at the bigger picture. The child does not have to master a target skill in its entirety to be showing improvement. Even the slightest changes can be crucial steps in the right direction, as these small steps come together to create positive change over time. Figure 18.3 shows examples from each domain.

These small, but meaningful moments may not seem that impressive from the outside, but they can represent major leaps in the child's progress. Remember, JASPER is specifically targeting core challenges of ASD, so each of these small improvements should be celebrated! Here are some of our favorite examples:

- A child with minimal eye contact looks up to share when something unexpected happens.
- A child first begins to vocalize or make sounds with communicative intent.
- A child who normally says only one word begins saying two.
- A child who typically insists on one type of toy shows flexibility and chooses another.
- A child accepts a new expansion that was previously rejected.

As sessions progress, the overall interactions may become more flexible, natural, and fun. Though these may seem to be small steps, they can be quite significant developmental milestones for the child and signify progress toward the child's goals.

18.4 JASPER Training

In training, we cover the basics of each strategy, help you choose targets, and provide feedback as you practice with a child. Learning JASPER is like learning any new skill. It requires practice and experience. While this book should help you understand the basics, you will not be fully prepared until you practice. Training, feedback, and self-reflection are critical components of this process. Those who would like to become JASPER-certified clinicians must receive certification through official JASPER trainings. Our introductory course is typically a 40-hour, hands-on training that will help you become familiar with JASPER goals and strategies. The training is a mix of didactic content with live coaching and clinical practice with several children throughout the week. This is the initial step to becoming a JASPER-certified interventionist. After becoming certified as a one-on-one JASPER interventionist, you may pursue additional training to become certified in peer-to-peer intervention, to train caregivers, or to train others in your community, such as teachers.

18.4.1 Fidelity

JASPER trainees are rated based on both their use of the strategies and the quality of their application. Trainees must submit videos with three different children of varying ability levels. For each video, they must achieve a score of 90% or higher, showing that they can successfully implement

Meaningful Signs of Progress

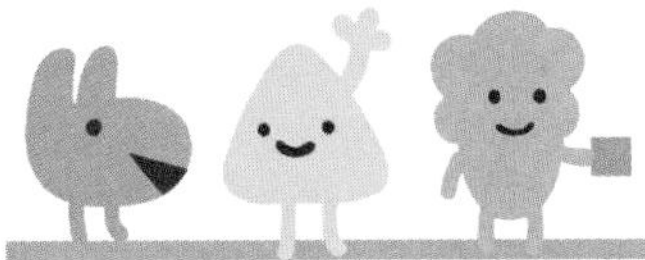

ROUTINES

- Child is able to choose a routine to start
- Routines include clear base steps
- Child initiates and follows expansions
- Duration of each routine increases
- Routines become more flexible
- Routines or steps of routines that were challenging become more fluid

PLAY SKILLS

- New play acts, play acts at different levels, emerging play skills
- Child-initiated expansions
- Play acts used in a new context or with new materials

JOINT ATTENTION AND REQUESTING GESTURES

- New or noteworthy emerging gestures
- Gestures used in a new context
- Gestures combined with language and/or eye contact
- Successful programming opportunities
- Success in fading supports or prompts while programming

LANGUAGE

- New or noteworthy words or phrases, including word approximations
- Words used for a new function or in a new context
- Advance in MLU
- Decrease in repetitive or odd use of language

ENGAGEMENT

- Decrease in challenges with engagement
- Successful strategies to reengage
- Moments of increased motivation and joint engagement

REGULATION

- Decrease in dysregulation
- Successful strategies to support regulation and respond to dysregulation
- Success responding to specific functions of behavior
- Greater ease in transitions

TROUBLESHOOTING

- Success with ACT framework
- Ability to fade support
  - Shift toward relying primarily on core strategies
  - Fewer adult models
  - Fewer directive prompts

FIGURE 18.3. Meaningful signs of progress.

the strategies according to our guidelines. This includes balancing and tailoring the strategies according to the child. Evaluation of skills is broken into the following categories: setting up and rearranging the environment, balancing imitation and modeling, establishing play routines, expanding play routines, programming for social communication, promoting language, and supporting engagement and regulation.

18.4.2 Improving Your Approach

There is a lot going on in a JASPER session. Your initial attempts will not be perfect. You must continue troubleshooting and seeking support to meet the child's needs. As you review your sessions, look for opportunities you may have missed and areas to improve. Notice your overall style, such as your pace, timing, and tone of voice. Were there moments when you were too passive or overly active? Did you miss any opportunities to respond to the child? Did you find an appropriate balance in the strategies (e.g., imitating vs. modeling, restarting vs. expanding)? Notice your level of confidence and style of communication as well. Like any new endeavor, this takes practice. The important thing is to learn from what you did well, as well as from possible missteps, and make adjustments for next time.

Master Each Strategy

As you begin learning JASPER, it may help to layer the strategies incrementally at first. Prioritize mastering strategies in the order they are presented in the book. Begin by setting up your environment and choosing developmentally appropriate and motivating toys. Once you are in session, focus on imitating the child and responding to communication and language. Then try to layer the support by modeling language and gestures on your turn, and modeling play acts when the child needs support. As you get more comfortable, you can try establishing the base as you maintain the previous steps of imitating and modeling play and communication. Once you feel confident in these roles, you can start thinking about expanding and try a programming opportunity or two. Next, begin thinking about engagement and regulation. What do you notice in the child's behaviors? Are there ways to set the child up for success? It is often the case that you must manage these challenges along the way. This is difficult to do as you are still mastering the basics. If possible, it helps to work alongside another trained JASPER clinician, who can guide you through the more complex, individualized aspects of the intervention while you are still learning. Once you feel confident with the core strategies, begin troubleshooting and responding to challenges— dysregulation, diminishing engagement, repetitive behaviors, and challenges with play and communication. Build in flexibility and diversity, work toward goals, and set new targets as the child masters new skills. As you get more comfortable with the child and the strategies, you will become more skilled at balancing all of these components together.

Look at the Big Picture

In order to truly progress, you must be able to step back and look at the bigger picture. There will be ups and downs in the child's progress, as well as your own. You and the child will have both good days and bad days, times of stagnation and times of growth. It is up to you to monitor all of this and determine when changes are required. Despite occasional ups and downs, the goal is to have an upward trend of growth.

Refocus on the Child in Front of You

As you are learning to balance each new JASPER strategy, it is common to feel overwhelmed or even distracted. In these moments, it is necessary not to lose focus on the child in front of you. It is okay to pause and collect yourself during session. Things may not go perfectly, but it is important to keep trying. Choose a strategy, acknowledge the child's reaction, and respond accordingly. When challenges arise, remember the child is not to blame. Instead, it is your responsibility to take a breath, troubleshoot, and find a solution.

Build a JASPER Community

If possible, we recommend building a community of JASPER experts around you. This can be a tremendous help as you learn the intervention and will remain a valuable resource as you grow.

We have learned that it can be just as effective to have informal discussion and feedback from a peer who has reached fidelity as it is to receive systematized intensive booster training from a specialized JASPER trainer (Shire, Worthman, Shih, & Kasari, 2021). By sharing creative routines and expansions, troubleshooting challenges, and brainstorming strategies together, you will help children reach their full potential.

18.5 Beyond the Basics

While the purpose of this book is to introduce JASPER in the context of interventionist and child interactions during toy play, JASPER research has also been extended to other contexts.

18.5.1 JASPER in the Community

Though not the focus of this book, the strategies contained in the book can be used throughout the day and across activities. JASPER has been successfully implemented with parents, caregivers, teachers, and paraprofessionals, one-on-one and in some cases in peer groups. Published research reports have extended JASPER to daily activities such as chores, dinner time, and story time (Kasari et al., 2014a), and very recent studies have adapted JASPER to peer interactions (called jasPEER; Shire et al., 2020a). We have studies teaching parents or caregivers (Kasari et al., 2010, 2015, 2014b), and we have taught teachers and paraprofessionals to use JASPER in small groups (Chang et al., 2016) or one to one (Lawton & Kasari, 2012; Goods, Ishijima, Chang, & Kasari, 2013; Shire et al., 2017). Following up with interventionists who received JASPER training in community settings 1 year later, we see sustained implementation of the intervention strategies and similar outcomes for children (Shire et al., 2019). Telehealth approaches, where JASPER was implemented either partially or fully remotely, have also been successful in training professionals and improving child outcomes (Shire, Worthman, Shih, & Kasari, 2020b; Shire et al., 2021).

18.5.2 JASPER across Cultures

In research trials, JASPER has been successfully delivered to families in their home languages, including English, Korean, Vietnamese, Russian, and Spanish (Kasari et al., 2014a, 2014b, 2015). The original JASPER intervention trial was also replicated by an independent research group and delivered in Norwegian (Kaale et al., 2012). Clinically, JASPER has been used internationally and implemented in several countries (e.g., Canada, Russia, Vietnam, Kazakhstan, Belgium, Macedonia, Japan, Romania).

18.6 Common Questions

In the following section, we address some common questions related to training, tracking progress, and implementation.

Can I record data during the session?

We highly discourage taking detailed notes during the session. This distracts from the child's engagement and inhibits your ability to support the child as you ought. If you are interested in a more thorough data analysis and are unable to video-record the child, you can request that another interventionist observe your sessions and record data live, so you are able to remain focused on the child.

Can I use JASPER with other interventions?

JASPER has been successfully added, blended, and sequenced in interventions (Kasari et al., 2006, 2014a, 2014b). We recognize that children need many different types of interventions, in combination or in sequence. We would encourage you to use the best evidence to create a comprehensive program for individual children (eclectic but informed—Kasari & Smith, 2013).

How does JASPER support long-term progress and generalization?

In our research studies, children are able to generalize skills they have learned with the interventionist to new interactions with their caregivers (Kasari et al., 2006, 2012, 2014, 2015) or to teachers in the classroom (Kasari et al., 2015). Some models program generalization separately from intervention sessions. In JASPER we have not found this to be necessary for a few reasons. First, if goals for the child are at her developmental level and integrated naturally into the session, the child is more likely to actually learn the skill. (Arguably a child who cannot generalize a skill may not have actually learned the skill.) Second, we systematically provide space for the child to initiate skills throughout the interaction. Children are expected and encouraged to initiate ideas and to communicate those ideas rather than be passive responders to adult instruction. Third, JASPER works within natural play routines with toys, where generalization may be more seamless. Thus, JASPER sessions act as a practice ground to learn new skills in a structured and supportive environment. As we develop flexible play routines and emphasize building lasting engagement, children are already learning skills within a natural context. This makes it easier and more likely for children to generalize these skills across environments that they come into contact with.

Is JASPER the same as other NDBIs?

There are a number of differences and similarities between JASPER and other NDBI models. The similarities are often in how we describe our interventions, yet if you dig deeper and note how we define common terms and apply similar strategies, there are distinct differences. Learning one model of NDBI will not easily translate to another model without training to reach fidelity. Why should you try JASPER?

1. In JASPER, play is carefully assessed for mastered and emerging levels, and this information feeds into the development of play routines that become the "topic" of the interaction, as well as a target for growth.
2. JASPER is structured in such a way that several strategies are layered to support the child's regulation and engagement throughout play routines that mirror the style of play in typical development.
3. The goal in JASPER is to foster child initiations to help the child become an independent and competent player and communicator.
4. Research evidence for JASPER has been consistently replicated, demonstrating improvement in the core social communication challenges common to children with autism, whether delivered by interventionists, caregivers, or teachers.

18.7 Conclusion

Like every good intervention, JASPER is still evolving. We continue to learn from children, families, and communities how best to adapt our program to meet the various needs of children with ASD. JASPER works best within a community of support where ideas, moments of success, and frustration can be shared and validated. There are always additional factors to consider, exceptions to the rules, and children who break the mold. We are continually inspired by each child we encounter. We hope you find this book useful in your practice.

FORM 18.1. **Intervention Log**

Child: _____ Adult: _____

SESSION DETAILS	TARGETS	PLAY	GESTURES	LANGUAGE	ENGAGEMENT	REGULATION
Session #: Date: Duration:	Play: Req. gesture: JA gesture: Language: Engagement: Regulation:		Requesting: JA:			
Session #: Date: Duration:	Play: Req. gesture: JA gesture: Language: Engagement: Regulation:		Requesting: JA:			
Session #: Date: Duration:	Play: Req. gesture: JA gesture: Language: Engagement: Regulation:		Requesting: JA:			

jasper

Data Collection Sheet

Child: _____ Adult: _____

Instructions:

- Use the following charts to measure the child's progress over time.
- Track the session date along the horizontal axis and the child's skills or states across the vertical axis.

HIGHEST PLAY LEVEL INITIATED:
Record the child's highest initiated (not imitated) play level during session

Thematic
Sociodramatic
Multi-scheme sequence
Doll as agent
Substitution without object
Substitution with object
Single-scheme sequence
Conventional combination
Child as agent
Physical combination
Pretend self
General combination
Presentation combination
Take-apart
Discriminate act
Indiscriminate act

Session date

JOINT ATTENTION:
Select the child's target skill below. Record the number of times the skill is used each session.

☐ Respond
☐ Look
☐ Show
☐ Point
☐ Give
☐ Coordinate skills

+9 times
7–8 times
5–6 times
3–4 times
1–2 times

Session date

REQUESTING:
Select the child's target skill below. Record the number of times the skill is used each session.

☐ Look
☐ Reach
☐ Point
☐ Give
☐ Coordinate skills

+9 times
7–8 times
5–6 times
3–4 times
1–2 times

Session date

(continued)

LANGUAGE:
Track the child's mean length of utterance once per week.

You should expect language progress to be gradual, rather than seeing significant increases in session to session.

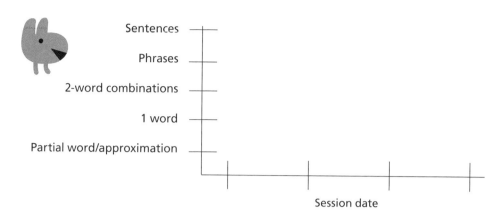

Sentences

Phrases

2-word combinations

1 word

Partial word/approximation

Session date

AVERAGE DURATION OF JOINT ENGAGEMENT:
Record the average duration the child spends in a state of joint engagement.*

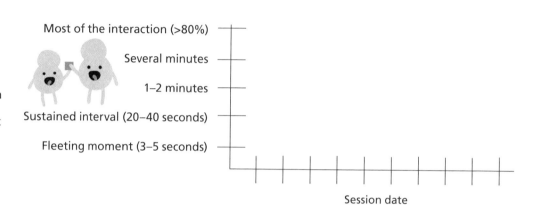

Most of the interaction (>80%)

Several minutes

1–2 minutes

Sustained interval (20–40 seconds)

Fleeting moment (3–5 seconds)

Session date

AVERAGE DURATION OF REGULATION:
Record the average duration the child spends in a regulated state throughout the session.

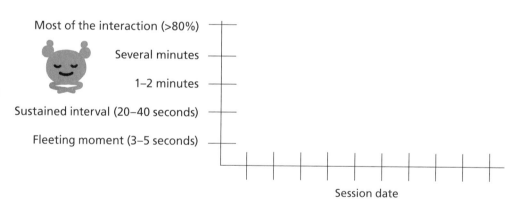

Most of the interaction (>80%)

Several minutes

1–2 minutes

Sustained interval (20–40 seconds)

Fleeting moment (3–5 seconds)

Session date

Note: These scales are created in reference to a 45- to 60-minute session. If your session is longer, please adjust accordingly.

*While you will see variability session to session, data shows that a 20% increase (+2 out of 10 minutes) from baseline is connected to change in JA and language (Shih, Chang, Shire, & Kasari, 2017).

APPENDICES

Strategies Checklist

SET UP THE ENVIRONMENT

- ☐ Choose developmentally appropriate toys (Ch. 6)
- ☐ Choose appropriate play area: table, floor, or combination (Ch. 7)
- ☐ Stay face-to-face (Ch. 7)
- ☐ Limit distractions in the room (Ch. 7)
- ☐ Set up routine options (Ch. 7)
- ☐ Manage the environment (Ch. 7)
  - ☐ Refill toys as needed
  - ☐ Group similar pieces together
  - ☐ Clear clutter
  - ☐ Reset the environment after the restart
- ☐ Prepare the environment for expansions (Ch. 7, 11)

ESTABLISH AND MAINTAIN THE ROUTINE

- ☐ Establish the base (Ch. 5, 10)
  - ☐ Manage the environment (Ch. 10)
  - ☐ Imitate productive play acts (Ch. 9, 10)
  - ☐ Model when the child needs support (Ch. 9, 10)
- ☐ Restart the routine (Ch. 5, 10)
  - ☐ Reset the materials (Ch. 10)
  - ☐ Support the next steps (Ch. 10)
- ☐ Expand the routine (Ch. 5, 11)
  - ☐ Prepare the environment for expansions
  - ☐ Imitate productive play expansions
  - ☐ Model expansions as needed
  - ☐ Use both horizontal and vertical expansions

FOSTER COMMUNICATION

- ☐ Use commenting language (Ch. 6)
- ☐ Match the child's MLU (Ch. 6)
- ☐ Leave room on the child's turn (Ch. 5, 10, 12)
- ☐ Use language and gestures on your turn (Ch. 12)
- ☐ Imitate and expand appropriate communication (Ch. 12)
- ☐ Model language and gestures (Ch. 12)
- ☐ Program for joint attention and requesting skills (Ch. 13)
- ☐ Include AAC as needed (Ch. 14)

IMPROVE ROUTINES OVER TIME

- ☐ Use the ACT framework to troubleshoot (Ch. 8)
- ☐ Encourage flexibility (Ch. 11, 17)
- ☐ Increase the complexity and diversity of play and communication (Ch. 11, 12)
- ☐ Bridge routines (Ch. 11)
- ☐ Fade support (Ch. 8)
  - ☐ Fade environmental support
  - ☐ Fade models and prompts
  - ☐ Primarily use core strategies

SUPPORT ENGAGEMENT AND REGULATION

- ☐ Support transitions (Ch. 8)
  - ☐ Use visual supports
  - ☐ Use AAC device (Ch. 14)
  - ☐ Set clear expectations
- ☐ Modulate positive affect
- ☐ Address dysregulation and interfering behaviors (Ch. 16)
  - ☐ Identify the function of the behavior

- ☐ Balance core strategies (Ch. 5–14)
  - ☐ Create a supportive environment (Ch. 7, 8)
  - ☐ Be an equal and active play partner (Ch. 5, 10)
  - ☐ Balance imitating and modeling (Ch. 9)
  - ☐ Foster communication (Ch. 12–14)
- ☐ Use the ACT framework to troubleshoot engagement and regulation (Ch. 15–16)

- ☐ Consider a conditional strategy (Ch. 15, 16)
  - ☐ Use person engagement
  - ☐ Include a well-mastered routine
  - ☐ Require appropriate requests
  - ☐ Follow through on expectations
  - ☐ Redirect
  - ☐ Actively ignore

Exercise Answers

Chapter 2

Exercise 2.1. Engagement States

- 1-C; 2-E; 3-A; 4-F; 5-D; 6-B

Exercise 2.2. Initiation or Response?

- Responses: 2, 4; Initiations: 1, 3, 5

Exercise 2.3. Play Levels

- 1-K, 2-D, 3-I, 4-H, 5-M, 6-L, 7-A, 8-C, 9-E, 10-F, 11-J, 12-N, 13-O, 14-B, 15-G, 16-P

Exercise 2.4. The Difference between Joint Attention and Requesting

- Joint Attention: 1, 3, 6; Requesting: 2, 4, 5

Chapter 3

Exercise 3.1. SPACE Language Level

- The child's language level is one word. The child used a variety of one-word and two-word utterances. Although two-word utterances were the most complex level of verbal communication the child produced, the child's language level is one word, because it is the most frequently occurring length of utterance with a total of eight one-word utterances and one two-word utterances. (We count memorized phrases such as "Old MacDonald" as one word.)

Exercise 3.2. SPACE Play Acts

- The child demonstrated *three or more types* of general combination play acts, and *two types* of pretend-self acts. We do not count every instance of a play act; rather, we identify types. So, when the child stacks three blocks, there are three play acts (of stacking) but only one type of play (one general combination action).

Chapter 4

Exercise 4.1. Mastered and Target Gestures

1. Mastered: eye contact to request; target: reach to request
2. Mastered: reach to request and point to request; target: give to request
3. Mastered: The child has not mastered any gestures; target: look and reach to request. You should include the look in addition to the reach, because the child showed no instances of eye contact to request.

4. Mastered: JA point; target: JA show. The JA show is still emerging, because the child is holding the object inward instead of outward toward the adult.
5. Mastered: JA point; target: JA give. Since the child showed an emerging JA give, you can target this skill before the JA show.

Exercise 4.2. Mastered and Target Length of Utterance

1. Mastered: one-word utterances; diversity target: flexible and diverse one-word utterances; complexity target: two-word combinations
2. Mastered: two-word combinations; diversity target: flexible and diverse two-word combinations; complexity target: phrases

Exercise 4.3. Mastered and Target Play Skills

1. Mastered: take-apart; target: presentation combination. The child has mastered simple play (discriminate acts and take-apart) but only one act of each presentation and general combination. Even though the child showed one pretend-self act, you should target presentation and then general combination before moving to presymbolic skills.
2. Mastered: child as agent; target: physical combination. You must go back to fill in the physical and conventional combinations before you can target symbolic play. Because the SPACE is a snapshot of the child's mastered and emerging skills, we may be seeing splintered skills due to the child's interest in some available materials over others. Over your first few sessions, you should adjust your targets if you see the child has mastered physical and conventional combinations given more varied opportunities.

Chapter 5

Exercise 5.1. Components of a Routine

1. True. Routines can have a range of base steps depending on the child's ability.
2. False. A routine can start with only one expansion or include several expansions.
3. False. You can restart at any time in the routine: after the base steps, after an expansion, when the child needs to return to an easier step, or when a natural moment arises.
4. True. There is no maximum duration for a routine, as long as the routine remains motivating and continues growing. One of our goals is to sustain the routine for longer periods of time.
5. False. The child does not have to finish any of the steps or components of the routine before moving on to something else. You can follow the child to the next routine at any point.

Exercise 5.2. Qualities of a Play Routine

1. False. While you should have some play steps in mind, the routine should not be overly controlled or structured. The goal is not to play in a particular sequence. The routine should remain flexible and responsive to the interests of the child.
2. False. While you will have goals to expand the child's play level in each routine, the specific play acts should remain flexible and should follow the child's interests.
3. True. You should provide choices for the child in order to promote initiations and to ensure you can maintain the child's engagement throughout the session.
4. True. The steps can be repeated in a different order. This helps the child practice flexibility.
5. False. You should not follow the child's actions when they are rigid, repetitive, or significantly below the child's developmental level. In these cases, you should provide support.

Exercise 5.3. Equal and Active Roles

1. Passive. Although providing access to materials is important, it should not define your turn in the interaction. If you are not playing with the child and are only arranging toys, then you are not maintaining an active role in the interaction. (Instead, take your turn in stacking.)
2. Equal and active. You can maintain a reciprocal role in the interaction by imitating the child's play act and responding to the child's language.
3. Directive. Instead of redirecting the child to the previous step, you should imitate the child's new play idea.
4. Equal and active. This interaction supports the child's play and communication and leaves room for the child to initiate.
5. Directive. Even though the child responds positively, the adult should provide the child with more space to initiate the next steps in the play.

Chapter 6

Exercise 6.1. Choosing Toys

1. C: The child demonstrates indiscriminate acts and should have toy options that allow for acts at the next play level, discriminate acts.
2. B: The child demonstrates one presentation combination act and should have toy options that could be used for a wider range of presentation combination acts.
3. D: The child demonstrates some presentation combination acts, a conventional combination act, a general combination act, and a pretend-self act. This child should have toy options that could be used for a variety of combination and presymbolic acts.
4. A: The child demonstrates general and physical combination acts, and doll-as-agent acts. The child should have toy options that allow for a variety of presymbolic acts and combinations as well as symbolic acts.

Exercise 6.2. Adult Language Level

- 1-A, 2-E, 3-D, 4-B, 5-C (Note: 1 and 5 are both appropriate answers for A and B; however, "Baby" is the better word to model for A, since the child's word approximation starts with the *buh* sound.)

Chapter 7

Exercise 7.1. Choosing the Environment

- 1-B, 2-A, 3-C

Chapter 8

Exercise 8.1. Support Transitions

Note: These are just some of the possible approaches you might take to begin session. There are multiple appropriate ways to support each child.

1. B: Using a "first, then" visual will show the child that he will see his dad again and is more concrete than offering only a verbal reminder. The child may need more gradual steps to separate, and so you may need to begin by inviting Dad to join session.
2. D: Adding a visual support such as an all-done bin helps clarify the expectation of cleaning up without the adult needing to increase the use of verbal prompts and input (which may cause further dysregulation).
3. A: The child has an established routine to signal that he is going to learn. You can mimic his school routine of hanging up his backpack before moving into session if he needs this familiar cue as he adjusts to this new environment.

4. C: Help the child calm down and regulate before ending the session. You do not need to place any additional demands since you have already told the child you are finished. However, you should add in something fun and comforting so you can end on a positive note.

Exercise 8.2. Using Prompts in JASPER

1. True. In JASPER, we follow a least to most prompting hierarchy to support the child to use a skill as independently as possible.
2. False. In general, you should use a prompt one time. If the prompt was not successful, increase support to help the child follow through.
3. False. A suggestive prompt provides an idea for the child but does not mandate following through with the idea. In contrast, once you provide a directive prompt, you should help the child follow through with the expectation.
4. True. Consider prompting in the context of your other goals for the child (e.g., spontaneous initiations) and plan to fade prompting quickly over time.
5. False. Verbal prompts and gestural prompts are considered "directive" prompts and used as a *conditional* strategy in JASPER. They are used less frequently and only after a foundation of core strategies have been considered. Environment and model prompts are *core* strategies to JASPER.

Chapter 9

Exercise 9.1. Appropriate Use of Imitation

1. No. We do not imitate the tapping because this is likely a rigid, repetitive, or sensory action.
2. Yes. The child's play act is not traditional, but it is creative and appropriate.
3. Yes. It is appropriate to imitate the play act, even using slightly different materials.
4. No. We would not imitate throwing the plane, as we do not want to encourage throwing toys.
5. No. Because the child is playing out the role of the chef, it would be more appropriate to play out the role of a customer to continue the story of the routine. A more fitting response is to pretend to eat the hamburger and say, "Thank you! I'm hungry!"

Exercise 8.3. Setting Expectations

1. No. The direction has several steps that the child may not understand. Instead, provide one clear direction and help her follow through.
2. Yes. By helping the child follow through with the instruction, you limit extraneous verbal input and reinforce the child for sitting without causing more dysregulation.
3. No. Try to avoid asking the child if she wants to play. By asking a question, you are inviting the child to say no. Instead, you can use other strategies to support the start of the session, such as saying "Let's play!" or offer the child a specific choice like "Play blocks or animals?"

Exercise 9.2. Appropriate Use of Modeling

1. No. Although it is right to model in this scenario, the play level of the modeled step is too high (symbolic) given that the child is playing with a toy that is typically for presentation combination steps. Instead, you should model a developmentally appropriate play act.
2. Yes. We recommend modeling an appropriate play step when the child starts lining up cars, because this is likely a rigid and repetitive action.
3. No. In this case, you should model with the sandwich, because the child showed interest by looking at this toy.
4. No. The model had too many actions (two-step

model). Instead, you should choose one action to model and wait to see if the child will respond.

5. Yes. You should follow the child's toy choice and model an appropriate step.

Exercise 9.3. Imitate or Model?

1. Imitate. This is an action at the child's mastered play level and is productive, so we would imitate.

2. Model. The child demonstrates a play act significantly below her play level by rolling the bus (simple play), so this is not the time to imitate. Instead, model an action the child could use at her mastered level (e.g., add figures into the bus).

3. Model. Tossing figures is not an appropriate act, and you should not imitate. Instead, model an appropriate action the child could take with the figures (e.g., walking the figures into the school or sitting them down on chairs at the school).

4. Imitate. The child's play act is at his target level (symbolic play). Imitate to reinforce the target skill by playing out your role in the child's idea (e.g., pretending your figure is a student).

Chapter 10

Exercise 10.1. Identifying an Established Base

1. Established. The child is showing signs that she is comfortable with this base by coordinating eye contact and restarting the routine by stacking the boxes after they crash.

2. Unstable. The child needs a lot of support (modeling, handing him a piece) to take his turn.

Exercise 9.4. What Comes Next?

1. B: Imitate. Although the child's idea is unconventional, it is still creative, productive, and increases the play level (symbolic play with a substitution). Do not model a new play step (A) or reject the child's action in order to model a new action (C).

2. C: The child's actions are repetitive and too low in terms of play level, so you should model an appropriate next step. You should not immediately take the toy away without giving the child an opportunity to play with it appropriately (A), nor should you imitate the repetitive action (B).

3. Unstable. These steps do not provide a solid foundation for the routine. The actions are disjointed and are not connected by a common theme or story. There is no repetition in steps, so the child is unlikely to initiate or have a clear sense of what you are doing together, and there is no room for the routine to grow.

Chapter 11

Exercise 11.1. Expanding Routines

1. C: Put expansion options into the environment to let the child initiate the next idea. You should try to put these materials in place *before* the child is ready to expand, so she does not start to lose engagement.

2. C: Follow the child's initiation by stacking the pizza. While this might seem like an odd next step to us, this is an appropriate expansion idea for a child at a general combination play level.

3. D: You can either model a productive step with the doors to help connect the child's idea to the routine and bring it back up to an appropriate play level (B), or you can add in new materials to suggest a more productive expansion step (C). You would not imitate by repeatedly opening and closing the doors, because this step is likely repetitive and leading to object engagement.

Chapter 12

Exercise 12.1. Imitating and Expanding Communication

1. Yes. You should notice the child's eye contact and respond with a gesture and language. (You are not required to respond with a gesture every single time, especially if you have many opportunities to respond with gestures throughout the routine.)

2. Yes. You should imitate and expand the child's language (while also imitating the child's productive play act).

3. No. Instead of directly imitating the child, it would be more appropriate to play out your role instead by saying something like "I'm the robber. I will run away!" This is a more appropriate language expansion for a child who speaks in sentences.

4. No. Instead of giving the child a direction to put more animals in, you should expand the phrase with a comment and gesture (e.g., JA point and say, "Tiger goes in the zoo") or comment while imitate on your turn (e.g., "Lion goes in the zoo!").

5. No. Rather than imitating the vocalization, you should respond with the full word "ball."

Chapter 13

Exercise 13.1. Creating Programming Opportunities

1. B: Hold up a brush and a shirt. Offering the child a choice is an appropriate way to evoke a requesting point and does not disrupt the flow of the routine too much as it provides expansion options. Limiting access to the doll (A) is not an appropriate prompting strategy in this case because it stops the routine and disrupts the child's engagement.

2. B: Put something silly, like a piece of cheese, onto the cake. Adding something unexpected or silly to the routine and then pausing creates an explicit opportunity for the child to notice something and react. Raising the volume of your models (A) is not an appropriate strategy and may cause the child to have unnatural intonation toward his peers.

3. B: Place a few of the puzzle pieces into a sealed container so the child has the opportunity to request for you to open it. Choosing a puzzle that the child will not be successful with (A) may cause dysregulation and will not allow you to take equal and active roles since the adult would need to prompt or assist in each turn.

4. A: Attach a piece of orange with a piece of banana. Build an unexpected combination of fruits as an expansion to your routine to create the opportunity to share about a funny or novel topic. Pause to ensure the child has space to gesture, comment, or look to share with you. Do not shake the container of pieces

(B) or otherwise recruit the child's attention, as this creates a prompted response that is led by the adult.

5. A: Pause expectantly as she tries to reach the top. Rather than jumping in to help, you are allowing the child the opportunity to request. Do not verbally prompt her to give you the block (B), as this is too much support and she has not had the opportunity to initiate the skill.

Exercise 13.2. Prompting and Programming

1. False. You should not physically prompt the child to make eye contact. Rather, you should use your environmental arrangement (e.g., stay face-to-face, orient toys in between you and the child) to encourage engagement. Choose a specific gesture target to program and prompt for and use your response to reinforce instances of eye contact that occur.

2. True. The child may use a different or emerging skill in response to your opportunity (e.g., vocalizing in place of a point to request). Prioritize engagement and respond by imitating and expanding to model the target skill for the child.

3. False. After providing the opportunity, pause expectantly for the child to respond. After the child has had time to initiate a response, you may choose to prompt the target skill.

4. True. If your first prompt was not successful, increase your level of support to help the child achieve the

target skill (e.g., start with a general verbal prompt; then move to a specific verbal prompt).

5. True. Consider your overall goal of child initiations, and plan to fade your level of prompting to encourage independence.

6. False. Programming and prompting should be used in select, salient moments in the routine. When used too frequently, these strategies conflict with maintaining an equal and active role and the adult becomes overly directive.

Chapter 14

Exercise 14.1. Incorporating a Speech-Generating Device

1. False. While you should prepare the SGD with words relevant to your routines, you may choose to say a word that is not on the device. It is important to keep your communication and pacing natural throughout the routine, so make a mental note to add recurring words to the device later on.

2. True. In the same way that you verbally model content words, it is important to program words that can be used flexibly throughout routines.

3. False. In order to limit distractions, you can use a system with "Guided Access," remove other applications, and limit scrolling to help the child learn to use the device for communication. For some children, you may need to establish a solid base routine and then introduce the SGD. This means there may be moments when the child does not have access while

you are building a solid routine before reintroducing the device and helping the child use it productively.

4. True. Similar to building up to an understanding of symbolism in play, children need to build an understanding of symbolic representations in images. Some children may need the icons to use real photos of the objects in your routines, while others can navigate icons of drawings or symbols.

5. False. You should pair your SGD use with verbal language models and gestures when appropriate. This provides the child with multiple modes of communication models to learn from.

6. True. Although this can be tough to remember at first, especially if you have routines that move between the table and floor, it is important that the child has access to the SGD throughout each routine so that it's possible to communicate freely.

Chapter 15

Exercise 15.1. Supporting Engagement

1. A: Your initial toy choices are far below the child's mastered level. Choose toys within the child's range of mastered and target play so the child does not become bored or unengaged. Leaving room on the child's turn (B) and moving in front of the child (C) will do little to support engagement if you do not have appropriate toy choice to begin.

2. B: After taking 10 turns each, the child is likely ready to move on but does not know what to do next. Instead of continuing to imitate (A), introduce a new, exciting expansion step to keep the routine going. You can model appropriate language as well (C), but this alone will not substantially increase engagement.

3. A: Despite trying to maintain the routine by expanding

with new steps for the blender and fruit, the child is losing interest. The routine may have run its course, and you should introduce another toy set into the environment to see if this is more motivating to the child. The problem is likely not with establishing the base (B; as you are already taking turns), and moving in front of the child (C) will not be enough to gain the child's engagement.

4. A: Use consistent and immediate imitation to take an active role in the routine and model being a fun and engaging play partner. Do not immediately jump to removing the toy (B) without trying less intrusive strategies first. While you can modulate your affect (C), you should first take an active role in the play.

Exercise 15.2. Responding to Fragile Engagement

1. D: You could either lower the play level (B) or build in person engagement (C) to establish engagement and then transition into steps at the child's mastered level. (You may also choose to add in other toy options if the child no longer seems interested in the cake.)

2. B: Reduce the number of toy choices so it is easier for the child to establish the base. While you do not want to completely remove the child's ability to choose toys, try to include toys that are related so you can build on the child's initiations to create a coherent routine. If there are too many different toys options present, the child may have a difficult time staying engaged and establishing a stable base.

3. D: By handing the child pieces and narrating what she is doing, you are sliding into a passive role and expecting the child to support the interaction on her own. Instead, you should pair your comments with your play turns, so you are taking a more active role. This shows the child what a joint engaged state feels like. You should also ensure the child continues to have access so she can freely play and engage with you in an equal and active role.

4. C: Introduce a well-mastered routine to reduce the cognitive demand of playing at a higher level, and focus on connecting with the child. Once you have established joint engagement, begin including horizontal and vertical expansions to balance familiarity with some challenge and creativity.

Chapter 16

Exercise 16.1. Supporting Regulation

1. A: It can be frustrating, and ultimately dysregulating, if the child cannot communicate her ideas. Use strategies to support the child's communication, such as incorporating an SGD and programming specific opportunities to increase the child's communication skills. Supporting transitions (C) does not seem to be a current challenge, and adding more structure to the environment (B) may cause the child more frustration if she has limited opportunities to convey her needs or ideas.

2. C: The routine has become too difficult, because there are too many vertical expansions. You should balance moments of increasing demand by including both horizontal and vertical expansions (B) and choosing moments to return to the base (A) for the child to play at his mastered level.

3. A: The child needs a clearer expectation of where she should be. Add structure to your session using furniture (e.g., bookshelf, turn a table on its side, place foam pad or carpet down) to create a clearer environment, and consider including a visual schedule to clarify expectations. Providing the child more space and time to wander the room (B) can lead to increased dysregulation and take away from opportunities to be engaged and learning. Increasing your affect (C) may increase dysregulation as you add to her already-elevated state.

4. B: Support the pace of the routine and consider your timing of imitation, modeling, and expanding to support regulation. Increasing the demand by programming for communication (A) or adding more directions (C) are not appropriate strategies here as they may help the child comply with you but will not help the child engage in a more active role.

Exercise 16.2. Responding to Dysregulation

1. A: The function of this behavior is likely attention seeking. You should ignore the behavior and continue to model a new productive step. Do not reinforce the child's inappropriate bid for attention by stopping the routine and picking up all the toys (B), singing (C), or reprimanding him (D). Increasing the amount of attention you give in response to the child's dropping toys might further reinforce the behavior.

2. C: The function of this behavior is likely access. When the child requests the ship, remind her it is available after you play together and redirect her to something else. You do not want to completely ignore each request (A), as this can cause further dysregulation. However, if she repeatedly asks, you may respond to only the first couple of instances and then continue to redirect her. Because you set a clear expectation and you know it will not lead to a productive interaction, you do not need to bring the ship back (B). Lowering play level (D) is not an appropriate strategy since this

is not the cause of the child's frustration and may lead to boredom or further dysregulation.

3. D: The function of this behavior is likely escape. You may start by teaching the child to appropriately communicate that he is no longer interested in those toys (B). However, if the child begins to do this with each toy set, this is becoming a new form of escape. You may also use a visual schedule (C) to help communicate the expectations. You should not end the session (A), as this reinforces this type of communication to escape.

Chapter 17

Exercise 17.1. Determining When to Respond

1. Continue monitoring: The behavior is not currently interfering. Continue monitoring for signs that the behavior is increasing.

2. Continue monitoring: Allow the child to hold the peg as long as it does not become too distracting.

3. Provide support: This behavior is not resolving on its own, and the child is missing out on valuable time to learn. Reconsider your toy choice and increase support.

4. Provide support: The child's preferences are making it difficult to have any productive play acts together. If you continue with this pattern, it will be difficult to build a routine and communicate together. Increase support to help the child engage.

5. Continue monitoring: It is okay if the child takes small breaks and then resumes engagement with you and the toys. In these moments, you can imitate and expand the child's communication as long as it does not significantly distract from the routine, take too much time away from the session, or lead to escape behaviors.

Exercise 17.2. Responding to RRBs

1. B: Since you have already tried other strategies and the child has solid language skills, use a behavioral statement like "We're playing together" to remind him of the expectation that you can take turns. While your turns do not need to be one to one, you should still be able to share your ideas and help him learn to play and engage with a partner. You should not lower the play level (A), since this will likely lead to boredom or further object engagement. Increasing your pace (C) will likely cause the speed of the routine to rapidly increase and become unmanageable.

2. C: You should try using suggestive prompts, such as holding your piece on after adding the topping (A) or quickly modeling two to three times to create a clear visual of what the next step can be (B). Often, this increase in support helps the child understand that you are adding an additional step and that she can join you in trying it out.

3. A: Set up a clear next step. For example, put out road pieces so you can drive the cars somewhere else, add figures to the cars (for presymbolic players), or have materials out for a "carwash." By preparing the environment, you can get ahead of the child's repetitive rolling while still incorporating his interest. Increasing your affect and volume (B) or verbally prompting the child (C) may get the child's attention but will hinder your goal of creating a fun play interaction with an equal and active role.

Caity's Toy Box

Child: Ernie

Age: 2 years
Mastered play level: General combination and pretend self
Target play level: Child as agent
Target JA gesture: Showing
Target requesting gesture: Combine pointing and single words
Target language level: Two to three words

Routine: Blocks
Toys in routine: Foam blocks, figures, ramp, boat with seats

    Base step: Build the foam blocks into a structure
- The adult and Ernie take turns stacking the foam blocks into a rectangle structure.
- The adult models JA shows by showing different colored blocks to Ernie before putting them on the structure.
- The adult says, "Build blocks!"
- Then when all the blocks are on the structure, Ernie smiles and says, "Big!"
- The adult responds and expands saying, "Big blocks!" and points to the blocks.

Expansion step 1: Add people to the structure
- The adult and Ernie take turns adding figures onto the structure.

Expansion step 2: Slide people into the boat
- The adult places a ramp from the structure into the boat, and Ernie initiates sliding people into the boat. The adult imitates and they put each person into the boat.

Expansion step 3: Sit people in seats on the boat
- The adult and Ernie take turns placing each person on a chair in the boat.

Restart: Tip over the boat
- The adult pushes the boat toward the blocks and tips it over.
- Ernie looks at the adult, crashes the blocks, and then points at the boat and says, "Oh no!"
- The adult responds by pointing and saying, "Oh no, they fell!" and then quickly resets the materials so that they can begin building the blocks or putting the people into the bus again.

Child: Ridge

Age: 3 years
Mastered play level: Discriminate acts and take-apart
Target play level: Presentation combination and general combination
Target JA gesture: Coordinated joint looks and JA points
Target requesting gesture: Give
Target language level: One word

Routine: Cars
Toys in routine: Two large cars and two small cars

    Base step: Push the car back and forth
- The adult and Ridge push the large car back and forth.
- The adult says, "Ready, set . . . " and pauses; Ridge says, "Go!"

- The adult pushes the car to Ridge.
- Ridge pushes car back to the adult and says, "Go!"

Expansion step: Car drives up wall
- The adult drives the car up the wall; says, "Up!" and then pauses holding her car up on the wall.
- Ridge points to the car and approximates "Down!"
- The adult responds and expands with "Slide down!" and pushes the car down the wall and waits.

Expansion step: Stack the cars

- Ridge initiates "building" cars by putting a smaller car on top of a big car.
- The adult imitates and puts another car on top and they continue back and forth.

Expansion step: Push the car tower
- The adult then pushes the car tower to Ridge.

Restart: Cars crash
- Ridge knocks down cars and looks at the adult.
- The adult responds and expands by saying, "Crash!", points to the fallen cars, and restarts the routine with the base step of rolling the cars.

Child: Madeline

Age: 4 years
Mastered play level: Multi-scheme
Target play level: Sociodramatic
Target JA gesture: Combine gestures with language
Target requesting gestures: Pointing and giving
Target language level: Sentences (fluent language with more variety)

Routine: Shopping
Toys in routine 1: Dollhouse, furniture, two doll-sized shopping carts, five to six small figures, magnetic tiles, cash register, pretend food

Base routine: The dolls wake up, brush their teeth, go potty, and wash their hands. The adult and child establish the base by taking turns acting out these steps with each figure.

Expansion step 1: Drive to the supermarket
- Madeline talks for the doll, saying, "Come on, Mommy, let's go to the farmers market."
- Madeline answers with the other doll: "Okay, let's go to the car." She then gives the doll to the adult and says, "You be the girl."
- The adult takes her role as the girl and says, "Don't forget your seatbelt!" as the doll buckles in.
- They put the rest of the dolls in the car and drive to the pretend food and shopping carts.

Expansion step 2: Shopping [station preset with block shelves, different foods, shopping carts, money, cash register, and shopping bags]
- They both have their dolls push the shopping carts and collect different food items from the shelves. The adult and child comment on the different items. The adult models a JA show gesture paired with a comment about some items she chooses. The child then notices a shelf full of ice cream and excitely uses a JA show while saying, "Let's buy chocolate chip!"

Expansion step 3: Checkout
- The adult models being the cashier: "Okay, are you ready to check out?"
- Madeline uses doll to answer, "Yes, we are!" They scan each of their groceries, pay, pack their groceries into the car, and drive home.

Expansion step 4: Cook lunch [add table, chairs, plates, and cutlery to the home station]
- The child initiates putting the food on the table and the dolls dish themselves up lunch, eat, and drink water.

Restart: The dolls brush their teeth, go potty, and wash their hands before expanding to other home activities or driving to a new station to build a new routine (e.g., the garden).

References

Adamson, L. B., Bakeman, R., & Deckner, D. F. (2004). The development of symbol-infused joint engagement. *Child Development, 75*(4), 1171–1187.

American Psychiatric Association. (2013). *Diagnostic and statistical manual of mental disorders* (5th ed.). Arlington, VA: Author.

Bailey, D. B., Hatton, D. D., Mesibov, G., Ament, N., & Skinner, M. (2000). Early development, temperament, and functional impairment in autism and fragile X syndrome. *Journal of Autism and Developmental Disorders, 30*(1), 49–59.

Bakeman, R., & Adamson, L. B. (1984). Coordinating attention to people and objects in mother–infant and peer–infant interaction. *Child Development, 55*(4), 1278–1289.

Beukelman, D. R., & Mirenda, P. (2013). *Augmentative and alternative communication: Supporting children and adults with complex communication needs.* Baltimore: Brookes.

Bruner, J. (1983). *Child's talk: Learning to use language.* New York: Norton.

Capps, L., Kasari, C., Yirmiya, N., & Sigman, M. (1993). Parental perception of emotional expressiveness in children with autism. *Journal of Consulting and Clinical Psychology, 61*(3), 475–484.

Chang, Y. C., Shire, S. Y., Shih, W., Gelfand, C., & Kasari, C. (2016). Preschool deployment of evidence-based social communication intervention: JASPER in the classroom. *Journal of Autism and Developmental Disorders, 46*(6), 2211–2223.

Cole, P. M., Martin, S. E., & Dennis, T. A. (2004). Emotion regulation as a scientific construct: Methodological challenges and directions for child development research. *Child Development, 75*(2), 317–333.

Cooper, J. O., Heron, T. E., & Heward, W. L. (2007). *Applied behavior analysis* (2nd ed.). Upper Saddle River, NJ: Pearson Education.

DeMyer, M. K., Barton, S., DeMyer, W. E., Norton, J. A., Allen, J., & Steele, R. (1973). Prognosis in autism: A follow-up study. *Journal of Autism and Childhood Schizophrenia, 3*(3), 199–246.

Feldman, R., Dollberg, D., & Nadam, R. (2011). The expression and regulation of anger in toddlers: Relations to maternal behavior and mental representations. *Infant Behavior and Development, 34*(2), 310–320.

Fisher, W. W., Piazza, C. C., & Roane, H. S. (Eds.). (2011). *Handbook of applied behavior analysis.* New York: Guilford Press.

Frost, L. (2002). The picture exchange communication system. *Perspectives on Language Learning and Education, 9*(2), 13–16.

Georgiades, S., & Kasari, C. (2018). Reframing optimal outcomes in autism. *JAMA Pediatrics, 172*(8), 716–717.

Goods, K. S., Ishijima, E., Chang, Y. C., & Kasari, C. (2013). Preschool based JASPER intervention in minimally verbal children with autism: Pilot RCT. *Journal of Autism and Developmental Disorders, 43*(5), 1050–1056.

Graziano, P. A., Reavis, R. D., Keane, S. P., & Calkins, S. D. (2007). The role of emotion regulation in children's early academic success. *Journal of School Psychology, 45*(1), 3–19.

Grolnick, W. S., Kurowski, C. O., McMenamy, J. M., Rivkin, I., & Bridges, L. J. (1998). Mothers' strategies for regulating their toddlers' distress. *Infant Behavior and Development, 21*(3), 437–450.

Gross, J. J., Carstensen, L. L., Pasupathi, M., Tsai, J., Götestam Skorpen, C., & Hsu, A. Y. (1997). Emotion and aging: Experience, expression, and control. *Psychology and Aging, 12*(4), 590–599.

Gulsrud, A. C., Hellemann, G. S., Freeman, S. F., & Kasari, C. (2014). Two to ten years:

Gulsrud, A. C., Jahromi, L. B., & Kasari, C. (2010). The co-regulation of emotions between mothers and their children with autism. *Journal of Autism and Developmental Disorders, 40*(2), 227–237.

Developmental trajectories of joint attention in children

with ASD who received targeted social communication interventions. *Autism Research, 7*(2), 207–215.

Jahromi, L. B., Bryce, C. I., & Swanson, J. (2013). The importance of self-regulation for the school and peer engagement of children with high-functioning autism. *Research in Autism Spectrum Disorders, 7*(2), 235–246.

Jarrold, C., Boucher, J., & Smith, P. K. (1996). Generativity deficits in pretend play in autism. *British Journal of Developmental Psychology, 14*(3), 275–300.

Kaale, A., Fagerland, M. W., Martinsen, E. W., & Smith, L. (2014). Preschool-based social communication treatment for children with autism: 12-month follow-up of a randomized trial. *Journal of the American Academy of Child and Adolescent Psychiatry, 53*(2), 188–198.

Kaale, A., Smith, L., & Sponheim, E. (2012). A randomized controlled trial of preschool-based joint attention intervention for children with autism. *Journal of Child Psychology and Psychiatry, 53*(1), 97–105.

Kasari, C., & Chang, Y. C. (2014). Play development in children with autism spectrum disorders: Skills, object play, and interventions. In F. R. Volkmar, R. Paul, S. J. Rogers, & K. A. Pelphrey (Eds.), *Handbook of autism and pervasive developmental disorders* (4th ed., pp. 264–267). Hoboken, NJ: Wiley.

Kasari, C., Freeman, S., & Paparella, T. (2006). Joint attention and symbolic play in young children with autism: A randomized controlled intervention study. *Journal of Child Psychology and Psychiatry, 47*(6), 611–620.

Kasari, C., Gulsrud, A., Freeman, S., Paparella, T., & Hellemann, G. (2012). Longitudinal follow-up of children with autism receiving targeted interventions on joint attention and play. *Journal of the American Academy of Child and Adolescent Psychiatry, 51*(5), 487–495.

Kasari, C., Gulsrud, A., Paparella, T., Hellemann, G., & Berry, K. (2015). Randomized comparative efficacy study of parent-mediated interventions for toddlers with autism. *Journal of Consulting and Clinical Psychology, 83*(3), 554–563.

Kasari, C., Gulsrud, A. C., Wong, C., Kwon, S., & Locke, J. (2010). Randomized controlled caregiver mediated joint engagement intervention for toddlers with autism. *Journal of Autism and Developmental Disorders, 40*(9), 1045–1056.

Kasari, C., Kaiser, A., Goods, K., Nietfeld, J., Mathy, P., Landa, R., . . . Almirall, D. (2014a). Communication interventions for minimally verbal children with autism: A sequential multiple assignment randomized trial. *Journal of the American Academy of Child and Adolescent Psychiatry, 53*(6), 635–646.

Kasari, C., Lawton, K., Shih, W., Barker, T. V., Landa, R., Lord, C., . . . Senturk, D. (2014b). Caregiver-mediated intervention for low-resourced preschoolers with autism: An RCT. *Pediatrics, 134*(1), e72–e79.

Kasari, C., Paparella, T., Freeman, S., & Jahromi, L. B. (2008). Language outcome in autism: Randomized comparison of joint attention and play interventions. *Journal of Consulting and Clinical Psychology, 76*(1), 125–137.

Kasari, C., & Smith, T. (2013). Interventions in schools for children with autism spectrum disorder: Methods and recommendations. *Autism, 17*(3), 254–267.

Konstantareas, M. M., & Stewart, K. (2006). Affect regulation and temperament in children with autism spectrum disorder. *Journal of Autism and Developmental Disorders, 36*(2), 143–154.

Lawton, K., & Kasari, C. (2012). Brief report: Longitudinal improvements in the quality of joint attention in preschool children with autism. *Journal of Autism and Developmental Disorders, 42*(2), 307–312.

Lifter, K., Sulzer-Azaroff, B., Anderson, S. R., & Cowdery, G. E. (1993). Teaching play activities to preschool children with disabilities: The importance of developmental considerations. *Journal of Early Intervention, 17*(2), 139–159.

Lillard, A. S. (2015). The development of play. In R. M. Lerner (Ed.), *The handbook of child psychology and developmental science* (pp. 425–468). Hoboken, NJ: Wiley.

Lillard, A., Pinkham, A. M., & Smith, E. (2011). *Pretend play and cognitive development*. In U. Goswami (Ed.), *The Wiley–Blackwell handbook of childhood cognitive development* (pp. 285–311). Malden, MA: Wiley–Blackwell.

Lovaas, O. I. (1987). Behavioral treatment and normal educational and intellectual functioning in young autistic children. *Journal of Consulting and Clinical Psychology, 55*(1), 3–9.

Mazefsky, C. A., & White, S. W. (2014). Emotion regulation: Concepts and practice in autism spectrum disorder. *Child and Adolescent Psychiatric Clinics of North America, 23*(1), 15–24.

Morris, A. S., Silk, J. S., Morris, M. D., Steinberg, L., Aucoin, K. J., & Keyes, A. W. (2011). The influence of mother–child emotion regulation strategies on children's expression of anger and sadness. *Developmental Psychology, 47*(1), 213.

Mundy, P., Delgado, C., Block, J., Venezia, M., Hogan, A., & Seibert, J. (2003). *Early Social Communication Scales (ESCS).* Coral Gables, FL: University of Miami.

Mundy, P., & Newell, L. (2007). Attention, joint attention, and social cognition. *Current Directions in Psychological Science, 16*(5), 269–274.

Mundy, P., & Sigman, M. (1989). Specifying the nature of the social impairment in autism. In G. Dawson (Ed.), *Autism: New perspectives on diagnosis, nature, and treatment* (pp. 3–21). New York: Guilford Press.

Mundy, P., Sigman, M., & Kasari, C. (1990). A longitudinal study of joint attention and language development in autistic children. *Journal of Autism and Developmental Disorders, 20*(1), 115–128.

Mundy, P., Sigman, M., Ungerer, J., & Sherman, T. (1986). Defining the social deficits of autism: The contribution of non-verbal communication measures. *Journal of Child Psychology and Psychiatry, 27*(5), 657–669.

Paparella, T., Goods, K. S., Freeman, S., & Kasari, C. (2011). The emergence of nonverbal joint attention and requesting skills in young children with autism. *Journal of Communication Disorders, 44*(6), 569–583.

Raver, C. C., Blackburn, E. K., Bancroft, M., & Torp, N. (1999). Relations between effective emotional self-regulation, attentional control, and low-income preschoolers' social competence with peers. *Early Education and Development, 10*(3), 333–350.

Romski, M., Sevcik, R. A., Barton-Hulsey, A., & Whitmore, A. S. (2015). Early intervention and AAC: What a difference 30 years makes. *Augmentative and Alternative Communication, 31*(3), 181–202.

Rutherford, M. D., Young, G. S., Hepburn, S., & Rogers, S. J. (2007). A longitudinal study of pretend play in autism. *Journal of Autism and Developmental Disorders, 37*(6), 1024–1039.

Rutter, M. (1983). Cognitive deficits in the pathogenesis of autism. *Journal of Child Psychology and Psychiatry, 24*(4), 513–531.

Schreibman, L., Dawson, G., Stahmer, A. C., Landa, R., Rogers, S. J., McGee, G. G., . . . Halladay, A. (2015). Naturalistic developmental behavioral interventions: Empirically validated treatments for autism spectrum disorder. *Journal of Autism and Developmental Disorders, 45*(8), 2411–2428.

Shih, W., Chang, Y. C., Shire, S., & Kasari, C. (2017, Spring). *Does joint engagement mediate intervention outcomes of joint attention in young children with ASD in preschool classrooms?* Paper presented at Gatlinburg Conference on Research and Theory in Intellectual and Developmental Disabilities, San Antonio, TX.

Shih, W., Shire, S., Chang, Y. C., & Kasari, C. (2021). Joint engagement is a potential mechanism leading to increased initiations of joint attention and downstream effects on language: JASPER early intervention for children with ASD. *Journal of Child Psychology and Psychiatry.* [Advance online publication] *https://doi.org/10.1111/jcpp.13405*

Shire, S. Y., Chang, Y. C., Shih, W., Bracaglia, S., Kodjoe, M., & Kasari, C. (2017). Hybrid implementation model of community-partnered early intervention for toddlers with autism: A randomized trial. *Journal of Child Psychology and Psychiatry, 58*(5), 612–622.

Shire, S. Y., Shih, W., Bracaglia, S., Kodjoe, M., & Kasari, C. (2020a). Peer engagement in toddlers with autism: Community implementation of dyadic and individual Joint Attention, Symbolic Play, Engagement, and Regulation intervention. *Autism, 24*(8), 2142–2152.

Shire, S. Y., Shih, W., Chang, Y. C., Bracaglia, S., Kodjoe, M., & Kasari, C. (2019). Sustained community implementation of JASPER intervention with toddlers with autism. *Journal of Autism and Developmental Disorders, 49*(5), 1863–1875.

Shire, S. Y., Shih, W., Chang, Y. C., & Kasari, C. (2018). Short Play and Communication Evaluation: Teachers' assessment of core social communication and play skills with young children with autism. *Autism, 22*(3), 299–310.

Shire, S. Y., Worthman, L. B., Shih, W., & Kasari, C. (2020b). Comparison of face-to-face and remote support for interventionists learning to deliver JASPER intervention with children who have autism. *Journal of Behavioral Education, 29,* 317–338.

Shire, S. Y., Worthman, L. B., Shih, W., & Kasari, C. (2021). *Randomized comparison of implementation strategies for early intervention practitioners: Community JASPER implementation.* Manuscript in preparation.

Shumway, S., & Wetherby, A. M. (2009). Communicative acts of children with autism spectrum disorders in the second year of life. *Journal of Speech, Language, and Hearing Research, 52*(5), 1139–1156.

Sigman, M., & Ungerer, J. A. (1984). Cognitive and language skills in autistic, mentally retarded, and normal children. *Developmental Psychology, 20*(2), 293–302.

Skinner, B. F. (1957). *Verbal behavior.* New York: Appleton-Century-Crofts.

Smith, T. (2001). Discrete trial training in the treatment of autism. *Focus on Autism and Other Developmental Disabilities, 16*(2), 86–92.

Sofronoff, K., Attwood, T., Hinton, S., & Levin, I. (2007). A randomized controlled trial of a cognitive behavioural intervention for anger management in children diagnosed with Asperger syndrome. *Journal of Autism and Developmental Disorders, 37*(7), 1203–1214.

Thompson, R. A., & Goodman, M. (2010). Development of emotion regulation: More than meets the eye. In A. M. Kring & D. M. Sloan (Eds.), *Emotion regulation and psychopathology: A transdiagnostic approach to etiology and treatment* (pp. 38–58). New York: Guilford Press.

Tomasello, M., & Todd, J. (1983). Joint attention and lexical acquisition style. *First Language, 4*(12), 197–211.

Trentacosta, C. J., & Izard, C. E. (2007). Kindergarten children's emotion competence as a predictor of their academic competence in first grade. *Emotion, 7*(1), 77–88.

Ungerer, J. A., & Sigman, M. (1981). Symbolic play and language comprehension in autistic children. *American Academy of Child Psychiatry, 20,* 318–337.

Ungerer, J. A., Zelazo, P. R., Kearsley, R. B., & O'Leary, K. (1981). Developmental changes in the representation of objects in symbolic play from 18 to 34 months of age. *Child Development, 52*(1), 186–195.

Vygotsky, L. (1978). Interaction between learning and development. In *Mind and society* (pp. 79–91). Cambridge, MA: Harvard University Press.

Index

Note. *f* or *t* following a page number indicates a figure or table.